the PSYCHOLOGY of DEAFNESS

the
PSYCHOLOGY
of
DEAFNESS

Understanding Deaf and Hard-of-Hearing People

McCay Vernon
Western Maryland College

Jean F. Andrews
Lamar University

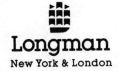

Longman

New York & London

The Psychology of Deafness
Understanding Deaf and Hard-of-Hearing People

Longman, 95 Church Street, White Plains, N.Y. 10601
A division of Addison-Wesley Publishing Co., Inc.

Associated companies:
Longman Group Ltd., London
Longman Cheshire Pty., Melbourne
Longman Paul Pty., Auckland
Copp Clark Pitman, Toronto

Acknowledgments to Gallaudet University, where the exhaustive literature search
for this book began when Dr. Vernon was awarded the Powrie V.
Doctor Chair for 1979–1980.

We thank Dr. Carol Sigelman for references;
Tom Penegore, James R. Burke, and Stuart Hays for photography; and
Mrs. Donna K. Jones, Mrs. Helen D. Martin, and Mrs. Paula Batts
for typing.

Executive editor: Raymond T. O'Connell
Production editor: Carol Harwood
Text design: Kevin Kall
Cover design: Kevin Kall
Cover photos: Patsy Lynch, Chun Louie
Text art: Susan J. Moore
Production supervisor: Joanne Jay

Library of Congress Cataloging-in-Publication Data
Vernon, McCay.

   The psychology of deafness : understanding deaf and hard-of
-hearing people / McCay Vernon, Jean F. Andrews.

      p.   cm.
   Bibliography: p.
   Includes index.
   ISBN 0-8013-0322-2

      1. Deafness—Psychological aspects.   2. Deaf—United States.
3. Deaf—Means of communication.   4. Deaf—Education—United States.
5. Hearing impaired—United States.   I. Andrews, Jean F.
II. Title.
HV2395.V47   1989
362.4'2'019—dc19   89-2255
                                                           CIP

ABCDEFGHIJ - DO - 99 98 97 96 95 94 93 92 91 90

To Edith Vernon. Her life as a deaf person gave a knowledge, empathy, and motivation to my work in deafness that could have come from no one else.

Contents

Tables

Introduction

Hearing loss isolates people from other people and from knowledge. The very essence of the disability of hearing impairment is its effects on communication and the resulting impact of communication on behavior. The consequence is a severe form of cognitive deprivation and the alteration of interpersonal relationships. It is these consequences that comprise a psychology of deafness.

Because hearing loss is now the most prevalent chronic health problem in the United States and in most scientifically advanced countries, it affects more people than heart disease and multiple sclerosis combined. It has been estimated that over 15 million Americans have hearing impairments which interfere with their communication (Boone, 1987; Schein, 1987). Despite the pervasiveness of the problem, relatively little attention has been directed toward understanding its psychological implications. For those people and their families and friends, this indifference is a tragedy. The magnitude of the problem will be compounded over the next few decades because the percentages of our population in older age ranges is rapidly increasing. In general, all adults have some hearing loss by age 30, and the rate doubles or triples as one moves from one age group to another.

To address these psychological implications, we take the view that deafness is a psychological variable which influences the behavior of deaf persons such that their life experience differs in some consistent ways from that of those who are not deaf. Through an analysis of relevant theoretical and empirical literature along with the authors' clinical experience in education, psychodiagnostics, research, and psychotherapy with deaf persons, the psychological aspects of hearing loss are described in this book.

The definition of hearing loss that has the greatest significance for psychological purposes is that it is an auditory loss in which the individual cannot hear sufficiently to understand conversational speech. The book focuses on prelingual and profound deafness, along with issues that concern those with severe and mild losses and those with partial hearing. Chapter 12 deals exclusively with the hard-of-hearing population. The effects of a hearing loss are pervasive and create psychological stress no matter what the extent of the loss.

PLAN OF THE BOOK

This book is divided into five sections. Each begins with an overview and ends with a summary and review questions to focus the reader's attention on significant issues. While all the chapters have the unifying theme examining deafness as a psychological variable, each chapter is self-contained and can be used by professionals in specialities such as education, mental health services, medicine, interpreting, and others.

Chapter 1 of the first section describes the characteristics of the American deaf community. It cannot be overemphasized that such information is important for those who work with deaf children but have little or no experience interacting with deaf adults. Chapters 2 and 3 deal with the causes or etiologies of deafness and explain how knowledge of these causes helps professionals and families understand the behavior of people with hearing losses.

In Section II, chapters 4 and 5 focus on communication and are linked to chapter 1 in content. Chapter 4 states that American Sign Language, commonly referred to as ASL, is the main identifying characteristic of the the deaf community and that it has been misunderstood and repressed throughout history. The historical and linguistic roots of ASL are traced and its significant contributions to education, special education, and psychology are described. Chapter 5 describes other forms of communication used by deaf people, some of which we believe are more useful than others. It is shown why speech and speechreading are rarely effective communication systems by themselves because of the ambiguity of speechreading. There is a display of photographs comparing and contrasting several manual systems, along with a description of the advantages and disadvantages of each system.

Section III is the heart of the book. It explains how overwhelming is the stress that deafness imposes on its victims and families. The intense emotional reactions parents experience at the time their child is diagnosed as deaf, along with the psychodynamics underlying these feelings, are described in chapter 6. Chapters 7 and 8 are linked with the common theme of the adjustment reactions of deaf persons. These reactions range from unique behavioral patterns to severe personality disorders and mental illness of psychotic and nonpsychotic origins. From this information, model services and methods of psychotherapy are recommended. Chapter 9 describes how the attitude of hearing people toward deafness is a major handicap faced by deaf children and adults. A detailed discussion is presented on the "authoritarian personality"—a personality type that tries to control and dominate deaf persons rather than facilitate their growth and development.

Chapter 10, on psychological evaluation is closely linked to chapters 2 and 3 on causes and chapter 6 on diagnosis. It presents information aimed at reducing the common occurrence of misdiagnosis with deaf children. The role of the psychologist is defined and general principles basic to psychodiagnostics with deaf persons are given. The components of a comprehensive psychological evaluation are outlined, which include assessments not only on intelligence and adaptive behaviors but also on personality, language and communication, academic achievement, and vocational interests and aptitudes. Case studies are given from the first author's numerous years of experiences as a practicing clinical psychologist administering psychological evaluations to deaf persons. It is explained how misdiagnosis often results in irreversible psychological and educational damage.

Chapter 11 describes a bilingual/bicultural approach to helping deaf children learn. Chapter 1 on the deaf community and chapter 4 on American Sign Language will help the reader understand this approach. It focuses on setting up an environment in which the deaf child can extract the rules of both languages—ASL and English—to function in the worlds both of hearing and of deaf people. The discussion includes a description of how language develops and how deafness affects communication competence. Six goals are suggested for setting up a bilingual/bicultural environment in the school. It is recommended, finally, that future research in classroom ethnography is needed to direct and evaluate deaf children's learning.

Chapter 12, the last chapter in Section IV, deals with the partial hearing or hard-of-hearing. Audiological considerations and audiological practices are reviewed, along with their psychological implications in depth, because these are frequently misunderstood by parents, professionals, and the lay public. The psychological factors and coping mechanisms are described of this group of people who feel marginal—feeling affiliation with neither the deaf community nor the hearing world. Early identification and therapy are recommended, followed by adequate support services in the educational system.

Whereas the first twelve chapters focus on improving service delivery to the deaf community, the final chapter, chapter 13, has a theoretical perspective and examines deafness as "an experiment in nature." We believe that deafness can be used as a frame of reference to help answer many psychological questions dealing with causes of diseases, language acquisition, and the nature of intelligence and human learning.

Other features of this textbook which readers may find useful are the references after each chapter, an index, and a resource list of organizations, institutions, and publications serving deaf people and professionals.

AUDIENCE

This book is written to provide current up-to-date information about deafness to professionals working with deaf children, youth, and adults. While it will benefit upper undergraduate and graduate level students in a psychology of deafness class, the book is also useful to practicing clinical psychologists, medical professionals as physicians, otolaryngologists, pediatricians, nurses, nurses aides, speech pathologists, audiologists, social workers, interpreters, and vocational rehabilitation counselors.

Providing effective and responsible services to the deaf community is the goal of professionals working with deaf persons. We hope that *The Psychology of Deafness: Understanding Deaf and Hard-of-Hearing People* will be a valuable resource and will be used to meet this goal.

REFERENCES

Boone, D. R. (1987). *Human communication and its disorder.* Englewood Cliffs, NJ: Prentice-Hall.

Schein, J. D. (1987). The demography of deafness. In P. Higgins & J. Nash (Eds.), *Understanding deafness socially.* Springfield, IL: Charles C Thomas.

the
PSYCHOLOGY
of
DEAFNESS

SECTION I

Characteristics of
the Deaf Community
and Causes of Deafness

OVERVIEW

We begin this section by introducing the view that deafness is a psychological variable which influences the behavior of deaf persons such that their life experiences differ from those of the nondeaf population. In the first chapter, the idea that deafness is most comprehensively understood within a societal context is emphasized. The chapter discusses how individuals are enculturated into the deaf community, get their education, find employment, and spend their leisure time. The use of American Sign Language (ASL) among deaf community members is the community's chief identifying characteristic; this theme is explained in chapter 1 and will be more fully developed in chapter 4.

In chapter 2 and 3 the numerous causes, or etiologies, of deafness are discussed. In cases of genetic deafness, full communication of genetic information to the families concerned is a matter of great psychological significance and has important implications for prevention and treatment also. The importance of the genetic counselor is emphasized in chapter 2 and the components of effective genetic counseling are outlined. Chapter 3 covers nongenetic and viral causes of deafness. Knowledge of these causes helps professionals and families understand the behavior of people with hearing loss. Each etiology is detailed, along with its effects on intelligence, educational achievement, hearing, communication skills, and psychological adjustment.

CHAPTER 1
The Deaf Community: A Modern-day Picture

. . . the basic reason for becoming involved with deaf adults: we are your children grown. We can, in many instances, tell you the things your child would like to tell you, if he had the vocabulary and the experiences to put his feelings and needs into words. Frederick Schrieber, 1969 in Schein, 1981

Fred Schreiber, the late executive director of the National Association of the Deaf, gives a compelling reason why professionals need to concern themselves with the adult deaf community. Unfortunately, few hearing professionals who work in deafness have knowledge about the deaf community nor are they able to communicate with them. Rarely are members of the deaf community consulted about the education and rehabilitation of deaf adults and children. Instead, the deaf community has been subjected to societal rejection and domination by those who hear and control their institutions (Lane, 1984).

Even with outside pressure, deaf communities have existed and survived over the centuries despite threats of annihilation (see Lane, 1984, for the history of this struggle). An example of the political strength of the deaf community is the election of Dr. I. King Jordon, the first deaf person to hold the position of president of Gallaudet University. In March 1988 a hearing person with no knowledge of sign language or deafness held the title of president for four days. She resigned after a week-long "Deaf President Now" campaign initiated and led by the students and supported by the faculty and by organizations and schools for deaf students throughout the United States.

Although the Gallaudet revolt and its media coverage gave a positive and constructive view of the deaf community, it is rare that these impressions are available to the public. More often, expositions on deafness are steeped in sentimental stereotypes or restricted to descriptions of audiological and linguistic deficiencies.

This chapter draws on current work in literature, sociology, psychology, and linguistics in order to construct a modern picture of the deaf community.

DEAF PEOPLE—AN IDENTITY

If you were to ask an audiologist, a sociologist, and a linguist to identify "a deaf person," you would likely get different answers. An audiologist describes a deaf person as having a particular decibel loss across a continuum from mild to profound. Typically, those in speech and hearing science and audiology refer to persons in the profound range as "deaf" and to the others as "hearing impaired." Persons with mild or moderate losses are called "hard-of-hearing." Onset, or age when deafened, is another critical variable used in describing the deaf person. A person who is born deaf or loses his or her hearing before the age of 2, or before the "critical period" for language development, is called prelingually deaf, whereas those who lose their hearing in childhood or adulthood are postlingually deaf.

The sociologist and linguist, on the other hand, will identify the deaf person along attitudinal parameters or their use of American Sign Language. (Baker & Cokely, 1980; Higgins, 1980; Padden, 1980). Higgins, a sociologist, (1980) refers to deaf people as "outsiders in a hearing world." One achieves membership in the deaf community by accepting their values (i.e., use of American Sign Language), identifying with other deaf people, and having shared experiences getting educated and coping in the hearing world (Higgins, 1980). Thus, the range of measurable hearing loss in the audiological sense is not as important as is an acceptance of the values of the deaf community. Persons who are profoundly deaf with unintelligible speech may not be socially "deaf" and in fact may have rejected the deaf, choosing instead to interact only with hearing people or, more often, to be isolated. Postlingually deafened adults, too, may consider themselves more "hearing" than "deaf" in a cultural sense. On the other hand, hard-of-hearing persons who have intelligible speech and residual hearing may instead choose to be members of the deaf community. Hearing children of deaf parents may also consider themselves members of the deaf community.

PREVALENCE AND DEMOGRAPHICS

Prevalence figures of the deaf population vary because of the inconsistency in defining and measuring deafness (Higgins, 1980). The most recent census of deaf persons was conducted in 1971 by New York University (Schein & Delk, 1974). Hearing impairment was recognized as the most prevalent chronic physical impairment in the United States, with more than 13 million people having a significant hearing loss. Almost 2 million citizens are deaf, meaning they cannot hear to understand speech and of these about a half million youths have not yet entered the job market. Most of these figures are based on the white deaf population. (See Table 1.1.)

Minority Groups

Precise figures of minority deaf populations such as black, Hispanic, Native Americans, and Asian Americans are not available. (There are other nonwhite deaf persons, but even our limited information is available only on these four groups.)

Of the minority groups, the most information is known about the black deaf. Hairston and Smith (1983) report that approximately 2 million blacks have a hearing impairment serious enough to require medical or educational services. Of these, about 22,000 are profoundly deaf. The Office of Demographic studies reports that about 18 percent of deaf school-age children surveyed in the United States are black (Annual survey of hearing-impaired children and youth, 1983–1984). The adult black deaf population is harder to locate than other deaf persons because they generally do not affiliate with deaf organizations of white deaf people (Schein & Delk, 1974; Higgins, 1980). Additionally, many black families have trouble earning a living and coping with the world, leaving less time and energy to devote to their deaf child. And many do not know where to find help (Hairston & Smith, 1983).

Historically the education provided to the black deaf has been inferior. Hairston

TABLE 1.1. Distribution of Hearing-Impaired Population by Regions in the United States, 1971

United States and Regions	Hearing Impaired	Deaf	Prevocationally Deaf
United States	13,362,842	1,767,046	410,522
Northeast	2,891,380	337,022	83,909
North Central	3,683,226	541,465	135,653
South	4,280,177	562,756	123,260
West	2,508,059	325,803	67,700
	Rate per 100,000 Population		
United States	6,603	873	203
Northeast	5,977	697	173
North Central	6,563	965	242
South	6,807	895	196
West	7,170	931	194

(SOURCE: From *The Deaf Population* (p. 25) by J. D. Schein and M. T. Delk, 1974. Silver Spring, MD: National Association of the Deaf. Reprinted by permission.)

and Smith (1983) interviewed black deaf persons who attended schools before integration and found that for the most part, deaf youths were not encouraged to graduate and were given only vocational training in areas such as hairdressing, tailoring, and barbering. Few deaf students had black teachers as role models. Many states had totally segregated facilities. However, in these so-called "Negro schools for the deaf" some of the vocational instruction was very good because the instructors often taught at nearby black colleges. Black deaf students were not encouraged to go to college. In fact, Gallaudet University did not integrate until 1952. Even today, few schools for the deaf contain information on black deaf history and few deaf children are exposed to black deaf teachers (Woodward, 1985).

Most black deaf adults are from lower socioeconomic brackets, have much lower average incomes, have a far higher rate of unemployment, and receive less adequate medical care than the white deaf person (Schein & Delk, 1974). Hairston and Smith (1983), however, report that even though the black deaf are *under*employed, they usually are employed and have lower rates of unemployment than blacks in general.

Racial prejudice exists in the deaf community. Segregation is due mainly to the differences in educational, social, and cultural backgrounds and in communication. In many metropolitan areas there are separate black and white deaf communities (Hairston & Smith, 1983; Higgins, 1980). Clubs for the deaf are highly segregated in Washington, D.C., Baltimore, Atlanta, Cleveland, Chicago, and Los Angeles. Higgins (1980) attributes this racial prejudice not to deafness per se but to the generally low education level of deaf persons. Educational level is generally considered a predictor of racial acceptance.

A major source of separation between white and black deaf is the type of sign language used by the two groups (Woodward, 1976). Research shows that black deaf persons use different signs and have different signing styles than white deaf persons (Woodward, 1976). Historically, the black signing developed because, as a result of societal attitudes and educational segregation, black deaf children had their own signed dialect (Hairston & Smith, 1983).

Black deaf leaders believe the major problems faced by black deaf people are undereducation, underemployment, and an unfavorable self-image (Hairston & Smith, 1983). While black deaf clubs are formed chiefly for social and athletic purposes, one organization, Black Deaf Advocates (BDA), works for the rights of black deaf citizens. In their words:

> The major goal of BDA is to prepare Black deaf people for leadership roles—to train them in the art of planning, organizing, and implementing programs and goals—and to provide them with the opportunity to function as leaders or to interact with role models. This in turn would provide Black deaf leaders and potential leaders with the experience and confidence to interact with officials of the NAD (National Association of the Deaf) and its membership. Otherwise, it would be the same old story—token Black person joins the organization and is a good old fellow, outmaneuvered by sophisticated white members, smiling all the while. It is time for a different approach. (Hairston & Smith, 1983, p. 48)

Several national black deaf conferences have been held where workshops on education, social services, mental health, and other topics provide information to the black deaf community.

The Hispanic deaf are increasingly obtaining educational services, in 1978–1979 accounting for 9.4 percent of the deaf school-age enrollment (Maestas y Moores & Moores, 1984). The enrollment of Hispanic children in schools for the deaf has dramatically increased, especially in large metropolitan areas such as New York City and Miami. The limited information available on academic and affective functioning of the Hispanic deaf population shows underachievement (Maestas y Moores & Moores, 1984).

There is a higher incidence of reported multiple handicaps within both the black and Hispanic deaf school-age population than among corresponding whites. This has been attributed in part to misdiagnosis due to assessment procedures and professionals insensitive to cultural differences (Delgado, 1984), lack of early identification, parents' difficulties locating services, and communication and cultural differences between professionals and parents (Christiansen, 1987).

Other minority groups such as the Native Americans and Asian Americans have even more difficulty obtaining medical, educational, and rehabilitative services. For example, it is estimated that as high as 20 to 70 percent of Native American and Eskimo children living on reservations have lost their hearing because of otitis media, which results in permanent deafness without medical care (Christiansen, 1987). Reservation children are further isolated from educational and rehabilitative services because of geographic location. As with the Hispanic deaf population, professionals may have difficulty determining the needs of these children because of language and cultural differences with their parents.

Needs and Services of Minority Deaf.   Minority deaf people receive fewer services, obtain less education, have greater unemployment, and make less money than the white deaf population. Improving services for them requires great sensitivity among professionals. Minority families typically prefer to take care of their own handicapped children and often resist the help of professionals, whom they perceive as intruders and whom they may mistrust. Because the deafness is commonly diagnosed late, early years of language learning are lost. When the deaf minority children enter a program, they may have to learn three or more communication systems: sign, the family's language, and the teacher's language. Rarely do schools employ minority deaf adults who can serve as role models for these children. As they grow older, nonwhite deaf persons face discrimination from the white deaf population.

Currently, many middle-class white deaf children leaving residential schools and are being mainstreamed into public school. Another trend is increasing populations of nonwhite deaf children (i.e. Hispanic, black) enrolling in state schools for the deaf. As a result, there is increased public awareness of the needs of minority deaf children. For example, programs in Rhode Island and New York are addressing the needs of the Portuguese and Hispanic deaf populations (Christiansen, 1987).

Males and Females
A slightly higher percentage of males are deaf than females. Deafness affects females more adversely than males, however. For example, deaf females show higher unemployment rates, lower personal incomes, and lesser educational achievement than deaf males (Barnartt, 1987; MacLeod-Gallinger, 1985; Schein & Delk, 1974). Deaf women tend to marry less often and later than hearing women, probably because most marry deaf men. They also tend to have fewer babies, perhaps because they marry later and usually are in the work force (Barnartt, 1987). The unemployment rate for deaf women is higher than for both deaf men and hearing women. Ironically, educated deaf women have a difficult time finding jobs. They may be overqualified for traditional female occupations such as maids or waitresses but be underqualified for professional jobs such as managers or teachers (Barnartt, 1987). Deaf women, like hearing women, face discrimination in the workplace, especially in income. They are paid significantly less than deaf males, hearing white females, and hearing black females, even though they may have more education and job experience (Barnartt, 1987).

To be black, deaf, and female places a person in triple jeopardy in our society. These women have a lower employment rate and education level (Schein, 1968; Schein & Delk, 1974) than white deaf and black hearing females. Black deaf women have formed social support clubs in Washington, D.C., Cleveland, and other cities (Hairston & Smith, 1983).

COMMUNITY MEMBERSHIP

What are deaf persons feeling about their deafness? Individuals differ, of course, but it has been generally found that deaf people have mixed feelings. For example, in his sample of 75 deaf adults in the Chicago area, Higgins (1980) found deaf people to be ambivalent about their deafness. They derive a sense of belonging and wholeness from their fellow members of the deaf community, and these feelings of group solidarity sustain them even into old age (Meadow-Orlans, 1985).

Membership in the deaf community involves identification with deaf people, shared experiences in school and work, and active participation in group activities with other deaf people (Higgins, 1980). Most notably, deaf community members share frustrating experiences trying to communicate in the hearing world. According to Higgins (1980), some hearing individuals, such as educators, counselors, and spouses, can be "courtesy" members. However, only deaf persons can really know what deafness means. Neither social class nor sex nor religion are important attributes for membership; the major distinguishing criteria are communication skill and preference.

Sign Language

At the heart of the deaf community is American Sign Language (ASL) (Baker & Cokely, 1980; Higgins, 1980; Meadow, 1972; Padden, 1980; Stokoe, 1960), which differs from spoken English in significant ways (Klima & Bellugi, 1979; Stokoe, 1960). (See chapter 4.)

A minority of deaf adults do not use ASL. Some rely primarily on speaking and lipreading when communicating (Higgins, 1980). These "oral" deaf adults may know some signs and use them now and then but not with fluency and skill. The deaf oralists frequently belong to an oral association of the deaf and may reject the "manual" deaf community, preferring to associate with other oralists. Many oralists may have attended day classes or private residential schools where signing was prohibited. Some deaf adults function in both the oral and signing deaf communities, but they are a minority.

The overwhelming majority of deaf adults prefer to use ASL. They rely on signs and fingerspelling, rarely using speech and lipreading when communicating with other deaf people (Higgins, 1980). Some have negative attitudes toward the status of ASL as a language as a result of experiences in schools where the use of signing was punished and repressed. (This process, common in minority cultures, is termed "internalizing the values of the aggressor" and is exemplified in the black community by the status given to straight hair and light skin.)

Within the signing U.S. deaf community, further sign differentiations exist in relation to socio-educational, regional, and ethnic boundaries (Woodward, 1976). For example, the more education deaf people have, the more English signs and word order will be included in their communication, especially at professional conferences and meetings. Regional differences in signing exist too. A deaf adult from New York, for example, may have specific regional signs as well as a signing style different from that of a deaf adult from Kentucky. Many deaf adults can identify where other deaf people attended school by their signs, much as hearing people rely on accents (Higgins, 1980).

Woodward (1980) describes signing as being on a continuum ranging from the "L" variety, which is ASL used in intimate conversations with other deaf people, to the "H" variety, which approximates English syntax and is used in formal interactions such as at church, in school, and in conversations with hearing people. Deaf persons do not have native competence in English and will typically use what English they do have in their signing to accommodate their hearing conversational partners. What often results is a Pidgin Signed English (PSE)—ASL signs and phrases used in an approximation of English order. PSE serves as a linguistic and cultural interface that allows for interaction between the hearing and deaf communities. It also preserves ASL for deaf persons only, thus contributing to a positive social identity and keeping ASL intact from intrusive hearing people (Woodward, 1980). (See chapter 4 for a discussion of PSE.)

Recently educators have taken ASL signs and used them to invent manual systems to represent English for purposes of instructing deaf children. (See chapter 5.) However, deaf adults do not look favorably on these systems. For example, Higgins (1980) writes:

> The deaf community does not view these invented systems positively. Since ASL is an important element of the deaf community, tampering with sign language is resisted as it is considered to be tampering with the deaf community's identity. (Higgins, 1980)

The awkward and unesthetic nature of these systems adds to their lack of acceptance. Deaf adults have spoken and written negatively about these invented systems (Schreiber, 1969, cited in Schein, 1981) at conferences and in the publication, *The Deaf American* (Baker & Cokely, 1980).

ENCULTURATION AND SCHOOLING

Deaf persons begin using American Sign Language when they enter the deaf community. Meadow (1972) has suggested three periods when this might take place: (1) infancy, for deaf children of deaf parents; (2) at the time of enrollment in a residential school, usually for those from 5 to 13; and (3) upon graduation from high school.

Few deaf children are born into deaf families. In fact, only 3 percent have two deaf parents and 7 percent have one deaf parent. Thus the number of deaf children born into the deaf community is very small.

At any one time 29 percent of deaf children are attending one of the 61 state residential schools in the United States (Craig & Craig, 1986). However, over time a much higher percentage get some part of their education in residential schools, often during their teens. It is here where they learn sign language, not from their teachers but from their deaf peers. Receiving a name sign from a peer, teacher, or counselor is typically one of the initiation rituals. In the context of ASL, a name sign is a formalized gesture referring to the individual's proper name (Meadow, 1977). Usually it reflects some aspect of the person's personal appearance or behavior and in many cases has negative connotations. In an analysis of 86 name signs, Meadow (1977) found 17 percent to refer to a positive quality, 37 percent to have a neutral referent, and 45 percent to have a negative referent. For example, as Meadow (1977) points out, the name sign for someone who limps may be CRIPPLE. The effect of the name sign on the young deaf person's self-concept and self-esteem is obvious.

Approximately 68 percent of deaf children attend a public school, either in a self-contained classroom, in a day school, or mainstreamed in classrooms with an interpreter or resource teacher (Craig & Craig, 1986). Many of these children may not meet a deaf adult until they enter the work force or enter a postsecondary program.

Deaf "enculturation" often occurs when deaf youth meet deaf peers in any of the 100 special postsecondary programs which provide support services (Rawlings & King, 1986; Vernon, 1983a). There are about 8,000 to 11,000 hearing-impaired individuals in institutions of higher education. Not all of these students are receiving support services (i.e., interpreting and note-taking services) (Rawlings & King,

1986). For example, deaf students can enroll in programs that have extensive support services such as the federally established programs, Gallaudet University, and National Technical Institute for the Deaf. Or they may attend one of the four regional programs—St. Paul Technical Vocational Institute, California State University at Northridge, Delgado (New Orleans, Louisiana) Community College, or Seattle Community College—where they will have classes with many other deaf students. Alternately, students may enroll in programs where support services are nonexistent or very limited (Rawlings & King, 1986); here they may meet few or no deaf people.

Continuing education is the means by which deaf secondary graduates can reduce difficulties of unemployment and underemployment (MacLeod-Gallinger, 1985). The number and types of programs offering support services for deaf students have rapidly expanded in recent years (Rawlings & King, 1986), but motivation is a problem and attrition rates are high. For example, the National Technical Institute for the Deaf (NTID) had a projected attrition rate of 48 percent for the class of 1984–1985 (NTID Annual Report, 1984–1985).

Deaf youth who do not go to college may attend one of the seven rehabilitation centers and programs. In these settings, they meet deaf peers, may find marriage partners (95 percent of deaf persons marry other deaf persons), begin to use interpreting services, join a deaf organization, and may buy a TTD (Telecommunication for the Deaf) to contact friends and a decoder for their TV (Vernon, 1983b).

According to national achievement scores, parents can expect their deaf children to reach the equivalent of a third- or fourth-grade education of a hearing child (Allen, 1986). In chapter 10 we will discuss deaf children's academic achievement.

WORK

In the past, the steel and automobile and other manufacturing industries employed the majority of deaf people as machine operators, assemblers, and technicians. Fifteen percent of deaf workers were employed in the printing field. Today many of these positions have been replaced with computer operations. The computer field is now a large employer of deaf persons (MacLeod-Gallinger, 1985; Vernon, 1987). Deaf individuals are generally not found in personnel service occupations such as sales and management because of the communication difficulties.

Two recent reports provide a sampling of current occupational choices of deaf adults in the work force, one from graduates of secondary schools (MacLeod-Gallinger, 1985) and the other from NTID graduates (NTID Annual Report, 1984–1985). A survey questionnaire was sent from secondary schools to graduates in the classes of 1984, 1982, 1980, 1974, and 1964. A total of 748 deaf adults responded to questions about their labor force participation, employment status, occupation and earnings, job satisfaction, job search efforts, and continuing education activities. Of those who responded, 60 percent were under 25. Few black deaf responded to the job questionnaire. Responding males were largely employed as "operators, fabricators, and laborers"; females worked mostly clerically in "technical, sales, and administrative support" areas. Less than 8.5 percent of deaf males, compared with 25.2 percent of the national population, were employed in managerial and professional specialties. Similarily, only 9.4 percent of the deaf females held management and professional positions, compared with 23.1 percent of females in the national population.

The second report, conducted on 1,490 graduates from NTID, showed that 80 percent were employed in business and industry, 13 percent in government, and 7 percent in education (NTID Annual Report, 1984–1985).

Type of occupation has implications for earnings. It's no wonder that deaf workers make less than the national average: The higher paid salaries are in the managerial and professional areas, where deaf people are not employed as often as in the service fields. For example, MacLeod-Gallinger (1985) reports that deaf males and females earn, respectively, an average of $109 and $56 less per week than the national average. As was reported in past surveys (Schein & Delk, 1974), deaf females earn overall the lowest salaries, particularly black deaf females.

Two other trends were noted in the MacLeod-Gallinger (1985) survey. One was the increase of part-time employment among deaf adults and the other was increased requests for Supplemental Security Income (SSI)—an increase of almost 10 percent in the past three years—and requests for money from Vocational Rehabilitation.

Do deaf adults enjoy their work? From one deaf adult's point of view, work can be less than gratifying:

> You work in a factory. You have a break. You sit alone. At lunch you sit alone. For 50 years you are pretty much alone at work. When you retire and they give you a gold watch, you go out and celebrate alone. (Holcomb, 1977, pp. 51–52)

However, MacLeod-Gallinger (1985) reports that 74 percent of the respondents in the Secondary School follow-up survey expressed general job satisfaction, 19 percent were not sure, and only 7 percent responded as unhappy.

Underemployment and unemployment continue to be chronic problems in the deaf community. Today unemployment is higher than in the past because automation has eliminated many jobs previously filled by deaf persons. Vernon (1987) estimates 20 to 25 percent of deaf people represent the hard-core unemployed. Many are young, black, or Hispanic and live in urban areas. They draw SSI, are on welfare, or receive other government assistance.

Poor educational preparation contributes to this low income. Cross (1985) conducted a survey in Kentucky and found a strong relationship of employment and income to educational level. Nineteen questions were constructed regarding level of education, high school attended, current student status, employment status and income, welfare status and income, severity of hearing loss, and similar information. Cross found that as average income grows, the level of education increases, ranging from $6,800 for less than a high school education to $16,800 for those with a degree. Each level of education had a significant effect on income for the individual. Of those unemployed, 77 percent received some kind of welfare, with average payments of $3,675 per year. Medical cards were received by 50 percent of the unemployed, bringing the annual state welfare costs to over $4,000 per person. Cross (1985) concluded that more education for the deaf individual results in a higher standard of living and represents positive revenues for the state by way of increased taxes and reduced or eliminated welfare costs.

Another factor that restricts the employability of deaf persons is negative employer attitudes (Schein & Delk, 1974). Safety risks as well as difficulty communicating with and training deaf workers are common complaints of industries in regard to hiring deaf persons (Vernon, 1987). Employers are often reluctant to place a deaf person in a supervisory job, so promotions and hence salary increments are blocked. Deaf adults experience these barriers to professional positions even in deaf education, an area where they could make significant contributions (Vernon & Makowsky, 1969).

Marriage Patterns and Fertility Rates

As you would expect, because of the ease of communications and shared experiences of deafness, 95 percent of deaf people choose deaf spouses (Schein & Delk, 1974). These marriages are relatively stable. There is a higher divorce rate among marriages between hearing and deaf persons (Schein & Delk, 1974). Deaf women tend to have fewer babies than the hearing population, usually only one or two children (Schein & Delk, 1974). Because of this, and the fact that most deaf children come from hearing parents (Lane, 1984; Schein & Delk, 1974), deaf mothers are not contributing to the high number of deaf children.

Leisure Activities—Hobbies and Organizations

Recreational reading is a hobby of many deaf adults (Braden, 1986). In several surveys, deaf adults report that they purchased and frequently read newspapers and magazines covering a wide range of topics. Comics were also favorite choices. Books were read less frequently. The books that were read typically had a movie counterpart which the deaf adult viewed before or after reading the book. While the deaf population in general has low reading achievement (Allen, 1986), these surveys demonstrated that recreational reading is still pursued among deaf people.

Most deaf adults also belong to one or more religious, civic, or social organizations for the deaf community, and these play a vital role in their lives (Mindel & Vernon, 1971). Their leaders and members can offer important information about deafness to hearing professionals in the field.

One major organization is the National Association of the Deaf (NAD). It serves as an advocate for the educational, employment, legal, and social concerns for deaf people. Controlled exclusively by deaf people, this organization has over 18,000 members with 50 state associations in the United States. The NAD also has a youth division, called the Junior NAD, which has chapters in most state residential schools and aims to create leadership among deaf youth.

The NAD belongs to the World Federation of the Deaf, an international organization. The NAD's monthly magazine, *The Deaf American,* and its monthly newsletter, the *Broadcaster,* are widely circulated among deaf community members. The NAD also publishes books, periodicals, and educational materials in deafness. In addition, it has a credit union and runs summer camps for deaf children and youth.

The NAD established an active Legal Defense fund which helps deaf people fight for their civil rights. The organization has received grants from the federal government for research and demonstration projects for the benefit of deaf people. For example, currently it has a training program which instructs deaf persons in clerical work such as filing, typing, and mail room skills. The NAD also conducts film evaluations to determine which films should be captioned.

Another organization is the National Fraternal Society of the Deaf (FRAT). It was founded in 1901 by deaf adults in order to provide low-cost insurance protection, which had been denied to deaf persons at that time. Today the FRAT is licensed in 35 states and Canada, with about 106 lodges in principal cities. Along with insurance sales, the FRAT makes continuous efforts to protect the rights of deaf persons to drive cars and to get insurance. It works to eliminate job discrimination. It also performs civic duties such as donating clothing and incidentals to residents of homes for the aged deaf and to hospitals. It contributes food and toys to needy children. It offers scholarships, giving recognition and cash awards to deaf students and athletes. The FRAT provides consumer education and information to deaf people. It publishes a bimonthly magazine called *The FRAT.* National FRAT conventions are held every four years and local chapters hold regular business meetings and social events.

Numerous other regional and local deaf clubs exist. Within a large metropolitan area there may be two or three deaf clubs in operation, located in private homes, city buildings, YMCAs, church basements, schools, or bars. Some clubs own their own building. These organizations regularly meet for parties, bowling tournaments, card playing, picnics, sports events, fund-raising activities, special olympics, tours, and viewing of captioned films. Homecomings and reunions at residential schools provide another opportunity for deaf people to socialize together. Many graduates send each other yearly newsletters to maintain continuous contact.

Kyle (1986a, 1986b) reports that deaf adults in Great Britain frequently attend meetings at their local deaf club, and those with greater hearing losses go most frequently. The major difference Kyle found between the United States and Great Britain was that TDD's are much less common in Britain. In Great Britain TDD calls are metered by time and are therefore expensive. Therefore few British deaf people own them but instead will go to the club to communicate with other deaf people. In a poll of deaf club-goers, Kyle found that most deaf people go to the club by choice because they feel accepted there, not because they use it as a refuge from the hearing world.

Many changes have occurred over the years in deaf clubs in the United States (Vernon, 1983b). For example, in the past, the deaf club was the center of social activity and recreation for many deaf people, especially when they left the residential school. There deaf people developed leadership skills, met marriage partners, and had a social support system. Today, however, deaf clubs attract fewer members because home-centered entertainment such as captioned films, videocassette recorders, and TV has replaced the meetings. Mainstreaming, too, has contributed to the decline in membership. Thus many deaf youth lack contact with other deaf adults. Consequently, the average and below-average deaf person from the lower socioeconomic bracket is losing the kind of community they need for social support and guidance.

There are also deaf clubs for oral members only. The Oral Deaf Section of the Alexander Graham Bell Association is a national organization with about 312 members. This group promotes the teaching and using of speech and speech reading. Those who use manual communication are denied membership.

A recent trend in the deaf community is the establishment of state commissions for the deaf and hearing impaired (Vernon, 1983). These are set up to meet the major needs of deaf people in vocational training, interpreting, education, job placement, legal services, and mental health. There are currently 17 commissions, all administered either directly by the governor or by the Division of Vocational Rehabilitation.

A deaf organization for dramatic arts is the National Theatre of the Deaf (NTD) (Figures 1.1 and 1.2). Established in 1967 by Dr. Edna Levine and Dr. Boyce Williams, it is made up primarily of deaf actors, with some hearing actors. The NTD,

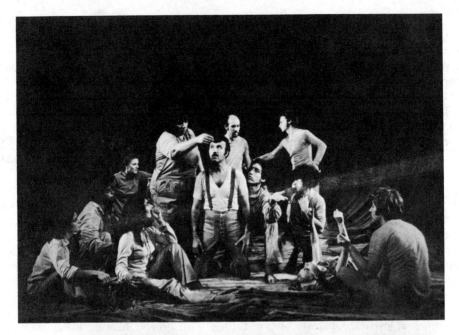

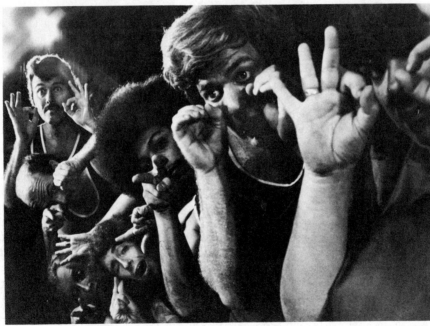

FIGURES 1.1. and 1.2.   Deaf actors performing in the National Theatre of the Deaf (Source: My Third Eye, an original piece created by the company. Photos by Jean Aare.)

which has won a Tony award, has performed on six continents. Their actors have appeared on Broadway, at New York City's Lincoln Center, on television, in theaters throughout the United States, on college campuses, and all over Europe. They have toured the People's Republic of China doing both stage and film work. The NTD also assists communities worldwide in setting up "deaf theater," making sign language within drama accessible to the hearing world. Typically at a performance both sign and spoken English are provided for the audience. The NTD runs a summer professional school funded by the U.S. Department of Education for those interested in acquiring acting skills. It also has a "Little theater of the deaf" which performs in schools both for deaf children and hearing children. Television and movie agencies who need deaf actors will often call the NTD for names. For example, deaf children recommended by the NTD have appeared on TV in "Dallas" and on a McDonald's hamburger commercial.

Sports-oriented deaf organizations are the American Athletic Association of the Deaf (AAAD) and the United States Deaf Skiers Association. The AAAD promotes state, regional, and national basketball and softball tournaments. It also promotes participation in the World Games for the Deaf and sponsors a Hall of Fame to honor deserving athletes. There are approximately 197 member clubs nationally and 20,000 individual members. Every four years an international deaf olympics is held. The AAAD publishes a newsletter called the *Deaf Spotlight.*

Deaf people are represented in almost every religious denomination (Schein & Delk, 1974). Many churches and synagogues will hold special services for deaf people. Religious oganizations have pioneered the providing of interpreting services for deaf people. Often a social hour will follow these services so that deaf people can meet and socialize with each other. Many religious places will have Sunday school for deaf children. Also, churches may conduct classes in sign language for interested hearing members who wish to communicate with deaf church members. There are some ordained ministers and priests who are themselves deaf. There are also national organizations of deaf people in the Baptist, Jewish, Catholic, and other major religious denominations. Still, in general, churches do not meet their obligation to deaf people, and as a result, many deaf persons are denied religious instruction and participation.

An organization that protects the legal rights of deaf citizens is the National Center for the Law and the Deaf (NCLD). It is partly funded by the NAD and is located at Gallaudet University in Washington, D.C. One of its primary objectives is to provide the deaf community with legal information that is both understandable and useful. It works to make legal terminology accessible to deaf persons. "Legalese" is confusing to deaf people because of their difficulty with the English language (only 10 percent of them read beyond the fourth grade). The problem is further compounded because legal jargon is often not easily translated into ASL. Consider one law—the Miranda Warning, which guarantees that all citizens be informed of their legal rights at the time they are arrested or questioned by the police. It is incomprehensible to a significant segment of the deaf population because of its lexical, syntactical, and conceptual complexity (Vernon & Coley, 1978). It is even difficult to translate into sign language because of the lack of existing signs for critical legal terms. The NCLD works on these kinds of problems and designs presentations, workshops, conferences, and materials to make legal issues understandable to the average deaf citizen.

The NCLD also offers educational programs to employers, teachers, hospital personnel, judges, lawyers, police officers, and court clerks. How to comply with federal and state laws for the handicapped in cost-effective ways is a frequent topic. The NCLD also provides legal information nationally to organizations, individuals, and service providers. The law center staff has written a book, *Legal Rights of Hearing-Impaired People* (DuBow et al. 1984). The organization has a legal services clinic which provides free counsel to Gallaudet University students and low-income deaf individuals in Washington, D.C. Other services the clinic provides are consumer information as well as information about government benefits and about legal rights.

The NCLD promotes legal careers of young deaf persons and encourages law schools to accept deaf applicants. It provides legal assistance to state legislators, associations, and commissions of the deaf in enacting state laws that provide equal access to deaf people. For example, significant progress has been made with state interpreter laws (Tucker, 1986). Legislative assistance has been provided by the law center to help make television and the telephone more accessible to deaf persons.

The organizations described above represent efforts of the deaf community to improve their quality of life and seek equal opportunity in society. There is another semi-organized activity that for many deaf people has a negative connotation: peddling.

Peddling is actually begging or selling. The deaf adult stands in a shopping center or airport, begs for money, and gives away cards with the manual alphabet or small items such as pens, needles, or key chains, on which is the message, "I am deaf and cannot work" (Higgins, 1980; Mindel & Vernon, 1971). Deaf peddlers usually work alone or in pairs. Some are controlled by a boss who manages a large operation. The deaf boss usually exploits deaf youth or deaf multi-handicapped adults. Peddlers have been known to make thousands of dollars without much work (Higgins, 1980; Mindel & Vernon, 1971).

Higgins (1980) has interviewed one boss, known as the "King" of the peddlers, who claimed that peddling was a legitimate form of selling and a reputable business. The deaf community, in contrast, does not view peddling favorably. It is considered deviant because it presents a false image to hearing people, suggesting that deaf people are incapable or unwilling to work and thus jeopardize employment opportunities for deaf people. Deaf sentiment is so strong that in 1934 the National Association of the Deaf passed a resolution condemning peddling, and the National Fraternal Society of the Deaf did the same in 1940 (Higgins, 1980).

Deaf Culture

Many professionals resist the belief that a deaf culture exists (Corwin & Wilcox, 1985). Even though the "deaf culture" expressed in written form and in the media is in its infancy (Corwin & Wilcox, 1985), there are many examples in literature, art, and drama which portray the daily patterns of everyday living, the frustrations, and the values of the deaf community (Rutherford, 1987, 1988).

The deaf community has shown repeated effort over the last 15 to 20 years in establishing national, regional, and local programs to develop the skills of deaf artists and provide them with a forum to display their work. These organizations disseminate information about the deaf culture or heritage and demonstrate artistic uses of sign language, especially in theater, dance, and poetry. In the past, these events were sponsored primarily by state residential schools or Gallaudet University, but deaf individuals around the country have also worked to set up organizations. While some of these organizations have ceased because of decreased federal funding, they have laid the groundwork for the future and undoubtedly fostered the appreciation of cultural events within the deaf community (Panara, 1987).

While literature, art, and drama entertain and inspire, they also preserve and transfer to the young the values and traditions of a culture. There are deaf actors, actresses, novelists, painters, sculptors, historians, scholars, and political leaders who produce writings and art forms to communicate values and traditions particular to the deaf community (see Panara & Panara, 1983, for biographies of deaf Americans, and Hairston & Smith, 1983, about black deaf Americans). For example, there is a rich folklore within the deaf culture which includes deaf stories, poetry, jokes, novels, and plays (Corwin & Wilcox, 1985). There are also rules of conversational etiquette which communicate values. For example, it is permissible to be blunt and to tell secrets because doing so facilitates and makes accessible communication (Hall, 1983), whereas in the hearing culture such behavior is considered rude.

There are plentiful examples of recorded and published literature, poetry, and drama in deafness. For instance, the speeches and stories of deaf adults have been made into movies and videotapes, many of which are located in the Gallaudet University library or can be purchased from the National Association for the Deaf, Gallaudet University Press, or T. J. Publishers. (See Appendix for addresses).

Jack Gannon's *Deaf Heritage* (1981) is a history of early deafness in America. Joanne Greenburg's novel, *In This Sign* (1970), is a classic which describes the deaf experience during the depression years. It was made into a TV screenplay entitled "Love Is Never Silent." Carolyn Brimley Norris wrote juvenile fiction—a mystery, *Island of Silence* (1983) and a novel, *Signs Unseen, Sounds Unheard* (1981). Douglas Bullard wrote the novel *Islay* (1986), which is a fantasy about a deaf man who establishes a state for deaf people where they rule themselves, use sign language, and are equal to hearing people. *Children of a Lesser God* (Medoff, 1980) is a play about a love story between a hearing man and a deaf woman and it has been made into a movie also. Another play, *Tales from a Clubroom,* is set in a deaf club and tells about living within the deaf community (Bragg & Bergman, 1981). Both novels and drama refer constantly to the struggles deaf people have in communicating and interacting in the hearing world from the deaf point of view with all of its resulting anguish and humiliations. Additionally, these literary works emphasize the positive aspects of the deaf community such as the feelings of group solidarity, the pride in using sign language, and the desire for human respect and dignity. There is the poetry of Dorothy Miles, which focuses on the beauty of sign language (1976). There are also paintings, drawings, and sculpture by deaf artists which express these same feelings and values. As the deaf community achieves greater visibility through the media, stage productions, and art exhibits, the output of this work will undoubtedly increase. (See Figure 1.3.)

ELDERLY DEAF COMMUNITY

The deaf community fosters a strong interdependence among its members even into old age. Elderly deaf people typically have lifelong friendships developed in childhood when they attended residential schools. Their social involvement will sustain them even after they have retired from the work force, especially those who

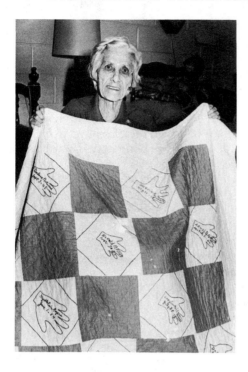

FIGURE 1.3. Deaf folk art: The hand-prints sewn on this quilt made by Myrtle Rodgers, a deaf woman from Waco, Kentucky, demonstrate the symbolic importance of hands.

worked in a hearing environment where they did not establish strong social ties. Many elderly deaf adults continue to use the state residential school to retain social contacts, congregating with classmates at homecomings, reunions, and other social and seasonal events (Becker, 1987).

The long-term support of the deaf community among its members is especially significant in old age, when people are dealing with chronic health problems and crises involving death of loved ones (Becker, 1987). There are some rest homes for the elderly deaf. These and senior citizens groups provide elderly deaf adults with recreational and social activities which the deaf clubs had provided for them when they were more mobile. The isolation which confronts the general population in old age is something deaf people have coped with growing up. Therefore, if they have a social network of elderly deaf friends, they do not seem to suffer this negative effect of aging as the normal population does (Becker, 1987). However, there are some elderly deaf persons who are in nursing homes where the staff do not use sign language with them. Those with little family support suffer the double isolation of old age and deafness.

A modern picture of the deaf community shows many constructive forces within it such as group solidarity, deaf pride, creative and artistic expression, and the linguistic knowledge of sign language. Yet, realistically it shows negative results too—undereducation, underemployment, and unemployment. The constructive forces, perhaps, are areas that could be utilized by professionals in deafness. Unfortunately, deaf adults are seldom consulted by hearing professionals making education and rehabilitation policy. This resource, if tapped, could yield improvement of services for deaf individuals.

REFERENCES

Allen, T. E. (1986). Patterns of academic achievement among hearing impaired students: 1974 and 1983. In A. Schildroth & M. Karchmer (Eds.), *Deaf children in America.* San Diego: College-Hill Press.

Annual survey of hearing-impaired children and youth. (1983–1984). Center for Assessment and Demographic Studies, Gallaudet Research Institute, Washington, DC.

Baker, C., & Cokely, D. (1980). *American Sign Language: A teacher's resource text on grammar and culture.* Silver Spring, MD: T. J. Publishers.

Barnartt, S. N. (1987). Deaf population: Women. In J. V. VanCleve (Ed.), *Gallaudet encyclopedia of deaf people and deafness.* New York: McGraw-Hill.

Becker, G. (1987). Deaf population: Aged. In J. V. VanCleve (Ed.), *Gallaudet encyclopedia of deaf people and deafness.* New York: McGraw-Hill.

Braden, J. (1986). Reading habits and preferences of deaf students beginning post-secondary program. *American Annals of the Deaf, 131*(3), 253–256.

Bragg, B., & Bergman, E. (1981). *Tales from a clubroom.* Washington, DC: Gallaudet College Press.

Bullard, D. (1986). *Islay.* Silver Spring, MD: T. J. Publishers.

Christiansen, J. B. (1987). Minorities. In J. V. VanCleve (Ed.), *Gallaudet encyclopedia of deaf people and deafness.* New York: McGraw-Hill.

Corwin, K., & Wilcox, S. (1985). The search for the empty cup continues. *Sign Language Studies, 48,* 249–268.

Craig, W., & Craig, H. (1986). Schools and classes for the deaf in the United States. *American Annals of the Deaf, 131*(2), 93–135.

Cross, P. R. (1985). *Relationship of employment and income to education level: A survey of hearing impaired in Kentucky.* Frankfort: Kentucky Commission for the Deaf and Hearing Impaired. Unpublished paper.

Delgado, G. L. (1984) Hearing-impaired children from non-native language homes. In G. L. Delgado (Ed.), *The Hispanic deaf: Issues and challenges for bilingual special education.* Washington, DC: Gallaudet College Press.

DuBow, S., Goldberg, L., Greer, S. Gardner, E., Penn, A., Conlon, S., & Charmatz, M. (1984). *Legal rights of hearing-impaired people.* Washington, DC: Gallaudet University Press.

Gannon, J. (1981). *Deaf heritage: A narrative history of deaf america.* Silver Spring, MD: National Association of the Deaf.

Greenburg, J. (1970). *In this sign.* New York: Holt, Rinehart and Winston.

Hairston, E., & Smith, L. (1983). *Black and deaf in America: Are we that different?* Silver Spring, MD: T. J. Publishers.

Hall, S. (1983). TRAIN-GONE-SORRY: The etiquette of social conversations in American Sign Language. *Sign Language Studies, 41,* 291–209.

Higgins, P. C. (1980). *Outsiders in a hearing world: A sociology of deafness.* Beverly Hills, CA: Sage Publications.

Holcomb, R. (1977). *Hazards of deafness.* Northridge, CA: Joyce Motion Picture Co.

Klima, E., & Bellugi, U. (1979). *The signs of language.* Cambridge, MA: Harvard University Press.

Kyle, J. G. (1986a, March). *British Sign Language research and the deaf community.* Paper presented to the Gallaudet "Deaf Culture" Seminar Series. Washington, DC: Gallaudet University Press.

Kyle, J. B. (1986b). Deaf people and minority groups in the U.K. In B. Tervort (Ed.), *Signs in life.* Amsterdam: Dutch Foundation for the Deaf.

Lane, H. (1984). *When the mind hears.* New York: Random House.

MacLeod-Gallinger, J. (1985). Secondary school graduate follow-up program for the deaf. Sixth Annual Report. Rochester Institute of Technology, National Technical Institute for the Deaf, Division of Career Opportunities.

Maestas y Moores, J., & Moores, D. (1984). The status of Hispanics in special education. In G. L. Delgado (Ed.), *The Hispanic deaf: Issues and challenges for bilingual special education.* Washington, DC: Gallaudet College Press.

Meadow, K. P. (1972). Sociolinguistics, sign language, and the deaf subculture. In T. J. O'Rourke (Ed.), *Psycholinguistics and total communication.* Washington, DC: American Annals of the Deaf.

Meadow, K. P. (1977). Name signs as identity symbols in the deaf community. *Sign Language Studies, 16,* 237–246.

Meadow-Orlans, K. P. (1985). Social and psychological effects of hearing loss in adulthood: A literature review. In H. Orlans (Ed.), *Adjustment to adult hearing loss,* San Diego: College-Hill Press.

Medoff, M. H. (1980). *Children of a lesser god.* Clifton, NJ: J. T. White.

Miles, D. (1976). *Gestures: Poetry in sign language.* Northridge, CA: Joyce Motion Picture Co.

Mindel, E., & Vernon, M. (1971). *They grow in silence.* Silver Spring, MD: National Association of the Deaf.

National Technical Institute for the Deaf (1984–1985). 1953–1984 Annual Report on Graduates and Employment. National Technical Institute for the Deaf, Rochester, NY.

Norris, C. B. (1981). *Signs unseen, sounds unheard.* Eureka, CA: Alinda Press.

Norris, C. B. (1983). *Island of silence.* Eureka, CA: Alinda Press.

Padden, C. (1980). The deaf community and the culture of deaf people. In C. Baker and R. Battison (Eds.), *Sign language and the deaf community: Essays in honor of William C. Stokoe.* Silver Spring, MD: National Association of the Deaf.

Panara, R. (1987). Cultural programs. In J. V. VanCleve (Ed.), *Gallaudet encyclopedia of deaf people and deafness.* New York: McGraw-Hill.

Panara, R., & Panara, J. (1983). *Great deaf Americans.* Silver Spring, MD: T. J. Publishers.

Rawlings, B. W., & King, S. J. (1986). Postsecondary educational opportunities for deaf students. In A. Schildroth & M. Karchmer (Eds.), *Deaf children in America.* San Diego: College-Hill Press.

Rutherford, S. (1987). *A study of American deaf folklore.* Unpublished doctoral dissertation, University of California, Berkeley.

Rutherford, S. (1988). The culture of American deaf people. In S. Wilcox (Ed.), Academic acceptance of American Sign Language. *Sign Language Studies, 59,* 129–147.

Schein, J. D. (1981). *A rose for tomorrow: Biography of Frederich C. Schreiber.* Silver Spring, MD: National Association of the Deaf.

Schein, J. D., & Delk, M. T. (1974). *The deaf population in the United States.* Silver Spring, MD: National Association of the Deaf.

Stokoe, W. C. (1960). Sign language structure: An outline of visual communication systems of the American deaf. *Studies in linguistics,* University of Buffalo, Dept. of Anthropology & Linguistics.

Tucker, P. T. (1986). Interpreter services: Legal rights of hearing-impaired persons. In *Oral interpreting: Principles and practices.* Baltimore, MD: University Park Press.

Vernon, M. (1983a) Postsecondary education federally established regional programs. Editorial in *American Annals of the Deaf, 128,* 1, 7.

Vernon, M. (1983b). Trends in the deaf community: Implications. Editorial in *American Annals of the Deaf, 128,* 1.

Vernon, M. (1987). Outcomes: Deaf people and work. In E. Mindel & M. Vernon (Eds.), *They grow in silence: Understanding deaf children and adults.* Silver Spring, MD: National Association of the Deaf.

Vernon, M., & Coley, J. (1978). Violation of constitutional rights: The language-impaired person and the Miranda warning.

Vernon, M., & Makowsky, B. (1969). Deafness and minority group dynamics. *Deaf American, 21,* 3–6.

Woodward, J. (1976). Black southern singing. *Language in Society, 5,* 211–218.

Woodward, J. (1980). Sociolinguistic research on American Sign Language. In C. Baker and R. Battison (Eds.), *Sign language and the deaf community: Essays in honor of William C. Stokoe.* Silver Spring, MD: National Association of the Deaf.

Woodward, J. (1985). Black deaf teachers—Short supply. *Perspectives for Teachers of the Hearing Impaired, 4,* 18–19.

CHAPTER 2
Genetics and Genetic Counseling

Genetics—*The lottery of life*   *Unknown*

This chapter deals with the nature of genetic deafness and with the issue of genetic counseling. Professionals who work closely with deaf children and their families, have a responsibility to understand hereditary deafness and the widespread psychological, audiological, and educational consequences of such a handicap for both victim and family.

PREVALENCE

Heredity accounts for 40 to 60 percent of childhood deafness (Shaver & Vernon, 1978). In about half of these hereditary syndromes, there are other defects as well (Konigsmark, 1972). Some involve the central nervous system and thus have direct psychological correlates (Vernon, 1976). In all cases of genetic deafness, the full communication of this information to the families not only is a matter of great psychological significance (Vernon, 1973) but also may contribute to the prevention and treatment of deafness and some of the severe syndromes of which hearing loss is a part.

There are over 150 different types of genetic deafness, with more being discovered every year (Shaver & Vernon, 1978). Over all, genetic deafness occurs in 1 per 2,000 to 6,000 births (Shaver & Vernon, 1978).

GENETIC TRANSMISSION OF DEAFNESS

Genetic deafness is transmitted in three major ways: dominantly, recessively, or through sex linkage (Shaver & Vernon, 1978). Figure 2.1 illustrates these processes and gives the basic probability information related to them. A full understanding of Figure 2.1 is essential for what follows in this chapter.

AUTOSOMAL DOMINANT DEAFNESS

There are more than 13 known forms of autosomal dominant genetic deafness (Shaver & Vernon, 1978). In dominant deafness, if one parent has a single gene for the condition, that parent will have the condition. In addition, there is a 50 percent chance of each child inheriting it. This is the usual situation in dominant pedigrees. However, if both parents have the same dominant form of deafness or if one parent

FIGURE 2.1. Basic genetic transmission (Source: Adapted from Fraser, F.C. (1971). Genetic counseling. *Hospital practice, 6,* 49—56.)

AUTOSOMAL DOMINANT CONDITIONS OF DEAFNESS

Counseling is relatively simple in autosomal dominant forms of deafness because of the clear relationship between the affected parents and the affected child. If neither parent is deaf, the deaf child probably represents a new mutation, and parents can be assured there is little risk to future siblings. However if the deafness is known to skip a generation occasionally or has a variable age of onset, the counseling must be more cautious.

One parent affected by deafness

50% of offspring will be deaf
regardless of sex

Both parents affected by deafness

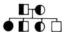

75% of offspring will be deaf
regardless of sex

AUTOSOMAL RECESSIVE CONDITIONS OF DEAFNESS

In autosomal recessive deafness the presumption following the birth of the deaf child is that both parents are carriers; they would be advised in counseling that the risk that a second child would be deaf is 1:4. Because of the recessive nature of the condition, a deaf individual cannot produce a child with recessive deafness unless the other parent is a carrier, but all his offspring will be carriers.

Both parents are carriers but not deaf

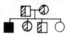

25% of offspring will be deaf
50% will be carriers regardless of sex

One parent deaf

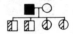

0% of offspring will be deaf
100% will be carriers

SEX-LINKED RECESSIVE CONDITIONS OF DEAFNESS

Counseling in X-linked disorders involving deafness usually depends on whether the mother is a carrier. If she has two or more deaf sons, or one deaf son and a deaf male relative (brother, father, maternal uncle) she must be considered a carrier. A single deaf son, however, may represent either a hitherto occult mutation in the mother's ancestors or a new mutation; sometimes special tests of the mother can settle this point. When the mother's carrier status is known and diagnosis is unambiguous, counseling can usually be given by the community physician.

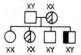

Sons: 50% will be deaf
Daughters: 50% will be carriers

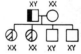

Sons: 100% will be normal
Daughters: 100% will be carriers

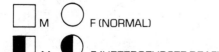

has two dominant genes for the same trait, the probability that offspring will manifest the disease increases to 75 and 100 percent respectively. Overall, about 10 percent of genetic deafness is dominant (Konigsmark, 1972).

Another important fact to remember in counseling families where there is a dominantly transmitted syndrome is that only those having the syndrome can pass it on. For example, a child who has a parent with Waardenburg's syndrome could rest assured that he does not carry the gene for the syndrome if he himself is not a Waardenburg. The problem is somewhat confused by the fact that dominant genes tend to be variable in their penetrance. For example, with Waardenburg's syndrome only two or three of the seven symptoms making up the disease may be clearly manifested.

RECESSIVE DEAFNESS

Ninety percent of genetic deafness is transmitted recessively (Shaver & Vernon, 1978). For an offspring to manifest recessive deafness, both parents must be carriers of the same gene for it. In such circumstances, each child has a 25 percent chance of being deaf, a 50 percent chance of having hearing but carrying the recessive gene for deafness, and a 25 percent chance of having hearing and not carrying the gene, that is, being a homozygous normal.

Often the recessive gene is passed on for many generations without being matched with another like it. Thus there is no deafness. When finally parents who have the same recessive gene have a deaf child, it can be extremely difficult to trace the genetic transmission, especially for one not aware of the complexities of recessive genetics. The result is often a confusion on the part of parents and professionals as to why the child is deaf.

In marriages between cousins or other relatives, recessive traits are especially likely to manifest themselves. Such consanguineous unions occur at a 9 percent rate among deaf persons as contrasted to a 1 percent rate among the hearing population (Rainer, 1968).

Because deafness can be caused by one of 30 to 40 separate recessive genes, couples who carry a recessive gene for deafness would run the risk of having a deaf child only if the "deafness" genes were in the same chromosome at the same loci (Shaver & Vernon, 1978). Were it not for this multiplicity of recessive genes transmitting deafness, the trait would be far more pervasive. However, the 50 or so "deafness" genes are centered in two or three chromosomes, and so their pairing is more probable than if they were evenly scattered over all 46 chromosomes (Nance, 1973).

SEX-LINKED DEAFNESS

In sex-linked genetic transmission, recessive traits are transmitted by women to half their sons and none of their daughters (Fraser, F. C., 1971). Half of their daughters are carriers. The male who has the trait transmits the recessive gene to all his daughters and to none of his sons. Thus, sex-linked recessive traits appear only in males except for extremely rare cases where they manifest themselves in a female carrier (Fraser, F. C., 1971).

Amniocentesis is important where sex-linked traits are suspected because this technique can determine the gender of the unborn child (Danes, 1970). Since the female generally does not have sex-linked disease, the issue of therapeutic abortion occurs primarily with male fetuses. In the rare case where the mother is a carrier and the father is affected, the female offspring can have the disease.

OTHER GENETIC FACTORS

Chromosomal aberrations sometimes cause deafness, as, for example, in the 13-15 Trisomy syndrome, which results in abnormalities of the central nervous system, eyes, hands, ears, heart, kidneys, and genitalia (Maniglia, Wolff, & Herques, 1970). However, the recurrent risk is low in most chromosomal defects (Fraser, F. C., 1968).

Mutant genes are another rare factor that can be a cause of deafness. In addition, deafness can be a multifactorial disease, that is, it can be caused by a number of genes and thus not follow simple Mendelian laws. In such cases, the probability of affected children must be based on empirical data gained from study of previous families with similar mutant conditions (Fraser, F. C., 1968). Rainer (1968) states that in families where both parents are deaf, 70 percent of the offspring are hearing. Where there is one deaf parent, the rate varies from 14 to 41 percent. Risk is obviously highest where one parent has a dominant form of deafness, such as Waardenburg's syndrome.

GENETIC SYNDROMES

About 50 percent of genetic deafness involves hearing loss and no other abnormality (Shaver & Vernon, 1978). The 13 major kinds of deafness in this category differ with regard to the audiometric pattern of the hearing loss, the time of onset, the site of lesion (middle ear or neural), the nature of genetic transmission (autosomal dominant versus autosomal recessive), and other factors (Konigsmark, 1972).

Of the 50 percent of cases where the deafness is combined with another abnormality, the following additional conditions are the most common.

The first is deafness and skin (integumentary) abnormality, including pigmentation disorders. Spotting of the skin (piebaldness), albinism, or a white forelock (part of Waardenburg's syndrome) are common examples. Other syndromes of this type include dermatitis, nail disorders, and hair abnormalities.

Deafness and eye disorders comprise another major group of genetic syndromes. Among the visual pathologies are retinal abnormalities, optic atrophy, and atypical lens and bulb conditions. Obviously, eye problems assume critical importance in deaf persons because those without hearing are forced to depend primarily upon vision. Usher's syndrome is the major syndrome involving the eye and ear (see discussion later in this chapter).

Deafness and associated nervous system disease represent another set of syndromes. Acoustic neuromes, cerebral dysfunction, and mental retardation are examples of the disorders in this group.

There are about 15 different hereditary forms of deafness with associated musculoskeletal defects such as facial deformities. Treacher-Collins syndrome and Klippel-Feil are examples of conditions in this category.

Deafness and renal disease comprise the final major group of syndromes. The most important condition here is Alport's syndrome.

There are several other possible groupings and also a number of isolated abnormalities which occur with genetic deafness. In most cases, these are thought to be due to different single genes affecting other systems as well as hearing.

GENETICS TODAY

The overwhelming implications of genetics in the area of deafness make it crucial that professionals not only know genetics but also have a familiarity with genetic counseling as it relates to deaf persons, their families, and those with whom they are considering marriage. This need is best understood in terms of what is happening in medicine today.

The detection, prevention, and treatment of genetic disorders is creating a revolution in the field of medicine similar to that following Pasteur's germ theory of infectious disease. For example, in 1951 there were 10 genetic counselors in the United States, and about the only therapeutic measure available to them was the recommendation that a couple avoid pregnancy. Furthermore, these counselors were able only to estimate the risk of a defective child in the broadest of generalities.

By contrast, today almost every medical center has a geneticist. Many genetic diseases can be diagnosed *in utero* early enough to permit therapeutic abortion. Often parents can be told whether or not they carry a given abnormal gene and pregnancies can be monitored. The list of treatable genetic conditions, though small, is growing.

Inherited diseases have come to the forefront, not because they are increasing, but because infectious diseases and their seriousness are on the decline, as the following statistics show (Danes, 1970). Infant mortality due to congenital malformations is about 5 per 1,000 births now, as it was in 1900. However, the overall infant mortality rate in 1900 was 151 per 1,000 births whereas today it is 20 per 1,000. Thus, in 1900, congenital malformations accounted for only 4 percent of infant mortality whereas today they account for 20 percent. Furthermore, while the incidence of congenital defects remains at 5 percent, vaccines, antibiotics, and better sanitation have decreased infectious diseases and their effects, thus placing greater relative importance on congenital conditions. This is particularly true in deafness, where scarlet fever, mastoiditis, diphtheria, polio, rubella, and complications of Rh factor used to be major causes of deafness but now less frequently result in hearing loss.

The increasing importance of genetics requires a tremendous re-education of physicians and professionals in deafness for a number of reasons. Historically, very few have known much about genetics. The doctor of the past studied a few diseases, such as polio and scarlet fever, which affected thousands of people. With the hereditary disorders of today, the situation is reversed. There are about 2,000 known genetic diseases, and the number is growing daily (Shaver & Vernon, 1978), but each affects only a small number of people. An incidence of 1 per 100,000 or per 1,000,000 is not uncommon (Danes, 1970). For example, cystic fibrosis is the most common serious hereditary disease among Caucasians, yet it affects only 1 per 2,000. Phenylketonuria affects 1 per 10,000, yet screening for it is mandatory (Danes, 1970).

Other genetic diseases affect only specific groups. Tay-Sachs is a terminal form of severe neurological degenerative mental retardation which occurs primarily among East European Jews. Sickle-cell anemia, a serious blood disease, affects mostly blacks. Thus in a typical practice a physician's chance of seeing many of these 2,000 genetic diseases is small (Danes, 1970). This is especially true for those 150 or so that involve hearing loss.

A third problem the physician faces with genetic diseases is that their treatment is highly specialized and expensive. Each of the more than 500 medical centers in the United States can specialize in only a few. A final problem is that therapeutic abortion is often the only "treatment," and such a solution involves a major ethical conflict for many.

THE NATURE OF GENETIC COUNSELING

The almost universal fallacy about genetic counseling is that it is a simple matter of computing the probabilities for a given disease and stating this bleak legacy to prospective parents. Nothing could be further from the truth. Good genetic counseling requires extreme sensitivity to human feelings, extensive knowledge of heredity, and a deep understanding of the medical-psychological involvements of a multitude of rare diseases. Even more important, the counseling entails an empathy for the psychological effects of the diseases on the child, his or her family, and society. The following case study illustrates the problem.

> David and Rebecca Wechsler, students in a school for deaf youth, have Usher's syndrome (congenital deafness and progressive blindness due to retinitis pigmentosa).
>
> Rebecca, at 19, has night blindness and narrowing visual fields characteristic of the disease. Her IQ is 101 but her academic learning has been retarded by her deafness and an aphasoic difficulty not uncommon in Usher's syndrome. She will leave school with a certificate of attendance and look for work or vocational training. An attractive woman, she has dated several of her class-mates. Because she is passive and naive, she has been seduced, but without resulting pregnancy.
>
> David, her brother, age 13 and with an IQ of 106, is in psychotherapy for fetishism and transvestism. David plays on the football team but has begun to have difficulty seeing at night and wears strong corrective glasses.
>
> The parents are intelligent, but personal problems have limited their educational and economic advancement. Mr. Wechsler is a school custodian and has a serious heart condition. He has never psychologically accepted his children's deafness and emotional conflicts, partly because of his own problems, which include a fixation on bondage themes in his sexual relations. Mrs. Wechsler has tried to keep the home together and meet the needs of the children, but her own unhappiness and fears of meeting people and coping with the competition of work and social interaction impair her efforts.

The case of the Wechsler family poses some of the many complex medical-psychological problems common to genetic counseling. For example, what should the predisposed patient be told, that is, do you inform a 13-year-old boy, already in psychotherapy for emotional disturbance, that he will become blind as well as deaf?

When and how do you tell Rebecca the prognosis for her vision? How do you explain the complex genetics of Usher's syndrome to Rebecca, when she knows little or no biology and reads at a third-grade level?

Do you arbitrarily sterilize both youths, as their ophthalmologist recommended, without letting them play any role in making the decision? What are the probabilities that they will mate with a person who is not a carrier of the Usher's syndrome gene, thus ensuring that their children will not have the disease but possibly perpetuating the gene for it? If informed of their disease and its genetics, should these two youths be given the right as adults to procreate if they wish? Should they be permitted to marry a known carrier, with the understanding that children from such a union would have a one in four chance of being born with Usher's syndrome and facing deafness and blindness? Is a normal expectancy of 25 years of good health, except for deafness, enough to justify the birth of a child who will eventually be deaf-blind? What about the religious convictions of those involved? And can society refuse citizens the right to bring children into the world who are likely to impose huge financial burdens upon institutions supported by that society?

Where is one to find a geneticist who is knowledgeable about rare conditions such as Usher's syndrome and who also understands the psychological and social implications of deaf-blindness? And if one is to be found, how would he communicate with David and Rebecca, who depend on sign language?

What about the wishes of the parents? Mrs. Wechsler adamantly wants grandchildren and plans to have them through David and Rebecca, her only offspring. What physician would sterilize these teenage children against their mother's will?

Whence does the money and time come for the genetic expertise needed in this case? There is probably one genetic counselor in the world sufficiently knowledgeable about Usher's syndrome and the psychological effects of deafness and blindness to provide the service needed; however, he is in Virginia and the Wechsler family is in Oregon.

The point is that there is more involved in this case than simply informing the family of the probabilities of the genetic transmission of Usher's syndrome. Such complexities characterize genetic counseling. Understanding these medical and psychological issues is an integral part of any comprehensive psychology of deafness.

COMPONENTS OF GENETIC COUNSELING

DIAGNOSIS

Certain basic services are provided in any complete genetic counseling program. The first is the diagnosis or confirmation of the presence of a hereditary disease. This usually demands laboratory tests such as sex chromatin determinations, blood grouping, chromosome examinations, and a variety of biochemical tests. Laboratories able to perform many of these tests are available only in large metropolitan areas, and some of the procedures are extremely expensive.

Equally important is the case history. It leads to the development of the family pedigree which, along with the laboratory findings, constitute the basic genetic data. These data are then used to establish the probabilities of the appearance of the disease in a given situation, probabilities which must then be communicated to the family. Finally, comprehensive genetic counseling services involve a follow-up of both the patient and his or her family. The process of communicating the findings to the family, the follow-up, screening, and other related functions are complex considerations.

FOLLOW-UP

The presence of a hereditary disease, including certain forms of deafness, immediately makes other family members high-risk cases. They too should be screened for the disease. For example, in the case of the Wechslers, other members of the family are certain to be carriers of the deaf-blindness syndrome. Some may actually have the disease and not yet know it. Unfortunately, in cases such as these where the genetic counselor is the bearer of bad news, his or her advice is often received with hostility, denial, and resentment (Fraser, F. C., 1971). For these reasons and because it is not always clear who is responsible, follow-up has tended to be a badly neglected aspect of counseling. Follow-up should become increasingly important as methods to detect heterozygous carriers improve and thereby remove much of the uncertainty in genetic counseling.

At present, follow-up counseling in deafness is almost nonexistent, despite the fact that genetic transmission is the major cause of hearing loss. The problem is illustrated in the current handling of Usher's syndrome. The government, instead of instituting preventive measures such as identification, follow-up, and counseling of families afflicted with this disease, has established expensive centers to diagnose and provide custodial care for the deaf-blind (Vernon, 1976). This is especially ironic because Usher's syndrome is the leading cause of deaf-blindness (Bettica et al., 1959). Follow-up offers little monetary incentive to physicians and other genetic counselors. In the case of deafness, this lack of follow-up is especially tragic because the high-risk population—deaf children—is highly centralized and readily accessible.

SCREENING

Screening is a major approach to prevention and is integral to adequate follow-up. Screening is feasible and relatively simple in the case of genetic deafness because, as was mentioned above, the high-risk population is small, easily identified, centralized, and available. Of the approximately 400 speech and hearing clinics in the United States and Canada, about 300 are in medical schools, hospitals, or colleges (Craig & Craig, 1981). The remaining 100 are in schools for the deaf or in private facilities (Craig & Craig, 1981). Thus, at preschool age most deaf children are identified and are patients at facilities likely to have access to people with some genetic knowledge.

The centralization of deaf youth continues to some extent when they reach school age. Then specialized educational requirements tend to concentrate the children in facilities representing large population centers or geographic areas. For example, in some states, the majority of deaf children go to a single residential school. Of the 60,000 or more deaf youths who are enrolled in special education programs in the United States and Canada, many are in one of 107 large residential or day schools (Craig & Craig, 1981). Most of the remaining ones are in day classes, mostly in metropolitan areas. In other civilized countries of the world there are analogous educational programs resulting in the same centralization of the deaf population.

Within this population of deaf youth, the high-risk group can be further narrowed by elimination of those known to have nonhereditary forms of deafness. Also a reasonably certain case for genetic deafness may be made for those students having deaf relatives.

The first phase of the screening procedure thus takes place at school. The screening of a relatively small population there will yield a very high number of cases whose cause of deafness is genetic and who may have additional disorders such as retinitis pigmentosa or nephritis.

The second phase of screening should involve the relatives of deaf persons. Carriers of some forms of deafness can be identified by new diagnostic techniques (Shaver & Vernon, 1978; Vernon 1976). Screening would also lead to the early identification of those with certain genetic diseases so that appropriate educational, medical, and rehabilitational plans could be made. Genetic counseling of carriers could then enable prospective parents among them to prevent the spread of serious syndromes.

Genetic screening, like genetic counseling, is a far more complex procedure than it seems. Families can be terrified by the information that they have a "killer" disease or are carriers of it. For example, large segments of the black community were panicked by the 1972–1973 screening program and the attendant public scare in connection with sickle-cell anemia. Many unaffected carriers mistakenly thought that they had a disease that would end in painful death. Some black elementary schoolchildren were led to believe that they would die any minute.

Thus genetic screening should include a careful explanation to the subject of at least three points: (1) the nature of the genetic deafness or syndrome, including whatever positive prognosis there may be for a proband; (2) the vast difference between having the disease and being a carrier; and (3) the data on the genetic transmission of the condition. There should be no genetic screening unless there is adequate counseling and overall follow-up.

PSYCHOLOGICAL ASPECTS
OF GENETIC COUNSELING

Frequently genetic counseling involves the communication of traumatic information to a person about his having a serious disease, whether a child will be born defective, and so on. The reactions and psychodynamics resulting from such information are, in many respects, similar to the reactions to other psychological traumas, such as the discovery that one's child is deaf. (See chapter 6).

The appropriate handling of these intense feelings requires great psychological skill on the part of the genetic counselor. He or she must understand the denial, hostility, fear, guilt and other feelings likely to be present at this time and be able to help in developing constructive ways of coping with them and with the situation. In the case of deafness, the counselor should understand what it means to be deaf. For example, the average hearing person, when asked if he would have children if he knew they would be deaf, answers "No." By contrast, deaf people who know through their own experience what deafness is, generally say "Yes." In fact, 32 percent of deaf parents express no preference at all as to whether their child should be born deaf or hearing (Rainer, 1968).

It is important to remember that the genetic counselor working with deafness is counseling not just for deafness but for other pathological conditions. For example, in conditions such as Alport's syndrome or the Jervell and Lange-Nielsen syndrome, the deafness, though serious, is a relatively minor component.

COUNSELING THE PREDISPOSED PATIENT

Suppose a patient is known to have a genetic disease, such as Usher's or Alport's syndrome, that manifests itself at a later stage of life. Is it best to tell the patient and bring on years of worry about something he or she may never live to see? How many of us would want to know the date we are to die if such a fact were available? In the case of the predisposed patient, should a close friend or family member be informed? If the condition requires no therapy, should the counselor just advise frequent checkups? With increased screening and improved genetic and laboratory diagnosis, the problem is going to arise with increasing frequency. For example, the use of improved diagnostic techniques which can detect Usher's syndrome early in childhood (Bergsma, 1973) also poses the problem of how much and when to tell a deaf child about his or her imminent blindness.

Usually, there is some action the predisposed patient can take to delay the onset of the disease, minimize its effects, and prevent its genetic transmission to others. For these reasons, some genetic counselors fully inform all patients, including those likely "to go to pieces" (*Medical World News,* 1972a&b). Some tell a close friend of the afflicted person.

The profound questions raised here have no simple answers. They do illustrate the need for great sensitivity and in-depth psychological skill in the genetic counseling process.

WHO SEEKS GENETIC COUNSEL?

Most of the people who seek genetic counsel about deafness are deaf couples, hearing children of deaf parents, consanguineous marital partners, or couples who already have one deaf child (Fraser, F. C., 1968, 1971). They generally want to know what the chances are of their having a child who is deaf or has an inherited deafness syndrome. Most people know little about the relationship of their family deafness to heredity (Rainer, 1968). Rainer (1968) reports that of deaf people who seek counseling, 45 percent want hearing children, 32 percent have no preference, 15 percent want deaf children, and 8 percent do not desire offspring.

Demands for genetic counseling are increasing, because of the public information available, new social options such as liberalized abortion, and modern techniques of early detection. Soon the question may not be "Should I have another deaf child?" but "Should I have this deaf child?"

THE REALITIES OF GENETIC COUNSELING

Most people connected with deafness are in favor of genetic counseling, at least to the extent of verbally supporting the idea. Ironically, the fundamental question of whether or not it has any effect is unanswered. One survey on genetic counseling in general indicated that most persons understood little or nothing of what was told to them (*Medical World News,* 1972). In other instances, they understood the arithmetic but not the reality, that is, they grasped the probabilities but not the consequences of a handicapped child in a family (Fraser, F. C., 1971). Obviously, these reactions mean that great effort needs to be made to help develop an understanding of this "reality." Prospective parents must be helped to see exactly what it means to have a deaf child, in terms of the specific conditions that would be encountered.

Generally, it takes about three sessions to explain hereditary deafness sufficiently well for couples to understand the risk of having a deaf child. The psychologically loaded information that may have to be communicated cannot properly be dealt with in such brief interaction. In one study (*Medical World News,* 1972a&b), those who had a defective child (not necessarily deaf), when followed up three to ten years later, remembered the risk figures and understood the odds of having another. The couples in this category fell into two groups, according to degree of risk. Of the "high-risk" cases (those with a 1 in 10 genetic probability of having a defective child), two-thirds chose birth control, adoption, or artificial insemination. Of the "low-risk" group (chances 1 in 20 or less), one-fourth did otherwise: When the genetic condition was one that caused death within the first few weeks of life or when it was treatable, like cleft palate, many took the chance. With serious chronic conditions, such as muscular dystrophy or severe retardation, they did not. Follow-up parental reaction to genetic counseling regarding the risk of deafness is not available.

QUALIFICATIONS OF THE GENETIC COUNSELOR

Ideally, a genetic counselor is a physician who has the medical knowledge to understand the various disease processes, the psychotherapeutic skill to cope with the tremendous emotional stress which is often a part of genetic counseling, and a thorough understanding of heredity. Such ideal persons are rare, and it is unrealistic to expect that they will be available in sufficient quantity to meet counseling needs in the foreseeable future.

Thus we have to settle for far less than the ideal counselor to deliver genetic information on deafness. Audiologists, psychologists, otolaryngologists, rehabilitation counselors, educators, psychiatrists, and other professionals working in deafness must become familiar enough with genetics to identify needs, provide rudimentary information, and guide those requiring help to qualified specialists, if they are available. If not, then an effort should be made to coordinate the best available services. For example, there may be an available geneticist who lacks a knowledge of deafness. In such a case, a team approach, with each member contributing a part of the total information needed, may be the practical solution.

TOOLS AVAILABLE TO THE GENETIC COUNSELOR

About the only preventive tool available to the geneticist in the past was advice not to have children. The situation has changed. A step forward has been *amniocentesis,* the analysis of the amniotic fluid surrounding the fetus. Such analysis can identify whether or not the unborn infant is a carrier of certain diseases, such as Hurler's syndrome. The gender of a fetus can be determined at 16 weeks or earlier through this technique.

The invention of the *fetoscope,* a device permitting the doctor to directly view the fetus *in utero,* is another step forward. Such a procedure makes possible the spotting of certain physical defects and safer blood sampling.

The liberalization of abortion is another development that provides an important tool. When coupled with the findings from amniocentesis and other data, abortion can be a major preventive step for parents and counselors who are not in opposition to it ethically.

Treatment is another tool. However, as yet very few diseases can be cured or ameliorated (Danes, 1970; Shaver & Vernon, 1978). Diseases such as diabetes and phenylketonuria, which require some missing product to be supplied, probably hold the best hope for a future cure. Usher's syndrome may also be such a condition (Vernon, 1969).

Preventing reproduction is more effective now than in the past. Advances in, or liberalization of sterilization, contraception, tubal ligation, the suppression of ovulation, and spermatogenesis have given couples greater control over conception. Adoption or artificial insemination are other possible alternatives.

Genetic screening and preventive counseling are also valuable tools of the genetic counselor. However, major impediments to these approaches remain: laws, religious beliefs, inadequate services, aversion on psychological grounds, fear, and ignorance.

Eugenics

Any in-depth discussion of genetic counseling eventually gets around to the concept of eugenics, which Charles Darwin (Zellweger, 1967), Adolph Hitler, and A. G. Bell (Mitchell, 1971), among others, have supported. There are real dangers in this area, centering around racism and physical superiority (Mitchell, 1971). Sickle-cell anemia screening laws, which are the first ever directed toward a specific race, have been criticized for this very reason.

It is one thing to inform people about their own genetic situation and probabilities or to help them cope with feelings about their circumstances. It is quite another to try to exercise control over an individual's family planning. Basic issues of human rights and the rights of society are involved at the deepest ethical and moral levels. To do as Alexander Graham Bell did and try to force upon deaf people a eugenic practice that represents a personal bias, would be a horrible injustice both to deaf people and to nondeaf persons thought to be carriers of the genes for hearing loss (Mitchell, 1971).

Future Needs

In order to increase the effectiveness of genetic counseling in regard to deafness, improvements are needed in several areas. The most important is in the identification of heterozygote carriers. This is of special value in conditions such as Usher's syndrome and Alport's disease. Detection of genetic conditions before gross clinical symptoms appear would also be a major step forward. Finally, progress is needed in the earlier detection of mutant genes in carriers.

A CLOSER LOOK AT THE MAJOR GENETIC SYNDROMES INVOLVING DEAFNESS

What follows is a description of nine major syndromes of concern to those involved with deaf persons or their families: their features, identification, diagnostic techniques, treatment, prevention, and research. The syndromes were selected from among the more than 150 which have been identified, for any of several reasons. Either they have a high prevalence, they represent conditions having psychological correlates, or they are syndromes of serious consequence. If identified and understood, they could be treated, prevented, or at least coped with more constructively.

USHER'S SYNDROME

The major features of Usher's syndrome are a congenital hearing loss, often profound, and a progressive blindness due to retinitis pigmentosa (Vernon, 1976). The visual loss is generally first diagnosed in the early teens or twenties, when the patient complains of night blindness. Most victims are forced to give up their professions at about 30 or 40 because of advancing sightlessness. Many become totally blind by 50 or 60 (Vernon, 1969). In severe cases, the visual loss is diagnosed during preschool years. There is apparently sometimes a central nervous system degeneration which may manifest itself in psychiatric illness, loss of olfactory sensitivity, aphasia, mental retardation, abnormal EEG readings, and other neuropathological and behavioral correlates. While it is a rare disease in the general population (three cases per 100,000), it is significantly more prevalent among those who are deaf. Approximately 3 to 6 percent of the genetically deaf are afflicted with this handicap (Vernon, 1976). Recent clinical findings suggest that some patients may retain considerable hearing and vision into their sixties and that many suffer no other correlates of the disease (Vernon, 1976).

Research indicates that heterozygote carriers of Usher's may be identifiable by complete auditory, visual, and vestibular diagnostic procedures (Kloepfer, Laguaite, & McLaurin, 1966). This is a hopeful, but tentative, finding relative to screening and prevention.

Usher's is more common in family pedigrees having cases of retinitis pigmentosa without deafness, a fact which, along with the variances of traits found in persons with Usher's, raises serious questions about its genetics and the possible embryological, toxic, or metabolic processes in its pathogenesis.

Commonly used techniques for diagnosing the disease (ophthalmoscopic examination and visual field testing) usually fail to detect the condition until it is in a relatively advanced stage and the patient is in his teens or twenties. More thorough techniques involving electroretinography and dark adaptation measures make much earlier diagnosis possible (Bergsma, 1973).

Although a wide variety of treatments have been tried, including surgery, endocrine therapy, vitamins, and transplants, at present the disease cannot be cured nor can its course be significantly altered. Therefore a premium is placed on prevention.

A program for prevention through high-risk diagnostic screening coupled with genetic counseling is both feasible and practical. The already existent centralization of the high-risk population ensures a yield from screening procedures of probably 3 to 6 percent. Thus prevention is strongly urged in view of the trauma and chronicity of the affliction. Following identification of cases of Usher's syndrome, relatives should be examined to determine if they are carriers.

Research into biochemical, genetic, metabolic, psychiatric, and other aspects of Usher's offers hope not only for greater understanding of this disease but also for findings of far greater generality. Usher's represents a centering of gross central nervous system pathology with major psychological correlates such as aphasia, memory pathology, psychosis, and mental retardation. An understanding of the pathogenesis of Usher's may give insight into causes of forms of these other conditions (Vernon, 1969).

ALPORT'S SYNDROME

Hearing loss, a progressive degeneration of the kidneys (nephritis), and eye defects (lens abnormalities) comprise Alport's syndrome (Miller, Joseph, Cozad, & McCabe, 1970; Turner, 1970). The kidney disease is often terminal, especially in males, who die before the age of 30 (Turner, 1970).

It is especially important that professionals in deafness know the syndrome, because early identification and counseling can be life-saving. For example, deaf women having the disease frequently do not know about it until well into pregnancy. The physiological stress of gestation in such persons can result in maternal death from nephritis or else greatly shorten the mother's life span following her child's birth.

The value of the current widespread use of renal transplants can be undermined if the genetic nature of Alport's disease is not understood. If the common practice of using a close relative as a donor is followed, there is a risk due to the probability that the donor may also have Alport's syndrome, or at least nephritis; the transplant would result in the replacement of one diseased kidney with another and leave both donor and recipient with the prospect of early death.

The hearing loss in Alport's syndrome varies greatly in degree and in time of onset. It may be congenital and profound or not appear until adulthood and be mild. The genetics of Alport's syndrome are not fully understood, but it appears to be a sex-linked dominant disorder (Miller, Joseph, Cozad, & McCabe, 1970; Patton, 1970). Deafness occurs in 50 percent of the cases (Miller, Joseph, Cozad, & McCabe, 1970). When deafness is not present, the disorder is known as Bright's disease. Ocular problems are present 15 percent of the time and are perhaps secondary to the renal disorder (Miller, Joseph, Cozad, & McCabe, 1970). The pathogenesis is not fully understood but is believed to be due to a genetically controlled enzyme effect (Turner, 1970).

Obviously, it is crucial that there be early detection, screening of relatives, and counseling of carriers and those having the disease. Among deaf people, it can be diagnosed by the presence of certain proteins in the urine. It is speculated that carriers may have a characteristic audiometric pattern.

Through early identification and recognition of the syndrome it may be possible to save the lives of some through renal transplants before extensive protein loss and toxemia occurs (Turner, 1970).

WAARDENBURG'S SYNDROME

There are six components in Waardenburg's syndrome, but it is rare for all six to be present in one individual case (Proctor & Proctor, 1967). Striking features are the white forelock and eyes of different colors (heterochromia of the iris). The most common traits are "wide-set" eyes (lateral displacement of the inner canthi), a broad nose at the root, and eyebrows that meet. Twenty percent of cases of Waardenburg's are deaf, and most others have milder hearing losses which may be progressive (Proctor & Proctor, 1967). The low and middle frequencies are most often affected. Cleft lip or cleft palate is not uncommon (Giacoia & Klein, 1969). In black or brown-skinned people there may be a patchy depigmentation of the skin of the face and forehead which tends to be cosmetically disfiguring (Fraser, G. R., 1964). (See Figure 2.2.)

In the first author's own clinical experience and research involving some 40 cases of Waardenburg's, there has been no observable intellectual or emotional aspect associated with the condition, except where the disfigurement of cleft lip or, in the case of black persons, abnormal skin pigmentation resulted in psychological problems (Conley & Vernon, 1975).

The prevalence of Waardenburg's syndrome in the deaf population is about 0.25 percent (Proctor & Proctor, 1967).

KLIPPEL-FEIL SYNDROME

In almost every school for deaf children there are one or two with what appear to be shortened necks and sometimes spinal curvatures. They have Klippel-Feil syndrome, a condition in which the bones of the neck (cervical vertebrae) are replaced by a skeletal mass of fused vertebrae. Females are most often affected (Palant & Carter, 1972). Though the hereditary pattern is not totally clear, the condition seems due to a recessive gene. Early diagnosis is important because it can lead to the prevention of complicating conditions often present, such as curvature of the spine (scoliosis).

JERVELL AND LANGE-NIELSEN SYNDROME

This is a rare syndrome, consisting of deafness and a functional heart disease, usually resulting in death during the teenage years (Fraser, Froggatt, & James, 1964). This condition can be identified by electrocardiograms. The pathognomic feature is a marked prolongation of the Q-T interval and large T waves. Once it is identified, steps can be taken to increase the life span significantly.

PENDRED'S SYNDROME

This is a combination of congenital deafness and goiter, the latter due to the lack of the enzyme required for normal iodine metabolism (Fraser, 1964). Pendred's syndrome accounts for about 10 percent of the cases of recessive deafness according to Konigsmark (1972). Except for the aforementioned disorders, general mental and physical development is usually normal. The deafness is most severe for high tones. Pendred's syndrome can be treated because it is due to a failure to metabolize iodine.

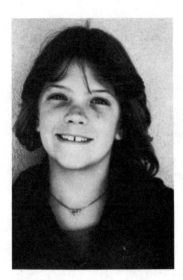

FIGURE 2.2.   This child shows several characteristics of Waardenburg's syndrome: wide set eyes and a broad nose at the root.

FIGURE 2.3.   This child shows several characteristics of Treacher-Collins syndrome: a receding chin, a downward slant of the eyelids, and an underdevelopment of facial and cranial bones.

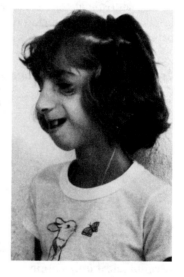

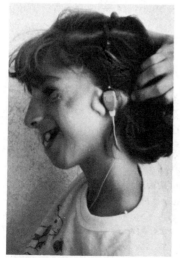

FIGURE 2.4.   The imperfect ossification of bones in Treacher-Collins syndrome can cause deafness, or hard-of-hearing because the middle ear bones do not form correctly.

Photos for Figures 2.2, 2.3, and 2.4 are courtesy of Dr. Karen M. Jensen, Department of Communication Disorders, California State.

The presence of a congenital hearing loss, a slash audiogram, and recessive genetic etiology should alert those working with deaf children to make a medical referral for a thyroid check.

HUNTINGTON'S CHOREA

Huntington's chorea is a genetic degenerative disease of the extra pyramidal nervous system characterized by progressive irregular jerking movements, mental deterioration, and death (Fraser, G. R. 1964). The condition is dominantly inherited, generally starts at about age 35, and proves fatal within 10 years. The deafness usually occurs in advanced stages of the disease, but it can be congenital and recessive (Proctor & Proctor, 1967).

LOCALIZED VON RECKLINGHAUSEN'S SYNDROME

This consists of bilateral acoustic tumors resulting in nerve deafness. Transmission is usually autosomal dominant, not sex-linked, but it is occasionally recessive (Konigsmark, 1972). Blindness due to tumors of the optic nerve may be present. Loss of balance resulting from the acoustic nerve tumors is often the first sign of the disease.

TREACHER-COLLINS SYNDROME

This is a facial deformity characterized by a markedly receding chin, a downward slant of the eyelids, and in general, an underdevelopment of facial and cranial bones known medically as mandibulo-facial dysostosis (Proctor & Proctor, 1967) (see Figure 2.3). The imperfect ossification can cause deafness because the middle ear bones do not form correctly (see Figure 2.4).

OTHER SYNDROMES

This cursory description of nine major genetic syndromes involving deafness hardly scratches the surface of the very important subject area of genetics and hearing loss. There are over 50 other deafness-linked syndromes, many of which have major psychological implications.

REFERENCES

Bergsma, D. R. (1973). Ophthalmic aspects of Usher's syndrome. Proceedings of Symposium on Usher's syndrome (pp. 12–18). Washington, DC: Gallaudet College Press.

Bettica, L. J., Keane, G. E., Bergman, M., Edgecomb, C. F., Lotz, J., & Goldberg, H. H. (1959). Communication—A key to service for deaf-blind men and women. In *A manual for professional workers,* Vol. I (pp. 35–59). Brooklyn, NY: Industrial Home for the Blind.

Conley, J., & Vernon, M. (1975). A study of behavioral characteristics of children with Waardenburg's syndrome. *Journal Academy of Rehabilitative Audiology, 3,* 60–68.

Craig, W. N., & Craig, H. (1981). Directory of programs and services. *American Annals of the Deaf, 120,* 261–276.

Danes, B. S. (1970). Genetic counseling. *Medical World News, 11*(45), 35–41.

Fraser, F. C. (1971). Genetic counseling. *Hospital Practice, 6,* 49–56.

Fraser, F. C. (1968). Genetic counseling and the physician. *Canadian Medical Association Journal, 99,* 927–934.

Fraser, G. R. (1964). Profound childhood deafness. *Journal of Medical Genetics, 1,* 118–151.

Fraser, G. R., Froggatt, P., & James, T. N. (1964). Congenital deafness associated with electrocardiographic abnormalities, fainting attacks, and sudden death. *Quarterly Journal of Medicine, 33,* 361–385.

Giacoia, J. P., & Klein, S. W. (1969). Waardenburg's syndrome with bilateral cleft lip. *American Journal of Diseases of Children, 117,* 346–348.

Kloepfer, H. W., Laguaite, J. K., & McLaurin, J. W. (1966). The hereditary syndrome of deafness and retinitis pigmentosa. *Laryngoscope, 76,* 3–15.

Konigsmark, B. W. (1972). Genetic hearing loss with no associated abnormalities. *Journal of Speech and Hearing Disorders, 37,* 89–99.

Maniglia, A. J., Wolff, D., & Herques, A. J. (1970). *Archives of Otolaryngology, 92,* 181–188.

Medical World News. (1972a). Genetic counseling: Is it heeded too little or too much? *Medical World News, 13,* 17–18.

Medical World News. (1972b). Genetic control—Threat or therapy? *Medical World News, 13,* 45–55.

Miller, G. W., Joseph, D. J., Cozad, R. L., & McCabe, B. F. (1970). Alport's syndrome. *Archives of Otolaryngology, 92,* 419–432.

Mitchell, S. H. (1971). The haunting influence of Alexander Graham Bell. *American Annals of the Deaf, 116,* 349–361.

Nance, W. E. (1973). Genetics and Usher's. *Proceedings of Symposium on Usher's Syndrome* (pp. 12–21). Washington, DC: Gallaudet College Press.

Palant, D. I., & Carter, B. L. (1972). Klippel-Feil syndrome and deafness. *American Journal of Diseases of Children, 123,* 218–221.

Patton, R. B. (1970). Chronic hereditary nephritis with nerve deafness. *Annals of Otology, Rhinology, and Laryngology, 79,* 194–203.

Proctor, C. A., & Proctor, B. (1967). Understanding hereditary nerve deafness. *Archives of Otolaryngology, 85,* 23–40.

Rainer, J. D. (1968). Genetic counseling in deafness. In G. T. Llody (Ed.), International Research Seminar on the Vocational Rehabilitation of Deaf Persons (pp. 338–342). New York: Department of Health, Education and Welfare.

Shaver, K., & Vernon, M. (1978). Genetics and hearing loss: An overview for professionals. *American Rehabilitation, 4*(2), 6–10

Turner, J. S. (1970). Hereditary hearing loss with nephropathy (Alport's syndrome). *Acta Otolaryngologica* (Suppl. 271).

Vernon, M. (1969). Usher's syndrome—deafness and progressive blindness: Clinical cases, prevention, theory, and literature survey. *Journal of Chronic Diseases, 22,* 133–151.

Vernon, M. (1973). Psychological aspects of the diagnosis of deafness in a child. *EENT Monthly, 52,* 60–66.

Vernon, M. (1976). Usher's syndrome: Problems and some solutions. *Hearing and Speech Action, 44,* 6–13.

Vernon, M. (1973). Overview of Usher's syndrome: Congenital deafness and progressive loss of vision. *Proceedings of Symposium on Usher's Syndrome.* Washington, DC: Gallaudet College Press. pp 1–11

Zellweger, Hans, M.D. (1967). Genetic counseling in clinical medicine. *Modern Medicine, 35* (7), 40–52.

CHAPTER 3
Other Causes of Deafness: Their Psychological Role

Half of us are blind, few of us feel, and we are all deaf.   *Sir William Osler*

There are four major reasons why causes of hearing loss are important in a comprehensive psychology of deafness. First, many of these diseases are also the leading etiologies of neurological damage and other organic pathologies which have direct effects on behavior (Karchmer, 1985; Vernon, 1982). Thus many deaf people are to some extent molded psychologically not only by the functional effects of their hearing, but also by organic disorders resulting from the condition that brought about the deafness. Second, any constructive approach to the prevention of deafness and the psychological problems associated with it is partly contingent upon an understanding of its causes. Third, without prevalency data, researchers are without knowledge of the base populations for which they need to develop appropriate programs and facilities. Fourth, an understanding of the condition causing a hearing loss is often valuable in differential diagnosis where factors such as site of lesion and possible central nervous system involvement need to be determined.

PREVALENCE AND ETIOLOGY

The leading causes of childhood deafness and their estimated prevalences are shown in Table 3.1. Medical factors have a strong influence over these prevalence figures, sometimes causing great fluctuations. For example, an epidemical disease such as rubella may result in high numbers of children deafened in one year and relatively few the next (Jensema, 1974). Vaccines and other scientific discoveries have greatly reduced the incidence of hearing loss due to certain conditions, such as complications of RH factor and rubella (Berkowitz, 1979; Harris, 1979). At the same time, other medical discoveries have caused more deafness by increasing survival rates for certain pathologies. Tuberculous meningitis illustrates the problem. In years past it was inevitably fatal, but with the advent of antibiotics, patients frequently survive the disease but are often left without hearing (Delage & Dusseault, 1979; Vernon 1967a). Similarly, medicine has raised the survival rate for premature infants, a significant percent of whom are deaf. Social-medical factors such as the dramatic increase in several types of sexually transmitted diseases that cause deafness in infants of infected mothers is another trend altering the numbers of deaf children and the psychological makeup of the deaf population (Vernon & Hicks, 1980).

PROBLEMS IN IDENTIFYING ETIOLOGIES

Determining the etiology of deafness in children is sometimes difficult, particularly because there is often a time lag between the onset of the hearing loss and its diagnosis. This lag almost always involves infants whose deafness was congenital or occurred within the first year or two. Such losses may not be recognized until the child is 2 or 3, or even of school age. The physician must then retrospectively consider factors such as family pedigree, medical history, and the site of auditory lesion in attempting to determine the cause. In some cases, several possible causal conditions may have been present, such as maternal exposure to rubella and deafness in the family, premature birth and meningitis, or other combinations. With infants who have this type of confusing history or who have no known abnormal medical background, the exact cause of deafness is frequently unknown.

Another problem in diagnosing etiology is the tendency of parents to ascribe deafness to an inaccurate adventitious factor rather than to state that the child was born deaf. This rather common tendency is sometimes the result of simple misinformation. Sometimes it is an unconscious denial by parents of their feelings of responsibility for their child's handicap (Vernon, 1973). In either case, it can lead to confusion about the actual cause of the hearing loss.

What follows is a discussion of the leading causes of childhood deafness. Background medical data will be given, but the emphasis will be on the psychological and education sequelae of the conditions.

PRENATAL RUBELLA

DESCRIPTION

Rubella is commonly known as German measles or three-day measles. In adults and children it is usually harmless, involving some fever, a rash, and other minor symptoms. However, when the rubella virus infects a pregnant woman, it frequently spreads immediately to the unborn fetus, where its effects can be traumatic. The virus invades developing embryonic tissue, and its toxins circulate throughout the rapidly multiplying cells of the fetus. The results are pervasive. The virus damages developing layers of embryonic tissue and reduces cell division. Consequently, the body parts that these cells were destined to form, such as the eye, brain, ear, and heart may be defective and there is often a general failure of the organism to thrive (Harris, 1979; Vernon & Hicks, 1980). These rubella-caused defects can be manifested at birth and even decades later.

Not only is rubella pervasive in its damage, it is elusive. Expectant mothers may have the disease with no awareness that they are ill. For example, in 40 to 50 percent of cases of prenatal rubella, the pregnant mothers have the disease subclinically, that is, their rubella is so mild that they are unaware of having it (Vernon & Hicks, 1980). The greatest danger to the unborn is in the first trimester of pregnancy. However, deafness and other problems can result if the fetus is infected at any time during gestation or even in the perinatal period (Harris, 1979).

Rubella is epidemical, occurring in cycles of about seven years. One of the worst epidemics swept the United States in 1963–1965, leaving in its wake many stillborn infants, spontaneous abortions, and 20,000 to 40,000 deaf infants (Harris, 1979; Vernon, 1969). Since then, vaccines have prevented any major epidemics.

TABLE 3.1. Prevalence Figures for Etiologies of Deafness Based on the Different Criteria Used in Defining Etiology (N = 1,468)

Cause of Deafness	Criteria	Number	Percentage
Heredity	Both parents deaf	79	5.4
	One or more deaf sibling(s)	190	12.9
	Deaf relatives other than parents or siblings	92	6.2
	Combination of family deafness and prematurity	11	.7
	Combination of family deafness and rubella	4	.3
	Combination of family deafness plus childhood illness and/or complications after pregnancy	8	.5
	Total	384	26.0
Rh factor	Rh factor and full-term	39	2.7
	Rh factor and prematurity	6	.4
	Possible Rh	9	.6
	Total	54	3.7
Prematurity	Birthweight 5 pounds 8 ounces or less and no other known cause of deafness	175	11.9
	Maternal rubella and prematurity	56	3.8
	Combination of Rh and prematurity	6	.4
	Possible prematurity	3	.2
	Combination of family deafness and prematurity	11	.7
	Combination of prematurity and meningitis	5	.3
	Combination of prematurity and tuberculous meningitis	1	.1
	Total	257	17.4
Meningitis	Auditory mechanism impaired by some form of meningitis (tuberculous meningitis excluded)	114	7.8
	Tuberculous meningitis	5	.3
	Possible meningitis	3	.2
	Combination of prematurity and meningitis	5	.3
	Combination of prematurity and tuberculous meningitis	1	.1
	Total	128	8.7
Rubella	Maternal rubella and full-term	73	5.0
	Maternal rubella and prematurity	56	3.8
	Possible rubella	5	.3
	Rubella and deaf relatives	4	.3
	Combination of rubella and other measles	1	.1
	Total	139	9.5
Unknown	No known cause of deafness given	447	30.4

TABLE 3.1. *(continued)*

Cause of Deafness	Criteria	Number	Percentage
Other causes and/or inadequate etiological reasons in addition to those listed above	Measles other than rubella	32	2.2
	Whooping cough	11	.7
	Head injury	11	.7
	High fever	8	.5
	Birth complications	8	.5
	Pneumonia	7	.5
	Polio	6	.4
	Maternal flu or virus	6	.4
	Combination of several diseases	6	.4
	Complications of gestation (no family deafness)	6	.4
	Adenoids and/or tonsils	5	.3
	Mumps	4	.3
	Mastoid	4	.3
	Functional	4	.3
	Encephalitis	3	.2
	Maternal kidney trouble	3	.2
	Ear infection	3	.2
	Scarlet fever	3	.2
	Virus (unspecified)	2	.1
	Maternal use of quinine during gestation	2	.1
	Anoxia	2	.1
	Chicken pox	1	.1
	Blue baby	1	.1
	Maternal scarlet fever during gestation	1	.1
	Combination of mumps and measles	1	.1
	Combination of whooping cough and measles	1	.1
	Combination of bone cancer and prematurity (cancer clearly established as the etiological factor)	1	.1
	Total	142	9.6

Note:—This table is an attempt to show the full range of possible prevalence figures for each etiology depending on the criteria used to establish the etiology. Therefore, the same criterion may appear under several etiologies, making it meaningless to add subtotals and expect the resultant figure to be the sample size. (SOURCE: Vernon, M. (1969). *Multiply handicapped deaf children: Medical, educational and psychological considerations.* Reston, Va.: Council of Exceptional Children. Reprinted by permission.)

However, many problems and unanswered questions remain regarding their use (Harris, 1979). For example, it is not yet known if these vaccines confer lifetime immunity. Protection may last only eight years (Harris, 1979). If the immunity does not continue for at least 20 years, there may in the near future be millions of women of child-bearing age coming down with rubella despite having been vaccinated in childhood. The result could be an entire reevaluation of the vaccine program (Harris, 1979).

EFFECTS OF VACCINE

The exact effect of the various rubella vaccines on the prevalence and nature of the deaf population is not clear at present, although it is known that they have reduced the number of rubella-deafened children (Jensema, 1974). The safety of the vaccines also has not been established with certainty. Research tends to indicate that those inoculated do not pass the disease to susceptible contacts (Sever, 1973). Another problem associated with the vaccine is that it requires an extremely well-organized medical delivery system sustained over time. Thus far, delivery has fallen far short of what it should be to make the vaccine effective (Fishbein, 1974).

At present we cannot be sure whether rubella will be virtually wiped out by vaccines, whether it will persist but at somewhat lower prevalence rates, or even whether it will increase. Extensive space has been devoted here to this essentially medical topic because it has such direct bearing on the nature and size of the deaf population in the future.

SEQUELAE OF RUBELLA

Intelligence

An average or better performance scale IQ is almost essential if a deaf child is to compete effectively in society, for example, graduate from an educational program for deaf youth (Vernon, 1973). Deaf students with IQs below 90 (based on performance scales) were found to have little chance of success even in a vocational program requiring a fourth-grade academic level as measured by the Stanford Achievement Test (Vernon, 1973). From the data reported in Table 3.2, several conclusions can be derived.

TABLE 3.2. IQ Distribution for 98 Post-Rubella Deaf Children (Mean IQ = 95.3, Standard Deviation = 16.8)

IQ Range	Number	Percent of Rubella Cases	Percent for General Population
130 or above	0	0.0	2.2
120–129	5	5.1	6.7
110–119	14	14.2	16.1
100–109	21	21.4	25.0
90–99	26	26.5	25.0
80–89	16	16.3	16.6
70–79	8	8.1	6.7
60–69	4	4.0	(2.2 who
50–59	3	3.0	score below
40–49	1	1.0	an IQ of 69)
Total	98	99.6	

(SOURCE: Vernon, M. (1969). *Multiply handicapped deaf children: Medical, educational and psychological considerations.* Reston, Va.: Council of Exceptional Children. Reprinted by permission.)

First, the mean IQ of 95.3 of the rubella group is significantly below the 100 IQ of the general population. About one-third of the rubella children are below 90, and 8 percent are mentally retarded—a sharp contrast to the 2.2 percent rate for the general population, and a conservative estimate when compared with figures offered by others (Ziring, 1978). The number of cases at the lower end of the intelligence continuum, coupled with the absence of cases having IQs above 130, characterizes the rubella distribution. Table 3.2 represents the major research findings on intelligence in post-rubella deaf children. Clinical reports and other research yield a similar picture (Chess, Fernandez & Korn, 1978). Thus, a major way in which rubella affects a psychology of deafness is to lower the intelligence of a significant percentage of its victims.

Educational Achievement

On the whole, post-rubella deaf children do not do as well educationally as their deaf peers (Vernon, Grieve & Shaver, 1980). Part of this academic retardation is accountable to intelligence levels. Brain damage and psychological factors account for other aspects of the problem. (See Table 3.3.)

The educational difficulties of post-rubella deaf children are illustrated by a study of 129 cases (Vernon, 1969) which revealed that, as a group, their educational achievements were considerably below those of other deaf youths and less than half that of the average hearing child. One representative analysis of the school records of this study group showed that 20.2 percent of the 129 were either ruled ineligible for school for educational reasons (mental retardation, behavior disorders, or learning disability) or dropped from school because of failure to make satisfactory educational progress (Vernon, 1969). Furthermore, of the 67 rubella youths 19 or older (graduation age), only one had passed college entrance examinations.

These data indicate that post-rubella youths as a group have a reduced probability of academic success compared to most deaf students (Vernon & Hicks, 1980).

TABLE 3.3. Educational Achievement of the Five Etiological Groups as Measured by Their Educational Quotients

Etiological Group	N	Mean Educational Quotient[a]	Standard Deviation
Hereditary	39	.6893	.1665
Rh factor	20	.5089	.1844
Premature	52	.4589	.1651
Meningitic	58	.4877	.1804
Rubella	66	.4553	.1362

$$^{a}\text{ Educational Quotient} = \frac{\text{Stanford Achievement Test Score}}{\text{Years in School}}$$

(SOURCE: Vernon, M. (1969). *Multiply handicapped deaf children: Medical, educational and psychological considerations.* Reston, Va.: Council of Exceptional Children. Reprinted by permission.)

Hearing

Relative to other children in educational programs for the deaf and hard-of-hearing, post-rubella youths have relatively large amounts of residual hearing (Hardy, Haskins, Hardy, & Shimizi, 1973). In a sample drawn from a residential school the mean hearing loss in the better ear in the speech range (500 to 2,000 Hz) was found to be 90 dB (ISO 1964) (Vernon, 1969). In general the audiograms are slightly cup shaped or relatively flat.

Overall there is a less direct relationship between pure tone hearing measures and actual usable hearing in post-rubella children than in any other etiological group (Vernon, 1969). Some post-rubella children with audiograms suggesting extensive residual hearing function as "deaf," while a few whose audiograms indicate profound losses are able to understand speech remarkably well. These discrepancies are not necessarily related to the degree of auditory training nor to the age at which training began; they are partly a function of the varied, almost idiosyncratic, way in which the rubella virus affects the auditory mechanism.

Communication Skills

Two communication problems appear more common among rubella-deafened children than others. First, they are more likely to be *aphasoid,* that is, to have abnormal difficulty with language, above that normally found in children with similar congenital hearing losses and IQs (Feldman, Lajoie, Mendelson, & Pinsky, 1971). Second, there is more *autism* among children with a history of rubella (Chess, 1977).

Aphasoid disorders and autism, along with the neurophysiological conditions contributing to these disorders, cause rubella-deaf children as a group to have greater difficulties with language than do other deaf youngsters. Speech (articulation) skills are usually not affected (Vernon, 1969). Ironically, there are isolated cases of rubella-deafened children who have exceptionally good language skills. Usually the functional hearing of these individuals far exceeds that expected on the basis of pure tone audiometry.

Psychological Adjustment

Research indicates that psychosis, behavior disorders, and general psychological maladjustment occur disproportionately among children with prenatal rubella (Trapp & Himelstein, 1972, pp. 379–96). Among the specific traits found were poor impulse control, excitability, rigidity, distractability, instability, and emotional shallowness (Chess & Fernandez, 1980; Vernon, 1969).

The overall clinical picture, in addition to test findings of the Bender-Gestalt, demonstrates that rubella causes neurological impairment which appears to underlie much of the psychological disturbance present.

It is important to realize that even though rubella does create disturbances in some individuals, the majority of prenatal rubella-deaf persons are within the normal range behaviorly. This fact is too frequently overlooked.

Recent research on rubella children deafened in the 1963–1965 epidemic indicates that late onset diabetes, other endocrine disorders, and additional physical problems are striking a disproportionate number of these youth as they enter their teenage years (Vernon & Hicks, 1980). This phenomenon may be due to latent viral activity and suggests that certain routine medical screening should be done, at least for diabetes.

MENINGITIS

DESCRIPTION

Meningitis is the leading postnatal cause of deafness among school-age children (Budden et al., 1974; Jensema & Mullins, 1974; Vernon, 1967a&b). Its overall prevalence of 8 to 12 percent as a cause of childhood deafness has remained fairly constant over the past 50 years (Jensema & Mullins, 1974; Trapp & Himelstein, 1972; Vernon, 1967a&b). However, the nature of the meningitic population has changed drastically.

The disease is an infection of the membranes surrounding the brain. It can be caused by a wide variety of living agents, including bacteria, viruses, fungi, microbacteria, and spirochetes (Vernon, 1969). About 3 to 10 percent of its survivors are deaf (Raivio & Koskiniemi, 1978).

In addition to being the ranking postnatal etiology of profound hearing loss, meningitis is a leading cause of brain damage (Raivio & Koskiniemi, 1978; Vernon, 1967a&b). Estimates of the percentage of postmeningitic patients having major neurological sequelae range from 15 to 71 percent (Keane, Potsic, Rowe, & Konkle, 1979). There is even greater danger when young children and infants are infected, because at these ages critical stages of neurological development and organization are occurring. Half of the victims of meningitis are under age 5, and a majority of these are below 2½ (Raivio & Koskiniemi, 1978; Vernon, 1967a&b). Prematures and newborns are particularly susceptible (Keane, Potsic, Rowe, & Konkle, 1979). Because of the difficulty of diagnosing premature infants, onset of treatment may be significantly delayed, and this delay increases the chances of serious residue (Vernon, 1969).

Intracranial pressure from accumulation of exudate, clotting or rupturing of blood vessels, and generalized hemorrhaging are often a part of the meningitic syndrome. These conditions result in severe neuropsychological sequelae (Vernon, 1969). Abnormalities in body physiology and biochemistry are also associated with meningitis, and they too have important psychological manifestations (Vernon, 1969).

EFFECTS OF ANTIBIOTICS

A critical factor in meningitis—age of onset of deafness—has changed dramatically since antibiotics have been used (Budden et al., 1974; Jensema & Mullins, 1974; Vernon, 1967a&b). Formerly the mean age of onset of those deafened by meningitis was late adolescence or adulthood. In figures reported in 1960 (Myklebust), the average age at onset was found to be 6½. Later data, however, reveal that the average post-meningitic deaf child lost hearing at 20 months (Budden et al., 1974; Jensema & Mullins 1974; Vernon, 1967a&b). The reason for this important change is that when the symptoms of the disease—headache, photophobia, stiff neck—can be verbalized, the physician can make an early diagnosis and institute treatment with antibiotics immediately. Consequently the patient survives, usually without serious residue. By contrast, the infant cannot describe symptoms, so the doctor is often unable to make the diagnosis until the child convulses, becomes phlegmatic, or develops an extremely high fever. By then the meningitis is advanced. Even if treatment results in survival, the chance of sequelae, such as deafness, is greater. This change in age of onset has major educational and psychological implications.

SEQUELAE OF MENINGITIS

Intelligence

In the only study reporting on the intelligence of post-meningitic deaf children, the mean IQ was found to be 95 (Vernon, 1969), significantly below the population average of 100. The study showed that when the disease was contracted in the first year of life, there was a fairly high probability of mental retardation or at least a lowered IQ (Table 3.4). These IQ effects tend to diminish when onset is after age 2.

Educational Achievement

Post-meningitic students as a group have academic achievement levels comparable to those of the post-rubella deaf but below those of the genetically deaf. As would be expected, those who are deafened after language acquisition and who are not aphasic generally do well in school.

As was implied earlier, the average meningitic deaf youth of today is much different from his counterpart of past decades. Instead of being a postlingually deafened student free of the intellectual sequelae of meningitis, he is more likely to be prelingually deafened and to have suffered some residue that affects his ability to learn. Schools serving deaf children once regarded post-meningitic students as a primary source of capable scholastic achievers who were relatively free of the crippling language retardation of congenital deafness. This is no longer so. For example, the male population of Gallaudet—the world's only liberal arts college for the deaf—used to be approximately 40 percent post-meningitic. This is no longer true.

Without the postlingually deafened meningitic student to depend upon, secondary and college programs for the deaf find their tasks more difficult. In fact, the greatest need may be for trade or technical education, not formal postsecondary academic offerings.

Thirty-four percent of post-meningitic deaf children have an IQ below 90, the level Brill (1962) found to be about the minimum required to complete a secondary

TABLE 3.4. IQ of Meningitic Deaf Children as a Function of Age at Onset of Meningitis

Age at Onset in Months	N	Mean IQ	Percent Mentally Retarded
0 to 6	19	92.52	5.2
7 to 12	26	91.50	34.6
13 to 24	17	94.82	5.8
25 to 30	5	101.00	—
31 to 36	7	97.28	14.2
37 to 48	9	104.33	—
49 to 72	8	112.12	—
Undetermined	1	50.00	100.0

(SOURCE: Vernon, M. (1969). *Multiply handicapped deaf children: Medical, educational and psychological considerations*, Reston, Va.: Council of Exceptional Children. Reprinted by permission.)

education. On the basis of Brill's norms, about 10 percent are of college-level intelligence. However, the prelingual onset of deafness in most meningitic deaf youths today and their one-third prevalence of multiple handicaps mean that college programs that in the past depended on meningitically deafened youths as a primary source of students can no longer realistically do this (Vernon, 1969).

Hearing

Post-meningitic children have the severest auditory losses among major etiologic groups of children in schools for the deaf (Vernon, 1967a&b). Their residual hearing in most cases does not permit them to understand speech, even with maximum amplification. Typically, audiograms have a slash pattern with islands of hearing at 250 and 500 and no response for other frequencies (Nadol, 1978; Vernon, 1967a&b).

Physical Handicaps

The prevalence of major disabilities in addition to deafness among the post-meningitic children was 38 percent (Table 3.5). Of these children, relatively few (8.6 percent) had more than one other handicap. Aphasia was the second most prevalent secondary disability, followed by mental retardation, psychological disturbance, and cerebral palsy. Most of the children with three or more major handicaps were cases of gross brain damage involving a syndrome of spastic hemiplegia, mental retardation, and psychosis.

Table 3.6 gives the prevalence of multiple handicaps associated with age at onset of meningitis. It is difficult to generalize from these data other than to say that the chances of three or more major handicaps striking a child are greater when meningitis occurs in the first year of life.

Approximately 15 percent of children afflicted by meningitis within the first two years of life did not walk until after 30 months of age. The reason is that the vestibular mechanism of these infants had been damaged, leaving them without normal capacities for equilibrium. In view of this combined balance–hearing problem, physicians, psychologists, audiologists, and others examining post-meningitic children should be alert to the possible significance of delayed walking in conjunction with the absence of speech. Instead of necessarily suggesting mental retardation, this symptom pattern may indicate a hearing loss and vestibular dysfunction. Rare but gross cases of misdiagnosis resulting in traumatic ramifications for the children and their families have occurred where deafness and vestibular pathology have mimicked (no speech and inability to stand or walk) the symptoms of mental retardation and led to institutional commitment (Sullivan & Vernon, 1979).

In sum, meningitis causes about 8 percent of the deafness in school-age children, males being far more often affected. Age of onset of deafness is now usually during the prelingual period (before the third birthday) in contrast to the past, when onset occurred at school age or later. Multiple handicaps are present in over one-third of the deaf post-meningitic youths, the most common secondary effects being aphasia, mental retardation, emotional disturbance, and spasticity. Those infected in the first year of life are most likely to have these residua (Vernon, 1969).

Communication Skills

The post-meningitic deaf had language inferior to that of those deafened genetically but better than that of rubella deaf children. This superiority is accounted for by

TABLE 3.5. Type and Prevalence of Multiple Handicaps Among Meningitic Post-Deaf Children (N = 92)

Multiple Handicaps	Number	Percentage
Deafness and one other major handicap		
Cerebral palsy[a]	2	2.2
Aphasia	12	13.0
Mental retardation	6	6.5
Major visual pathology	—	—
Emotional disturbance	5	5.4
Orthopedic	1	1.1
Total[b]	26	28.3
Deafness and two other major handicaps		
Cerebral palsy and aphasia	—	—
Cerebral palsy and mental retardation	1	1.1
Cerebral palsy and visual pathology	—	—
Cerebral palsy and emotional disturbance	—	—
Aphasia and mental retardation	—	—
Aphasia and visual pathology	—	—
Aphasia and emotional disturbance	1	1.1
Aphasia and orthopedic anomaly	—	—
Mental retardation and visual pathology	—	—
Mental retardation and emotional disturbance	1	1.1
Mental retardation and orthopedic anomaly	—	—
Other	1	1.1
Total	4	4.3
Deafness and three other major handicaps	4	4.3
Deafness and four other major handicaps	1	1.3
Grand total	35	38.0

[a] Most of the meningitic cases classified within the broad rubric of cerebral palsy were children having spastic hemiplegias.

[b] Data presented in the table are rounded off to one decimal place; however, the totals were computed on the unrounded figures. (SOURCE: Vernon, M. (1969). *Multiply handicapped deaf children: Medical, educational and psychological considerations.* Reston, Va.: Council of Exceptional Children. Reprinted by permission.)

those few post-meningitics who had late onsets of hearing loss (Vernon, 1969). On two other important communication variables, speech and speech reading, no significant differences were found between the meningitic and other etiological groups.

Aphasia, or aphasoid involvement, is a condition of particular importance in post-meningitics because of the prevalence of hemiplegias among them. The hemiplegias often involve dominant hemisphere cerebral damage, a kind of damage frequently associated with loss of speech and language.

Vernon (1969) found that 16.3 percent of the 92 meningitic schoolchildren studied were aphasic. Aphasics who became deaf at 37 months or older represent an especially interesting group. Verbal language had already been established in at least rudimentary form. Any aphasia with these youths was aphasia in the classic sense: a loss of language rather than a failure to develop it. Table 3.7 shows that meningitis

TABLE 3.6. Prevalence of Multiple Handicaps Associated with Various Ages at Onset of Meningitis in Deaf Children

Age at Onset of Meningitis (in Months)	Number	Major Disabilities								Total	
		Two Only		Three Only		Four Only		Five Only			
		N	Percent	N	Percent	N	Percent	N	Percent	N	Percent
0–6	19	1	5.3	2	10.5	1	5.3	—	—	4	21.1
7–12	26	9	34.6	1	3.8	2	7.7	1	3.8	13	50.0
13–24	17	3	17.6	—	—	1	5.9	—	—	4	23.5
25–36	12	5	41.7	—	—	—	—	—	—	5	41.7
37 plus	17	7	41.2	1	5.9	—	—	—	—	8	47.1
Unknown	1	1	100	—	—	—	—	—	—	1	100
Total	92	26	28.3	4	4.3	4	4.3	1	1.1	35	38.0

(SOURCE: Vernon, M. (1969). *Multiply handicapped deaf children: Medical, educational and psychological considerations.* Reston, Va.: Council of Exceptional Children. Reprinted by permission.)

TABLE 3.7. Prevalence of Aphasia in Children Deafened by Meningitis at 37 Months or Older

Age Range in Months	Total	Number Aphasic	Number Aphasic Without Recovery
37–48[a]	9	4	2
49–60[a]	6	2	1
61–72	3	0	0
Total	18	6	3

[a] In each of these groups there was one child for whom no data regarding aphasia were available. (SOURCE: Vernon, M. (1969). *Multiply handicapped deaf children: Medical, educational and psychological considerations.* Reston, Va.: Council of Exceptional Children. Reprinted by permission.)

that is serious enough to cause deafness in children over 37 months often causes this type of aphasia. More important, the organic components of the disease in some cases prevent relearning of language under existing techniques of teaching. Children with this problem have an overwhelmingly debilitating condition: a language disability due to both deafness and aphasia.

Among post-meningitic aphasics who were able to reacquire language, the learning process was like that of a congenitally deaf child. There was no spontaneous return of the language skills possessed prior to illness.

Psychological Adjustment

Although teachers' ratings indicate that post-meningitic children are relatively well adjusted overall, not being significantly below the genetic group on this variable and being above the maternal rubella sample, the percentage of postmeningitic students dropped from school for emotional disturbance (8.3) is rather high (Vernon, 1969). Psychological evaluations indicate that 29.3 percent had serious psychological maladjustments.

The nature of such disturbance falls into four general categories (Vernon, 1969). First, there are a few abnormally aggressive, asocial children who are violent and prone to attack others. These children sometimes become court cases. They often represent chronic brain syndromes and may wind up in mental hospitals or prisons.

The second type of post-meningitic child is characterized, in part, by hyperactivity, poor impulse control, and distractibility. It is possible that the organic factors underlying these problems and those of the group just described are similar. The difference may be in the degree of organic damage.

A third pathological behavior pattern noted was that of clear-cut organic psychosis. The youths having this condition are out of touch with reality, demonstrate bizarre behavior patterns, and are unable to reproduce Bender-Gestalt designs. Those who were tested by electroencephalography showed gross abnormalities (Vernon, 1967a&b).

The fourth type of disturbance was a reaction to aphasia. These aphasic children responded with overwhelming anxiety to their double handicap and its consequent psychoeducational problems. There was an ego disintegration of varying degrees, but generally very severe (Vernon, 1969).

TUBERCULOUS MENINGITIS

Tuberculous meningitis deserves separate discussion. It used to be invariably fatal until antibiotics were developed to which the tuberculin bacillus was sensitive (Vernon, 1967b). Thus in years past it was not a cause of deafness, but now it is (Trapp & Himelstein, 1972; Vernon, 1967b).

The disease is rare in the first six months of life but reaches a peak at about 2 to 4 (Vernon, 1967b). The mortality rate remains high (Delage & Dusseault, 1969; Trapp & Himelstein, 1972). The important consideration for a psychology of deafness is that cures are often hollow triumphs because of the pervasiveness of serious permanent residua among survivors (Kennedy & Fallow, 1979; Mackay, 1964, pp. 30–40; Vernon, 1967b).

The only study of deaf post-tuberculous meningitic patients available involved just seven cases (Vernon, 1967b). From these data, in addition to follow-ups of nondeaf tuberculous meningitic patients, it is clear that those deafened by the disease are likely to have other residua in addition to deafness (Haas et al., 1977). Neuromuscular pathology (hemiphegia and mild cerebral palsy), endocrine disturbances (sexual precocity), aphasia, and perceptual problems associated with brain damage appear to be the most common sequelae. Hearing losses are profound (Vernon, 1967a&b).

PREMATURITY

DESCRIPTION

Medical advances have raised the survival rate for prematurely born infants. For example, betwen 1933 and 1972 the mortality rate was reduced over 60 percent and this trend continues (Trapp & Himelstein, 1972; Vernon, 1969). Although many more infants now live through the catastrophic events of the perinatal stage, the prevalence of severe multiple handicaps among them has increased, and one of them is hearing loss. (Lubchenco et al., 1972; Trapp & Himelstein, 1972).

The full significance of prematurity and its possible ramifications in the area of deafness are further illustrated by the fact that the condition takes a higher toll of infant life than any other single factor. It also ranks as one of the leading causes of death among the general population, accounting for 10 percent of the total mortality (Trapp & Himelstein, 1972; Vernon, 1967a&b). A condition of this pathological magnitude, often involving the central nervous system, could logically be expected to cause sensorineural hearing loss and psychological disorders.

The total impact of prematurity is amplified by the fact that it is associated with other conditions causing deafness, such as prenatal rubella, complications of Rh factor, meningitis, and ototoxic medication. For example, 43 percent of rubella-deafened children were also born prematurely (Vernon, 1969). Fourteen percent of those with an Rh factor etiology were of low birthweight (Vernon, 1969). Thus a significant percentage of deaf premature infants face both the sequelae of low birthweight and residua from some other pathology such as rubella, complication of RH factor, or meningitis.

There are more than four times as many deaf schoolchildren as normally hearing children who were premature. Furthermore, within the very low birthweight categories (3 pounds, 4 ounces or less) this disproportion is even greater (Vernon, 1969).

In view of the fact that emotional, physical, and learning problems have been found to be much more common among premature children, especially those below 3 pounds, 4 ounces, it follows that among school-age deaf children there are probably significantly more of these problems than among the normally hearing (Lubchenco et al., 1972; Vernon, 1969).

SEQUELAE OF PREMATURITY

Intelligence

The mean performance IQ of prematurely born deaf children is 89.4. There is a 16.3 percent prevalence of mental retardation (Vernon, 1969). (See Table 3.8.) Many educational programs for deaf children will not include youngsters scoring below 70 in IQ, and those below 90 have trouble graduating (Brill, 1962). This means that many premature youngsters (16.3 percent) will not be accepted into programs for the deaf and that approximately 42 percent may never graduate.

Table 3.9 shows that as the birthweight of a premature deaf child drops, on the average his or her IQ diminishes appreciably. For example, the mean IQ for those below 3 pounds, 4 ounces is less than 80. With medical science saving more and more fetuses within extremely low birthweight classifications, these findings assume major psychological significance.

Educational Achievement

In view of the depressed IQ scores of the premature, it would be logical to expect a limited overall academic achievement for these youngsters. The data indicate this to be the case.

In a California study (Trapp & Himelstein, 1972; Vernon, 1969) 10.3 percent of prematures applying for admission to school were judged to have too little academic potential or achievement to be admitted even on a trial basis. Another 9.7 percent were dismissed from school for inability to achieve at the minimal standards. Thus, one out of five of these premature children was regarded as essentially unable to be educated in a regular program for deaf children (Vernon, 1969).

The academic achievement of those who were accepted was found to be low compared with that of other deaf children (Vernon, 1969). For example, relatively few premature children earned academic diplomas or passed entrance examinations to colleges for deaf students. A disproportionate number were given vocational diplomas indicating they met only the minimal requirements for graduation.

Hearing

In the only study done specifically on the auditory functioning of deaf prematures (Vernon, 1969), it was found that, although their hearing losses were profound, they had somewhat more residual hearing than would be expected in the population of a residential school for the deaf. In addition, many of the applicants who were found to have too much hearing for admission to the school were born prematurely, an indication that the low birthweight represents a prominent etiology of defective hearing at all gradations of loss.

The patterns of the audiograms of the premature did not yield the configuration of the typical nerve loss; that is, hearing did not decline linearly as frequencies

TABLE 3.8. IQ Distribution for 115 Premature Deaf Children

				IQ Categories				
	0–69	70–79	80–89	90–99	100–109	110–119	120–129	130 up
Premature	16.3	9.5	15.6	25.2	24.3	5.2	2.6	.8
Normal Distribution	2.2	6.7	16.1	25.0	25.0	16.1	6.7	2.2

Note: Mean IQ = 89.4; standard deviation, 19.0; mean IQ of 89.4 has a .0001 (one tailed) probability of being significantly different from the population mean IQ of 100. (SOURCE: Vernon, M. (1969). *Multiply handicapped deaf children: Medical, educational and psychological considerations.* Reston, Va.: Council of Exceptional Children. Reprinted by permission.)

TABLE 3.9. IQ Data on the Premature Deaf Group with Birthweight

Birthweight (Pounds, Ounces)	Number	Mean IQ	Standard Deviation	Percent Mentally Retarded	Probability that Mean Difference from Population Norms to IQ Is Due to Chance
4, 7 to 5, 8	49	95.28	16.67	8.1	.0239 (one tailed)
3, 5 to 4, 6	34	90.05	20.39	17.6	.0022 (one tailed)
2, 4 to 3, 4[a]	23	79.04	18.85	30.4	.001 level (one tailed)
1, 2 to 2, 3[a]	6	76.16	15.67	16.6	.05 level (one tailed)

[a] Student's t's (t-ratios) were used because sample size was below 25. Probabilities in the t-table are given at confidence levels, not absolute probabilities, which is why they are expressed this way in the table. (SOURCE: Vernon, M. (1969). *Multiply handicapped deaf children: Medical, educational and psychological considerations.* Reston, Va.: Council of Exceptional Children. Reprinted by permission.)

increased. Instead, the audiograms were typically relatively flat, having a slight asymmetric curving, with the thresholds at the extremes of the audiogram a little higher than those in the middle.

Physical Handicaps

Prematurely born deaf children are compared with other groups in Table 3.10 (p. 59). The 17.6 percent rate of cerebral palsy (including hemiplegia) is far above the 0.1 to 0.6 prevalence found in the general population. The findings of orthopedic problems and visual defects (all cases with glasses or medical diagnosis of serious visual pathology) also exceed expectancies for the general population. In addition to being familiar with the prevalence of physical anomalies among these children, it is important to know how they are distributed. The most striking finding is that slightly over two-thirds of premature deaf children are multiply handicapped. The disabilities other than deafness cover the full spectrum, including cerebral palsy, mental retardation, aphasia, visual pathology, and emotional disturbance. Thirty-three percent had one disability other than hearing loss, 27 percent had two additional handicaps, and 7.9 percent had three. The syndromes most frequently found were aphasia with emotional disturbance and aphasia with cerebral palsy. In cases where four or more major handicaps were present (7.9 percent), cerebral palsy and/or mental retardation were almost always involved.

Table 3.11 (p. 60) shows that as the birthweight of the premature child decreases, the probability of multiple handicaps rises sharply. This is particularly true of the more disabling conditions—mental retardation, cerebral palsy, and emotional disturbance.

It is obvious from these data that premature deaf children are characterized by one or more additional disability. Futhermore, these secondary involvements are critical conditions in the lives of these children and demand intensive psychological, educational, and medical attention if the children are to be adequately prepared to meet the demands of society.

Communicative Skills

Communication problems over and above those due solely to deafness are present in a significant percentage of prematures. For example, of five major etiologic groups, the prematures were judged the poorest in speechreading and only the Rh group, with their high rate of cerebral palsy, had lower ratings for speech intelligibility (Vernon, 1969). The rate of aphasoid involvement was also found to be highest among the premature. A comparison of written language samples shows them to be below the average deaf child in linguistic ability (Vernon, 1969).

Psychological Adjustment

It is clear from research on normally hearing prematures that low birthweight is correlated with various psychological and physical problems (Komich et al., 1973; Lubchenco et al., 1972). Schizophrenia, lesser behavioral disorders, and learning disabilities are among them.

The major psychological study of deaf prematures included psychological evaluations, teacher ratings, and examination of the school records of 117 cases (Vernon, 1969). Of these, 29 percent were diagnosed as having behavioral disturbances severe enough to jeopardize their capacity to function adequately in a school setting.

A majority of these disturbed cases fell into one of three broad pathological syndromes. The first was a schizoid pattern, which in some cases consisted of passive homosexual behavior and hallucinations (the seven cases diagnosed as psychotic were all schizophrenic). The second syndrome was one of immaturity, hyperactivity, explosiveness, and an anxiety-ridden impulsiveness. Many of the children with this syndrome were obviously brain damaged, having abnormal EEGs, positive neurological signs, and perceptual disabilities. The final syndrome involved a combination of an above-average performance scale IQ and an almost total aphasia. The frustration to which a school setting exposed these youngsters, their awareness of their ability to reason but not to remember, and the many other problems created by the double handicap of severe aphasia and profound deafness were shattering to the ego structure of these youths. In general, there seems to be a greater prevalence of disturbance as birthweight drops.

The premature reflected, a far greater prevalence of unsatisfactory adjustment than would be expected among the general population of deaf children or other etiological groups such as the genetic or post-meningitic deaf. Only the post-rubella group yielded evidence of more maladjustment. As was indicated earlier, 43 percent of the rubella children were also premature, a statistic that further emphasizes the relationship between prematurity and psychological disturbance.

OTHER ETIOLOGIES

COMPLICATIONS OF RH FACTOR

For years, complications of Rh factor were the fifth leading cause of deafness in children, accounting for about 3 to 4 percent of the overall total (Vernon, 1967a & b, 1969). However, medical advances in Rh immunization and prenatal transfusions have made the condition preventable or treatable in most cases (Sheig, 1974). The exact effects of these preventive measures on the role of complications of Rh factor as a cause of deafness are unclear because no recent prevalency studies are available, nor is it known how universal the delivery of the preventive services are.

When complications of Rh factor result in profound hearing loss, there may be

TABLE 3.10. Type and Prevalence of Multiple Handicaps Among the Five Etiological Groups

Multiple Handicaps: Deafness and One or More Additional Major Disabilities	Heredity (62 cases)		Rh (45 cases)		Prematurity (115 cases)		Meningitis (92 cases)		Rubella (104 cases)	
	N	%	N	%	N	%	N	%	N	%
Two Major Handicaps Only:										
Cerebral Palsy	—	—	9	20.0	4	3.5	2	2.2	2	1.9
Aphasia	—	—	5	11.1	16	13.9	12	13.0	11	10.6
Mental Retardation	—	—	—	—	4	3.5	6	6.5	2	1.9
Partial Sight	—	—	1	2.2	3	2.6	—	—	2	1.9
Emotional Disturbance	3	4.8	1	2.2	11	9.6	5	5.4	13	12.5
Orthopedic	—	—	—	—	—	—	1	1.1	1	1.0
Total	3	4.8	16	35.6	38	33.0	26	28.3	31	29.8
Three Major Handicaps Only:										
Cerebral Palsy/Aphasia	—	—	4	8.9	5	4.3	—	—	1	1.0
Cerebral Palsy/Mental Retardation	—	—	2	4.4	4	3.5	1	1.1	—	—
Cerebral Palsy/Partial Sight	—	—	1	2.2	1	0.9	—	—	—	—
Cerebral Palsy/Emotional Disturbance	—	—	—	—	2	1.7	—	—	—	—

	None									
	No.	%	No.	%	No.	%	No.	%	No.	%
Aphasia/Mental Retardation	—	—	—	—	2	1.7	—	—	—	—
Aphasia/Partial Sight	—	—	1	2.2	1	0.9	—	—	2	1.9
Aphasia/Emotional Disturbance	—	—	—	—	9	7.8	1	1.1	9	8.7
Aphasia/Orthopedic	—	—	—	—	—	—	—	—	1	1.0
Mental Retardation/ Vision	—	—	—	—	2	1.7	—	—	1	—
Mental Retardation/ Emotional Disturbance	—	—	—	—	1	0.9	1	1.1	1	1.0
Mental Retardation/ Orthopedic	—	—	—	—	2	1.7	—	—	1	—
Other	—	—	2	4.4	2	1.7	1	1.1	4	3.8
Total	2	—	12	26.7	31	27.0	4	4.3	18	17.3
Four Major Handicaps	1	1.6	4	8.9	9	7.9	4	4.3	4	3.8
Five or More Major Handicaps	—	—	—	—	—	—	1	1.1	3	2.9
Grand Total	4	6.5	32	71.1	78	67.8	35	38.0	56	53.8

(SOURCE: Vernon, M. (1969). Multiply handicapped deaf children: Medical, educational and psychological considerations. Reston, Va.: Council of Exceptional Children. Reprinted by permission.)

TABLE 3.11. Major Physical Defects Associated with Various Birthweights Among Premature Children

Birthweight (pounds, ounces)	Number	Cerebral Palsy *N*	Cerebral Palsy Percent	Mental Retardation (IQ below 70) *N*	Mental Retardation (IQ below 70) Percent	Aphasoid Disorder *N*	Aphasoid Disorder Percent	Visual Defect *N*	Visual Defect Percent	Visual Defect Type of Anomalies Reported
4, 7 to 5, 8	49	5	10.2	5	10.2	16	32.6	8	16.3	1 cross eye 1 blind (cataract)
3, 5 to 4, 6	34	4	11.7	6	17.6	10	29.4	8	23.5	2 strabismus 1 strabismus
2, 4 to 3, 4	23	5	21.7	7	30.4	9	39.1	10	43.4	2 blind 1 wandering eye 1 no upper gaze
1, 2 to 2, 3	6	3	50.0	1	16.6	3	50.0	4	66.6	1 blind 1 cross eye
Premature but exact birthweight unknown	3	3	100.0	none	none	3	100.0	1	33.3	

(SOURCE: Vernon, M. (1969). *Multiply handicapped deaf children: Medical, educational and psychological considerations.* Reston, Va.: Council of Exceptional Children. Reprinted by permission.)

extensive other central nervous system damage which has behavioral manifestations. These include high prevalences of cerebral palsy and lesser, but serious, coordination problems, aphasoid involvements, academic disabilities, a generally depressed IQ level, seizures, and atypical interpretation of sound. In 71 percent of these children, deafness is one of two or more disabilities. Educationally, in addition to the language and communication problems of deafness, there is a high percentage of aphasia.

Although there are serious physical and academic correlates of the organic pathology of erythroblastosis fetalis, the areas of the brain involved do not seem to be directly related to pathological emotional adjustment. Rh children seem better adjusted than at least three of four major etiological groups of deaf youths (Vernon, 1969).

It appears that the functional value of their residual hearing as measured by pure tone audiometry is less than that normally found in children with similar audiograms. There appears to be pathology of auditory preception or integration and symbolization of sound that reduces the effectiveness of the ability to respond to auditory input.

MEDICINE-INDUCED DEAFNESS

The rapid development of new drugs has resulted in some that are ototoxic; that is, a side effect may be hearing loss. For example, approximately 3 per 1,000 hospitalized patients experience deafness due to medication (Brazelton, 1970). Not all cases involve permanent losses. Among the major ototoxins are aspirin (salicylates), amino-glycoside antibiotics (examples are neomycin, kanamycin, and streptomycin), quinine, and thalidomide (Kaku, Farmer, & Hudson, 1973; Meriwether, Mangi, & Serpick, 1971).

One psychological consideration is that most drug-induced deafness occurs adventitiously, sometimes fairly late in life. Often it is associated with patients who take medication because of other problems such as rheumatoid arthritis (aspirin), kidney disorder (ethocrynic acid), or tuberculosis (streptomycin) (Meriwether, Mangi, & Serpick, 1971; Vernon, 1969). In some cases, medicines used during pregnancy may cause deafness in the child (Brazelton, 1970).

Thus far there has been no research on the exact psychologic sequelae of deafness caused by medication. One problem is that it is often difficult to know whether the disease or the drug used to treat it caused the deafness and any other problems (Vernon, 1967a & b, 1969). Frequently a medicine known to be ototoxic must be used because no other will save the patient's life. On some occasions, as with tubercular meningitis, even though the life may be saved, the sequelae of the disease or drug may be severe enough to leave the patient able to function only at a minimal level psychologically and physically.

NOISE-INDUCED DEAFNESS

Exposure to noise can cause hearing loss (Alberti, Morgan, & LaBlanc, 1974; Cantrell, 1974; Fishbein, 1971; Kryter, 1973; O'Neill, 1973). Noise also causes psychological and physiological effects, such as irritability, loss of equilibrium, cardiovascular disease, biochemical changes in blood and urine, and gastrointestinal motility (Cantrell, 1974). Russian research reports neurologic and psychiatric difficulties (Cantrell, 1974).

Usually noise does not cause total deafness. Furthermore, the hearing loss tends to appear in adulthood. However, because of the increasing noise level in our society, there will be more hearing loss from this cause. For example, snowmobiles (Bess & Poyner, 1974), powerful new industrial machines (Alberti, Morgan, & LeBlanc, 1974), modern amplified music (Chadwick, 1973), and huge trucks (Tyler, 1973) are all relatively recent environment factors which impair as a result of prolonged exposure. Even some of the incubators which save the lives of premature infants have been found to function at decibel levels that imperil the infants' hearing.

Psychologically, the person rendered hearing-impaired from noise has two dimensions to his or her adjustment. First are the psycho-physiological problems associated with noise: raised cholesterol levels, vasoconstriction, head noises, distractibility, anxiety, and others. Second are the reactions to the hearing loss itself, especially those of late onset.

Syphilis

Current lifestyles have brought about an increase in the rate of syphilis (Wiet & Milko, 1975), and there is a proportionate increment in its role as a cause of deafness.

Both acquired and congenital syphilis can result in profound hearing loss. However, it is more common in the latter. In the acquired form, onset of deafness occurs from a few years to advanced stages many years after infection (Wright, 1971). With congenital syphilis the disease is contracted from the mother (Paparella, Hohman, & Huff, 1971). Approximately 20 to 40 percent of the infants infected with the congenital form will eventually be deaf or hard-of-hearing (Wright, 1971). A survey of a large British eye, ear, nose, and throat clinic indicated that 3 percent of its cases of sensorineural deafness were due to congenital syphilis (Wright, 1971).

It is important to determine when syphilis is the etiology of deafness, because there are implications for psychology and rehabilitation. For example, neurological impairments are a late manifestation (hemiplegia or paraphegia). Mental retardation may occur, and there are sometimes convulsions. The presence of interstitial keratitis, saddle nose, or small, widely spaced, narrow, peg-shaped teeth are key diagnostic clues to congenital forms (Forfar & Arneil, 1974). However, the disease can be present without these symptoms.

Ataxia, confabulation, and organic brain syndromes are common late sequelae of advanced acquired syphilis. The organism causing syphilis can invade and damage almost any organ (Bergsma, 1973). The symptoms of Ménière's disease and of presbycusis can sometimes be easily confused with deafness due to syphilis unless appropriate medical tests are done (Paparella, Hohman, & Huff, 1971; Wright, 1971).

It is crucial for psychologists, audiologists, and other professionals to be aware of the symptoms—especially in children having the congenital form—so they can be referred for diagnosis and treatment. Prognosis is dependent in part on the promptness of effective therapy.

MÉNIÈRE'S DISEASE (ENDOLYMPHATIC HYDROPS)

This is a condition characterized by dizziness, progressive and sometimes fluctuating sensorineural hearing loss, tinnitus, and a feeling of fullness in the ear. There is generally a loss of discrimination out of proportion to the degree of hearing loss (Shaver, 1975). Treatment depends on the cause, but in most cases there is no cure (Pulec, 1973).

Psychologically, anxiety may be present because the patient never knows when he or she may experience a severe loss of balance, nausea, and tinnitus (Pulec, 1973). In severe cases, especially those where the tinnitus is unbearable, surgery can be performed (Pulec, 1973). The disease usually occurs in adulthood, creating the psychological problems of late onset deafness.

MUMPS

About .006 percent of bilateral childhood deafness is reported to be caused by mumps (Jensema, 1975). Considering the fact that about 60 to 80 percent of adults have had the disease, it is obvious that the percentage left deaf is minute (Jensema, 1975). In half the mumps cases, onset is before age 3, and in only 15 percent is it after 5 (Jensema, 1975). Thus, as a group, children deafened by mumps have a later onset of deafness than most deaf youngsters. They tend to be in day schools or part-time special education classes, and not to be multiply handicapped (Jensema, 1975).

OTHERS

There are a multitude of other factors that can cause deafness, many of which have psychological consequences related to other sequelae. Among these are measles (Jensema, 1974), tubercular mastoiditis (Birrell, 1973), chronic otitis media (English, Northern & Fria, 1973), typhoid, smallpox, vitamin deficiency (Kapur, 1966), hyperthyroidism (Rubenstein, Rubenstein, & Theodor, 1974), lack of oxygen at birth (Towbin, 1969), chromosomal abnormalities, cancer, cerebral palsy, multiple sclerosis, and osteogenisis imperfecta (Smith & Thebo, 1973). Along with syphilis there are other sexually transmitted diseases, including herpes simplex, cytomegalovirus, *B-strep,* and *C. Trachomatis,* all associated with hearing loss. These are increasing in prevalence (Vernon & Hicks, 1980), and there may well be an increase in the number of deaf children.

SOME EPIDEMIOLOGICAL CONSIDERATIONS

Race

Among black children hearing loss is considerably less prevalent than among whites (Schein & Delk, 1974). This is somewhat puzzling considering that blacks as a group get poorer medical care, a factor that is usually related to prevalence of deafness. For example, meningitis, complication of Rh factor, and prematurity are more common when preventative medicine is inadequate. However, complications of Rh factor and ABO incompatibility are rare among black and brown-skinned people (Vernon, 1969). Comparable data are not available for other ethnic groups.

Economic Integration

Another epidemiological consideration is that as deaf people are increasingly integrated into the society economically, their marriage and fertility rates tend to increase. This increase results in more deaf children (Brill, 1963; Fraser, 1971).

Diet

Populations that have a high intake of saturated fats tend to have a high incidence of arteriosclerosis, elevated cholesterol levels, and an associated higher incidence of hearing loss (Rosen et al., 1970). Russia and Finland are countries with such populations. Obviously there are psychological correlates of such an etiology, especially when arteriosclerosis is present.

Medical Services

A final epidemiological consideration is that in countries lacking adequate medical service, typhoid, polio, smallpox, and other diseases are major causes of deafness (Kapur, 1966). In technically advanced areas of the world such diseases have been almost completely eliminated. Until studies are done of children deafened by these etiologies, however, their full psychological significance will not be known.

SUDDEN PROFOUND HEARING LOSS

Some 15,000 persons per year in the United States experience a sudden profound deafness (75 dB or greater for average of three speech frequencies) (Byl, 1975). Usually the loss is permanent, especially in older patients, although some forms are treatable (Byl, 1975). Etiologies are varied, including such conditions as poor circulation (Byl, 1975), lightning (Wright & Silk, 1974), underwater diving (Pang, 1974), head injury (Podoshin & Fradis, 1975), acoustic neuroma (Higgs, 1973), hormones (Schiff & Brown, 1973), idiopathic sensorineural factors (Simmons, 1973), viral disease (Simmons, 1973), and the other conditions discussed elsewhere in this chapter.

In certain cases, such as head injury or circulatory failure, additional neurological damage may occur. Here too there may exist a need to consider the psychological problems of deafness and of central nervous system dysfunction.

REFERENCES

Alberti, P. W., Morgan, P. O., & LeBlanc, J. C. (1974). Occupational hearing loss—An Otologist's view of a long-term study. *The Laryngoscope, 84,* 1822–1834.

Bergsma, D. (1973). *Birth defects: Allos and compendium.* Baltimore: Williams & Wilkens.

Berkowitz, G. P. (1979). Management of Rh incompatible pregnancies. *Continuing Education, 10,* 95–100.

Bess, F. H., & Poyner, R. E. (1974). Noise-induced hearing loss and snowmobiles. *Archives of Otolaryngology, 99,* 45–52.

Birrell, J. F. (1973). Aural tuberculosis in children. *Proceedings of the Royal Society of Medicine, 66,* 331–338.

Brazelton, T. B. (1970). Effect of prenatal drugs on the behavior of the neonate. *American Journal of Psychiatrics, 129,* 95–100.

Brill, R. G. (1962). The relationship of Wechsler IQ's to academic achievement among deaf students. *Exceptional Children, 28,* 315–321.

Brill, R. G. (1963). Deafness and the genetic factor. *American Annals of the Deaf, 108,* 359–372.

Budden, S. S., Robinson, G. C., MacLean, C. C., & Cambon, K. G. (1974). Deafness in infants and preschool children: An analysis of etiology and associated handicaps. *American Annals of the Deaf, 119,* 387–395.

Byl, F. (1975). Thirty-two cases of sudden profound hearing loss occurring in 1973: Incidence and prognostic findings. *Transactions of American Academy of Ophthalmology and Otolaryngology, 80,* 298–305.

Cantrell, R. W. (1974). Prolonged exposure to intermittent noise: Audiometric, biochemical, motor, psychological and sleep effects. *The Laryngoscope* 1974, *84*(Suppl. I), 3–55.

Chadwick, D. L. (1973). Music and hearing. *Proceedings of the Royal Society of Medicine, 66,* 105.

Chess, S. (1977). Follow-up report on autism in congenital rubella. *Journal of Autism and Childhood Schizophrenia, 7,* 69–81.

Chess, S., & Fernandez, P. (1980). Neurologic damage and behavior disorder in children. *American Annals of the Deaf, 125,* 998–1001.

Chess, S., Fernandez, P., & Korn, S. J. (1978). Behavioral consequences of congenital rubella. *Journal of Pediatrics, 93,* 699–703.

Delage, G., & Dusseault, M. (1979). Tuberculous meningitis in children: A retrospective study of 79 patients with an analysis of prognostic factors. *Canadian Medical Association Journal, 120,* 305–309.

English, G. M., Northern, J. L., & Fria T. J. (1973). Chronic otitis media as a cause of sensorineural hearing loss. *Archives of Otolaryngology, 98,* 18–22.

Feldman, R. B., Lajoie, R., Mendelson, L., & Pinsky, L. (1971). Congenital rubella and language disorders. *Lancet, 14,* 978.

Fishbein, M. Quiet please. (1971). *Medical World News, 12,* 76.

Fishbein, M. A risk no child should take. (1974). *Medical World News, 15,* 60.

Forfar, J. O., & Arneil, G. C. (1974). *Textbook of pediatrics.* New York: Longman.

Fraser, F. C. (1971). Genetic counseling. *Hospital Practice, 6,* 49–56.

Haas, E. J., Modhaven, T., Quinn, E. L., Cox, F., Fisher, E., & Burch, R. S. (1977). Tuberculous meningitis in an urban hospital. *Archives of Internal Medicine, 137,* 1518–1521.

Hardy, M. P., Haskins, H. L., Hardy, W. G., & Shimizi, H. (1973). Rubella: Audiologic evaluation and follow up. *Archives of Otolaryngology, 98,* 237–245.

Harris, R. E. (1979). A protocol for rubella vaccine. *The Female Patient, 4,* 56–57, 60.

Higgs, W. A. (1973). Sudden deafness as the presenting symptom of acoustic neuroma. *Archives of Otolaryngology, 98,* 73–76.

Jensema, C. (1974). Post-rubella children in special educational programs for the hearing impaired. *Volta Review, 76,* 466–473.

Jensema, C. (1975). Children in educational programs for the hearing impaired whose impairment was caused by mumps. *Journal of Speech and Hearing Disorders, 40,* 164–169.

Jensema, C., & Mullins, J. (1974). Onset, cause and additional handicaps in hearing impaired children. *American Annals of the Deaf, 119,* 701–705.

Kaku, Y., Farmer, J. J., & Hudson, W. R. (1973). Ototoxic drug effects on cochlear histochemistry. *Archives of Otolaryngology, 98,* 282–286.

Kapur, Y. P. (1966). Hearing and infectious tropical and nutritional diseases. *Silent World, 1,* 27–76.

Karchmer, M. A. (1985). A demographic perspective. In E. Cherow, N. Matkin, & R. Trybus,

Hearing-impaired children and youth with developmental disabilities: An interdisciplinary foundation for service. Washington, DC: Gallaudet College Press.

Keane, W. M., Potsic, W. P., Rowe, L. D., & Konkle, D. F. (1979). Meningitis and hearing loss in children. *Archives of Otolaryngology, 105,* 39–44.

Kennedy, D. H., & Fallow, R. J. (1979). Tuberculous meningitis. *Journal of American Medical Association, 241,* 264–268.

Komich, M. P., Lansford, A., Lord, L. B., & Tearney, A. (1973). The sequential development of infants of low birthweight. *American Journal of Occupational Therapy, 27,* 396–402.

Kryter, K. D. (1973). Impairment to hearing from exposure to noise. *Journal of Acoustical Society of America, 53,* 1211–1234.

Lubchence, L. O., Detivoria Papadopoulos, M., Butterfield, L. J., French, J. H., Medcalf, D., Hix, I. E., Danick, J., Dodds, J., Downs, M., & Freeland, E. (1972). Long term follow-up studies of prematurely born infants. I. Relationship of handicaps to nursery routines. *Journal of Pediatrics, 80,* 501–508.

Mackay, R. P. (Ed.) (1964). *The yearbook of neurology and psychiatry.* Chicago: Yearbook Medical Publishers.

Meriwether, W. D., Mangi, R. J., & Serpick, A. A. (1971). Deafness following standard intravenous dose of ethracrynic acid. *Journal of American Medical Association, 216,* 795–798.

Myklebust, H. (1960). *The psychology of deafness.* New York: Grune and Stratton.

Nadol, J. B. (1978). Hearing loss as a sequela of meningitis. *The Laryngoscope, 88,* 739–755.

O'Neill, J. J. (1973). Hearing conservation. *Rehabilitation Record, 14,* 508.

Pang, L. Q. (1974). Sudden sensorineural hearing loss following diving and treatment by compression: A report of two cases. *Transactions of American Academy of Ophthalmology and Otolaryngology, 78,* 436–443.

Paparella, M. M., Hohman, A., & Huff, S., Jr. (1971). *Clinical otology.* St. Louis: C. V. Mosby.

Podoshin, L., & Fradis, M. (1975). Hearing loss after head injury. *Archives of Otolaryngology, 101,* 15–18.

Pulec, J. L. (1973). Ménière's disease: Etiology, natural history, and results of treatment. *Otolaryngolic Clinic of North America, 6,* 25–39.

Raivio, M., & Koskiniemi, M. (1978). Hearing disorders after Haemophilus influenza meningitis. *Archives of Otolaryngology, 104,* 340–344.

Rosen, S., Preobranjensky, N., Khechinashvili, S., Glazunov, I., Kipshidze, N., & Rosen, H. V. (1970). Epidemiologic hearing studies in the U.S.S.R. *Archives of Otolaryngology, 91,* 424–428.

Rubenstein, M., Rubenstein, C., & Theodor, R. (1974). Hearing dysfunction associated with congenital sporadic hypothyroidism. *Annals of Otology, Rhinology, and Laryngology, 83,* 814–820.

Schein, J. E., & Delk, M. T. (1974). *The deaf population of the United States.* Silver Spring, MD: National Association of the Deaf.

Schiff, M., & Brown, M. (1973). Hormones and sudden deafness. *The Laryngoscope, 84,* 1959–1981.

Sever, J. L. (1973). Present status of vaccines for rubella. *Archives of Otolaryngology, 98,* 265–268.

Sheig R. (1974). Neonatal jaundice. *American Family Physician, 10,* 158–164.

Shaver, E. F. (1975). Allergic management of Ménière's disease. *Archives of Otolaryngology, 101,* 96–99.

Simmons, F. B. (1973). Sudden idiopathic sensorineural hearing loss: Some observations. *The Laryngoscope, 83,* 1221–1227.

Smith, K. E., & Thebo, J. L. (1973). *Causes of hearing impairment in Kansas City: Pediatric cases.* (Mimeographed publication). Lawrence: Hearing and Speech Department, Kansas University Medical Center.

Sullivan, P. M., & Vernon, M. (1979). Psychological assessment of hearing impaired children. *School Psychology Digest, 8,* 271–290.

Towbin, A. (1969). Cerebral hypoxic damage in fetus and newborn. *Archives of Neurology, 20,* 35–43.

Trapp, E. P., & Himelstein, P. (1972). *Reading on the exceptional child* (pp. 379–396, chapter by M. Vernon) New York: Appleton-Century-Crofts.

Tyler, D. A. (1973). Noise and truck drivers. *American Industrial Hygiene Journal, 34,* 345–349.

Vernon, M. (1967a). Meningitis and deafness: The problem, its physical, audiological, psychological, and educational manifestation in deaf children. *The Laryngoscope, 10,* 1856–1974.

Vernon, M. (1967b). Tuberculous meningitis and deafness. *Journal of Speech and Hearing Disorders, 32,* 177–181.

Vernon, M. (1969). *Multiply handicapped deaf children: Medical educational and psychological considerations.* Reston, VA: Council of Exceptional Children.

Vernon, M. (1973). Psychological aspects of the diagnosis of deafness in a child. *The Eye, Ear, Nose, and Throat Monthly, 53,* 60–66.

Vernon, M. (1982). Multihandicapped Deaf Children: Types and causes. In D. Tweedie and E. Shroyer (Eds.), *The multihandicapped hearing impaired: Identification and instruction.* Washington, DC: Gallaudet College Press.

Vernon, M., Grieve, B. J., & Shaver, K. (1980). Handicapping conditions associated with the congenital rubella syndrome. *American Annals of the Deaf, 125,* 993–996.

Vernon, M., & Hicks, D. (1980). Relationship of rubella, herpes simplex, cytomegalovirus, and certain other viral disabilities. *American Annals of the Deaf, 125,* 529–534.

Wiet, R. J., & Milko, D. A. (1975). Isolation of the spirochetes in perilymph despite prior antisyphilitic therapy. *Archives of Otolaryngology, 101,* 104–106.

Wright, J. W., & Silk, K. L. (1974). Acoustic and vestibular defects in lightning survivors. *The Laryngoscope, 84,* 1378–1387.

Wright, M. I. (1971). *The pathology of deafness.* Baltimore: Williams and Wilkins.

Ziring, P. R. (1978). Psychiatric sequelae of the 1964–65 rubella epidemic. *Psychiatric Annals, 8,* 57–66.

SECTION I SUMMARY

In the introduction deafness was seen as a psychological variable that alters deaf people's behavior. Chapter 1 showed how deafness affects many of life's experiences such as schooling, language development, choice of leisure activities, employment, choice of marriage partners, and growing old. It described a culture within which are minorities such as black, Hispanic, and Native Americans with their own needs for services. It also discussed the rich source of art, literature, and drama that has grown and flourished from the deaf experience.

Chapter 2 discussed the genetic causes of deafness and emphasized how important it is to convey this genetic information to families involved. Nine major genetic syndromes involving deafness were discussed in detail along with the nature and role of genetic counseling. Finally, chapter 3 described the nongenetic or organic etiologies of deafness which have psychological consequences in intelligence, educational achievement, hearing, communication skills, and psychological adjustment of the deaf child.

REVIEW QUESTIONS

1. Describe the service needs of minority deaf populations (black, Hispanic, Native American).
2. When and where does "deaf enculturation" typically occur?
3. How might knowledge of genetic deafness contribute to the prevention and treatment of deafness?
4. Why does genetic counseling involve more than simply computing probabilities for a given disease and relaying this information to the parents?
5. Why are the causes of deafness important in a comprehensive psychology of deafness?
6. What are the leading nongenetic causes of childhood deafness and what are the psychological and educational sequelae of each condition.

SECTION II

Communication: Languages and Systems

OVERVIEW

A psychology of any group of people takes into account the language of the community. Thus a chapter is devoted to American Sign Language (ASL), and to communication issues introduced in chapter 1, on the deaf community. First the American and French roots of ASL are traced. Then its content and linguistic form are briefly covered. Next is a discussion of its educational uses in schools for deaf children, where it has been rejected for many years and erroneously referred to as "broken English." In contrast, sign language has been welcomed into hearing schools, where it is used in language arts classes as well as in clinics for exceptional children. Finally are descriptions of how researchers in linguistics and psychology have used ASL to study the acquisition and processing of language by humans and primates.

Even though the deaf community prefers ASL, other forms of communication have been imposed on them. Chapter 5 deals with speech, lipreading, amplication, and manual systems of representing English. Cued Speech, fingerspelling, the SEE systems, and Signed English are contrasted with ASL and are illustrated in photographs. While it is generally agreed that speech combined with a manual system is a better communication system than lipreading alone, there is controversy in the field as to which manual system is most useful. These concerns are addressed in this chapter. Finally is a brief discussion of writing and reading as useful forms of communication—an issue that will be expanded on in chapter 12 on education.

CHAPTER 4
American Sign Language: Its History, Culture, and Modern-day Uses

The Gesture
This, is the voice from silent hands;
This, is the voice not heard, but seen
Reaching across the empty space between
Words, and the action that the mind demands
When words are not enough; this is the gesture.   *Dorothy Miles, 1976*

Sign language has developed over the centuries and is used among deaf people all over the world. In the United States it is used in teaching not only deaf children but hearing children as well—both normal and exceptional. It is used in clinics and classrooms for language therapy. It is taught in public preschool, elementary classrooms, and high schools. College students choose to enroll in sign classes in preservice teacher-training and interpreter-training programs as well as programs for social workers and vocational rehabilitation counseling. Sign is often chosen as an elective or a foreign language requirement within a wide variety of majors and for Ph.D. degrees. Psycholinguists and psychologists, too, have studied sign language to examine topics such as theories of language, language acquisition in humans and primates, and language processing. This chapter will examine the historical roots of sign language and its modern uses in both education and psychology.

HISTORY OF AMERICAN SIGN LANGUAGE

The origins of American Sign Language, commonly referred to as ASL, can be traced linguistically through an examination of language variation and change (Stokoe, 1960; Woodward, 1978, 1980). ASL can also be traced historically by looking at documents written about the education of deaf children (Lane, 1984; Scouten, 1984).

LINGUISTIC ROOTS

According to linguists, sign language varieties have existed in America as long as there were deaf people around to use them (Woodward, 1978; Stokoe, 1960). These sign languages consisted primarily of *home signs,* gestural behaviors which develop among deaf people who are isolated from other deaf people. Home signs come about with the daily interaction of an isolated deaf person and other hearing persons.

Because transportation was poor and there was no public formal schooling, deaf people were isolated from each other, and so these home signs could not become standardized.

While there is no documentation on the structure of these sign varieties in America, there are records of two isolated deaf communities who used signs. Groce (1985) collected oral histories of islanders who lived on Martha's Vineyard about 70 or 80 years ago. A hereditary form of deafness in the Martha's Vineyard population resulted in a high percentage of deaf islanders. Groce's records reveal that sign language was used widely among both hearing and deaf citizens. The deaf members were easily integrated into the life on the island since all citizens used sign language from childhood.

Sign language was reported to be use also among people on an isolated area in the Caribbean—Providence Island (Woodward, 1978); This sign language did not follow oral syntax. Here also both hearing and deaf residents of the island used it for daily activities and so deaf citizens were integrated into everyday life.

Other linguistic evidence suggests the early existence of signs in America. Woodward (1978) examined cognates of words or signs to see if they were related to words or signs in other languages. He found that about 40 percent of signs in America used today are related to languages other than French Sign Language. Woodward theorizes that probably a number of sign languages or sign systems such as the varieties found on Martha's Vineyard and Providence Island existed in 17th- and 18th-century America before French Sign Language was introduced to America in 1817.

HISTORICAL ROOTS

Historical documents on the education of deaf children show that ASL is a hybrid of French Sign Language (FSL), which Thomas Hopkins Gallaudet and Laurent Clerc brought to the United States from Paris in 1816 (Lane, 1984; Scouten, 1984).

Thomas Hopkins Gallaudet (1787–1851), a student for the ministry, was employed by Dr. Mason Cogswell, a prominent physician in Connecticut, to teach his deaf daughter, Alice (1805–1830). Gallaudet first traveled to England to visit the Braidwood's School, which used the oral methods. He had hoped to combine the oral methods with signs and fingerspelling, which he had been studying from a book by the French educator Roch-Ambroise Sicard (1742–1822). When Gallaudet arrived in England, the Braidwood family refused to reveal their teaching techniques. However, Gallaudet did meet Sicard, who was on a lecture tour with his two deaf pupils—Jean Massieu (1772–1846) and Laurent Clerc (1785–1869) and Sicard invited Gallaudet to visit his school in Paris.

Prior to Sicard's tenure at the school in Paris, it was directed by its founder, Charles Michael de L'Epee (1712–1789), a French Roman Catholic priest. L'Epee is often called the "father of the deaf" because he started the first public school of deaf youths in Paris. L'Epee studied the French sign language of the Paris street youths then attempted to standardize it to conform to French syntax, inventing signs for articles and grammatical markers. L'Epee also used the Spanish manual alphabet that had been developed in the 15th century by Juan Martin Pablo Bonet. L'Epee frequently held public demonstrations to secure funding for his program: His students would write in French after he dictated to them in his French manual system, which was different from the sign language they used among themselves in communication. This system became known as the "French Method."

After L'Epee's death, his successor, Sicard, criticized his work, saying that the deaf youths did not really understand what they were writing. Sicard simplified L'Epee's method and then devised other methods by which the deaf students could compose sentences by themselves. He too held frequent demonstrations, where his star deaf pupils, Jean Massieu and Laurent Clerc, would perform by answering questions posed by Sicard in sign language. Both L'Epee and Sicard focused on manual signs that corresponded to French syntax rather than the natural sign order of the deaf community.

A contemporary critic of the French Method was a hearing student of Sicard's—Auguste Bébian (1789–1843). He criticized the use of these "methodological signs," which he considered cumbersome and complex. He recommended that teachers use instead the natural signs of deaf students. Bebian was fired from his position and later started his own school. Interestingly, Bebian's approach predates researchers today who advocate the use of American Sign Language rather than the manual codes of English in classrooms. Many years ago Bebian wrote about his observations, which, interestingly enough, concur with current linguistic analyses:

> . . . the more profoundly these signs decompose the sentence—thus revealing the structure of French—the further they get away from the language of the deaf, from their intellectual capacities and thinking. That is why the deaf never make use of these signs among themselves; they use them in taking word-for-word dictation, but to explain the meaning of the text dictated, they go back to their familiar language. (From R. Bebian in Lane & Phillip, 1984, p. 23).

Despite these controversies, the dominating method in the Paris school was the French Method. Thus when Gallaudet went back to Paris with Sicard, he received manual French lessons from Clerc and Massieu. Gallaudet invited Clerc to return to America with him and together they set up a school in Hartford, Connecticut, using the French Method. French Sign Language subsequently spread throughout the United States so rapidly that a national college—Gallaudet College—was established by an Act of Congress in 1864 for higher education for the graduates of the schools using the sign language method. In 1986 Gallaudet College became Gallaudet University.

Modern-day American Sign Language is therefore believed to be a mixture of Old French Sign Language brought over by Clerc with the varieties of sign languages already existing in the United States. This form, called Old American Sign Language, has evolved over the years into the American Sign Language used by the deaf community today (Baker & Cokely, 1980). Some linguists believe that ASL is still evolving as it becomes more integrated with signed English (Fischer, 1978).

CULTURE

PRIMARY USERS

ASL is used chiefly by about half a million deaf people in the United States, Canada, and Mexico. In addition, deaf people in Puerto Rico use a variation of ASL (Baker & Cokely, 1980). About 10 percent of the deaf population learn it from their deaf parents; the other 90 percent typically learned it when they enter residential schools where they meet other deaf children and adults. Those who attend public school may learn ASL when they take a job or enter a postsecondary program with other deaf adults. ASL is the only language that is typically not learned from parents but passed from child to child (Padden, 1980). This phenomenon has profound linguistic implications and also significantly influences deaf children's attitudes about sign language.

American Sign Language is different from sign languages in other countries just as spoken languages vary from country to country. For example, Great Britain, Italy, and Pakistan each has its own sign language. Sandager (1985) has described sign languages from 22 countries around the world. Thus the statement that sign language is universal is a myth, although its heavy component of mime gives sign languages more similarities to each other than is the case with spoken languages.

ASL: ITS FORM

American Sign Language (ASL) is a language just as is English, Spanish, French, Swahili, Latin, or German (Klima & Bellugi, 1979). It has a syntax and vocabulary as all languages do (Stokoe, 1960). Ironically, for years people in the field of deafness failed to recognize this fact. They referred to ASL as a system of mime and gestures, depreciating or denying its linguistic status. This naive position is still maintained by a few individuals, most of whom do not know American Sign Language but who oppose its use.

In ASL, the words or signs are formed by the hands, arms, face, and sometimes the entire upper body (Figure 4.1). A single sign can correspond to a single word, or one sign may represent a phrase or sentence. Fingerspelling is incorporated in ASL.

Advantages

The major advantage of sign language is that it is highly visible, that is, the signs are easy to see and to discern one from another. Thus it does not create the problems of ambiguity and confusion that often result from speechreading and the speech of most deaf people.

American Sign Language also has the advantage of being perhaps the most affective of all language systems. Because it is a "body language," feelings are communicated with amazing vividness. In fact, Broadway scenic designer and director David Hays calls it "the ideal language of theater" for this very reason.

Of course, ASL has obvious and important value when deaf people wish to communicate with each other.

Disadvantages

There are some major disadvantages of American Sign Language. One is that its grammar is different than that of English. In using ASL as an aid to learning English, these differences must be learned if there is to be a satisfactory carryover. Also, because ASL is not known by the majority of hearing people, its value as a communication tool is limited. For example, a deaf person cannot go to his or her family physician and expect to be understood using ASL. However, significant others in the life of a deaf person—family members, teachers, rehabilitation counselors, and so on—can realistically be expected to learn ASL. This is the key issue. ASL can then be used to communicate to deaf persons basic concepts such as mathematics, human values, career counseling, and so forth, which in turn enable the deaf person to be

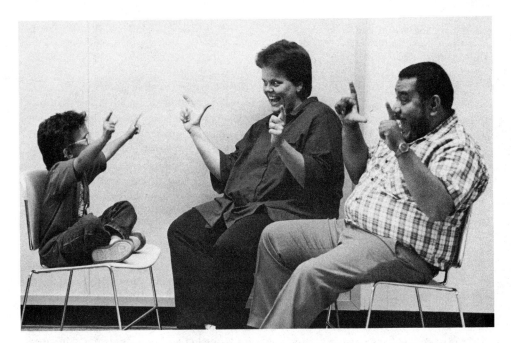

FIGURE 4.1.   American Sign Language (ASL) uses signs formed by hands, arms, face, and upper body.

more effective in coping with the "hearing world." If deaf people had to depend on speechreading, much of this vital information would not be learned.

While ASL is a language as English is, its linguistic structure is markedly different from that of English. This difference can be seen in the way both languages form lexical items. An English word is made up of phonemes which occur in a sequence, while an ASL lexical item—the sign—is composed of four parameters (hand configuration, movement, location, and orientation) which are executed simultaneously. ASL makes use of space and movement of gestures. Other differences exist in the way each of the languages incorporates morphemes and forms sentences. ASL uses nonmanual cues such as facial expressions, head tilts, body movement, and eye gazes to express grammatical relations (Baker-Shenk, 1985). While linguists have written extensively on the grammar of ASL, practitioners in education and rehabilitation rarely have this knowledge. Not understanding that ASL actually promotes and facilitates the language acquisition and development process, some mistakenly think ASL is "broken English" and try to discourage deaf children from using it. Nevertheless, most deaf adults who complete education/rehabilitation programs persist in using ASL for communication purposes. In fact, ASL is the chief identifying characteristic of the deaf community (Meadow, 1968; Baker & Cokely, 1980).

ASL: Its Content

American Sign Language is used to transmit all kinds of information just as is any other developed language. For example, college lectures on abstract topics such as philosophy and religion can be interpreted in American Sign Language. With the increased opportunities for deaf persons to enroll in postsecondary programs and technical fields, signs have been developed for instructional purposes (Kannapell, Hamilton, & Bornstein, 1969), for computer terminology (Jamison, 1973), and for medical terms (Garcia, 1983).

In the theater, plays such as *Hamlet* are performed in sign language. Plays are also written especially for production in sign. For instance, original dramas such as Bernard Bragg and Eugene Berman's "Tales from a Clubroom" not only have been written specifically to be performed using sign language, but also incorporate themes, values, and feelings of the deaf community. In "Tales from a Clubroom" the playwrights express deaf people's dislike of manual English. (See chapter 1 for references to these plays.)

ATTITUDES

As far back as 1779 the deaf educator-writer Pierre Desloges wrote about the negative attitudes of the public toward sign language: "Few people have adequate notion of our state, our resources, or our way of communicating with each other with sign language" (Desloges, 1779, cited in Lane & Phillip, 1984). Despite public misunderstanding, sign language has persisted through history and across continents (Lane & Phillips, 1984; Brill, 1984; Nash, 1987).

Most deaf adults have pride in their sign language and deeply resent educators and others who attempt to modify or change it (Higgins, 1980). When communicating with a hearing adult they will incorporate more English signs and speech to enable the hearing person to understand, but with a deaf adult they will usually "turn off voice" and use a pure form of American Sign Language. Deaf adults will differentiate among themselves as to who are the "signers" and who are the "oralists" (Higgins, 1980). The pejorative sign "think hearie" is often used by a deaf person to insult someone who doesn't agree with the values of the deaf community. On the other hand, there is a small minority of deaf adults who reject American Sign Language and think it is an inferior way of communicating. They reflect an incorporation of the negative attitudes of hearing educators who transmitted negative, punitive views on sign language when teaching them.

PIDGIN SIGN LANGUAGE

Only deaf adults, particularly native signers, are typically fluent in ASL. When the hearing parents, teachers, or professionals are signing, they generally change ASL to a grammar that is more similar to English (Kluwin, 1983; Erting, 1985). The result is a Pidgin Sign English. For example, instead of saying "me home," the ASL form of the concept, they sign "I go home" and they say "I am going home."

Thus, Pidgin Sign Language combines characteristics of both American Sign Language and English, depending on how much American Sign Language the hearing person knows. When more English is used, the system is called Pidgin Sign English (PSE). To elaborate further, when signing a sentence in PSE, the signer may omit the articles, "the" and "a," since ASL does not have these elements, but may retain grammatical structures of verb directionality found in ASL (Baker & Cokely, 1980).

Like other pidgins, PSE is a blending. While some linguists are currently debating whether it is a pidgin or actually "foreign talk," it is generally agreed that

Pidgin Sign Language contains natural ingredients of both English and ASL. PSE is accepted by the deaf community because it focuses on communication between deaf and hearing people (Baker & Cokely, 1980), it follows the meanings of ASL, and it does not attempt to drastically alter its structure as manual codes do (See discussion of manual codes in chapter 5).

USE IN EDUCATION

In Schools for Deaf Children

The acceptance of and pride in sign language felt by most of the adult deaf community is seldom shared by parents, administrators, and educators in schools for deaf children. In fact, most hearing teachers neither understand pure ASL nor use it (Allen & Woodward, 1986). Only about 35 percent of hearing parents use even a sign code such as Signed English with their deaf children (Jordan & Karchmer, 1986). This situation has been changing dramatically over the last 15 years, with more parents and professionals learning some form of manual communication.

How did ASL get into the schools? Historically, Clerc and Gallaudet introduced ASL to the educational establishment when they set up the American School for the Deaf in Hartford in 1817, As these methods spread throughout the United States from the 1800s to the early 1900s. many schools hired deaf teachers who used ASL with their students. Additionally, a high percentage of hearing teachers came from deaf families in which they learned ASL.

Manual versus Oral Controversy

During this time, another movement in the United States, based on the English and German methods, stressed the exclusive use of speech. ASL was not recognized as a language, and its use by deaf children was severely punished. This movement, led by the inventor Alexander Graham Bell, held that deaf people should be taught using only the "articulation" or "oral" method. This controversy had been going on during L'Epee's time in France and existed throughout Europe during the 1800s and 1900s. The first International Conference on Deaf Education upheld the oralism position. However, it was the Second International Conference, held in Milan in 1880, that had the most powerful impact on language policy in schools for the deaf worldwide. At this conference a resolution was passed supporting oralism and stating that manual communication was harmful to the speech, lipreading, language, and thinking of deaf people. As a result, many countries chose the oral only method and rigidly forbade signing (Brill, 1984). In the United States, deaf teachers were fired and the use of signs was strictly prohibited in most schools for the deaf. In some secondary-level residential programs there was a limited use of signs, but even there their use was concealed or denied when visitors came to the school (Moores, 1987).

From 1900 to about 1965 the main instructional method in schools for deaf children was the "oral" or "speech-only" method. However, studies in the late 1960s with deaf children of deaf parents showed that a primary language can be acquired with manual communication (see Table 4.2). Several of these studies showed that the use of signs facilitate rather than impede speech development as it was previously believed. Further, this research showed that children who had early manual communication performed better than the oral-only children on measures of academic achievement. While this finding motivated many schools to introduce the use of speech with signs (Jordan, Gustason, & Rosen, 1976), the controversy still persists in the field. Tables 4.1 and 4.2 (pp. 80–85) illustrate the amount of effort researchers in the field have put forth to examine this very heated argument.

In Schools for Hearing Children

In contrast to the controversy of sign language use in schools for deaf children, public schools have been enthusiastic and receptive to it. Signs recently have been used with preschool and elementary hearing children to develop expressive language as well as to teach beginning reading and reading readiness (Vernon, 1983). Typically, this does not mean using American Sign Language but ASL signs in English word order.

Language Increments

Manual signs have increased the use of adjectives and adverbs with nouns in the expressive language of four normally hearing kindergarten children (deViveiros & McLaughlin, 1982). The results showed that the frequency of use of English adjectives and adverbs increased after the manual sign teaching.

Reading and Spelling

Many case studies document the value of using fingerspelling and signs to teach beginning reading and spelling to hearing children. Significant gains were made by first- and second grade-students who used sign vocabulary to reinforce their sight word vocabulary (Wilson & Hoyer, 1985). Other studies show the effectiveness of teachers using signs and fingerspelling to reinforce spelling with first graders (Wilson, Teague, & Teague, 1985). The authors of these studies find that in order to apply these manual techniques, teachers do not have to learn the American Sign Language, but merely know the key vocabulary they wish to teach and fingerspelling learned from a book (Bornstein, Saulnier, & Hamilton, 1983; Bornstein & Saulnier, 1984; Greenberg, Vernon, DuBois, & McKnight, 1981).

Gifted Children

Signs and fingerspelling are particularly effective in teaching reading to gifted children. Studies of hearing children of deaf parents show that they are frequently "reading" by age 3 or 4 (Vernon & Coley, 1978; Vernon, Coley, & Ottinger, 1979).

In Programs for Exceptional Children

There has been a growing literature over the past 15 to 20 years which shows that sign language can facilitate communication and language skills in children with various exceptionalities such as learning disabilities, language delay, mental retardation, aphasia, autism, blindness, and combinations of disabilities. Usually the teacher or clinician uses both signs and speech in English word order.

The Nonvocal

Signing has been used with children and adult clients who are unable to speak because of mental, physical, or emotional disabilities (Bryen & Joyce, 1985; Musselwhite & St. Louis, 1982). It has been helpful with individuals ranging in age from 3 to adulthood. The success of these manual methods has been attributed to the fact that signing bypasses the oral-motor speech mechanism and is cognitively easier to carry out (Bryen & Joyce, 1986). Further, the iconicity of many signs is seen to facilitate learning (Griffith & Robinson, 1980). Sign language has even been found to facilitate the development of speech in some students (Bryen & Joyce, 1985). Thus, contrary to the past belief that signs impede talking, researchers are finding that using signs helps the nonvocal child, in some instances, to begin to vocalize and then drop the signs.

Mental Retardation

A review of 19 studies shows that mentally retarded subjects from age 3 to adulthood who were not able to learn speech were capable of attaining a receptive sign vocabulary and, to a lesser extent, sign production (Poulton & Algozzine, 1980). Delayed language development was facilitated when the subjects were taught to associate objects with the manual sign equivalent. Similar results were found with 15 nonverbal mentally retarded youths in the severe and profound ranges (Cirrin & Rowland, 1985); their communication abilities were increased with the use of signs.

Autism

In a review of data with over 100 autistic children it was found that youth were able to learn receptive and expressive signs and combine signs for communication purposes (Bonvillian, Nelson & Rhyne, 1981). In another study, Konstantareas, Hunter & Sloman (1985) used manual signs with a blind, autistic 10-year-old child. After an eight-month training program using primarily the tactile-kinesthetic and auditory modalities, this blind, low-functioning, nonverbal autistic child was able to acquire a functional sign vocabulary.

These are but a sample of the many studies that have been published about developing a communication system with nonvocal handicapped children.

Language Impairment

Signs are also used with children with language impairment who already have some basic language (nouns and verbs) but need intervention to develop more advanced structures such as function words. Signs have been used as gestural cues as an instructional strategy with children diagnosed with mild to moderate developmental delay, language impairment, learning disability, emotional disturbance, or hearing impairment (Musselwhite, 1986). Conventional signs were used to support the learning and remembering of communication skills. Teachers taught language forms, such as inflectional markers, pronouns, and auxiliary verbs, by giving the children the manual sign (or Signed English) marker for each and then using them in a communicative context. The gestural cues were faded out when the child mastered the language form in spoken form.

Another study applied signs with fourteen 3- to 11-year-old language-impaired children who were capable only of producing telegraphic speech (Konstantareas, 1985). Signs were used as prosthetic devices to facilitate the spontaneous verbalizations of functors as pronouns and prepositions. Here, signs are used not as the main vehicle for communication but as aids to more complex speech production for those who already have useful but limited speech. The sign is initially superimposed on the missing functor word, then eventually faded out once the child has acquired its spoken language equivalent. (See Table 4.3 on page 86 for additional studies.)

TABLE 4.1. Oralism Effects on Deaf Children

Studies	Subjects	Results
Corson, 1973	Deaf child/deaf parent oral communication/O; Deaf child/deaf parent sign & oral comm./SO; Deaf child/hearing parent	Both deaf of deaf +> deaf of hearing; O/deaf of deaf +> SO/deaf of deaf
Holdt,* 1975	11 oral/regional/86db; 54 state school/94db; 11 oral private/102; taught social studies rule and location	Auditory/oral +> total communication
Carson and Goetzinger, 1975	35 Students state school. Reception of nonsense syllables, signs	Total communication not superior to lipreading and audition
Kelliher, 1976	45 deaf/nondeaf pairs. Coopersmith's self-esteem & Meadow rating scale: T=total, S=self, P=peer, O=school, H=home	Hearing +> deaf in self-esteem T/S/P; Oral=TC self-esteem T/S/P/H/O; Degree hearing loss=self-esteem T/S/P/H; Degree hearing loss TC +> school self-esteem; All deaf + relationship/mother; Oral deaf + relationship/father/sibs
Clark et al.,* 1977	British Columbia	Oral +> TC vocabulary; Oral + TC reading comprehension; Oral = TC math/computation/concepts
Jensema and Trybus,* 1978	HI children communicate with parent, with teacher	Preschool +later use speech; SES +speech; Parent education +speech; Parent occupation +speech; – restricted environment +speech
Ogden, 1979	637 former students from 3 private oral schools	Graduates + success educationally and professionaly. Graduates attribute success to oral English. Student body and their families were a socioeconomically elite group.

Study	Description	Findings
Gray, 1980	26 prelingually profound deaf; 11 oral matched 13 TC on IQ, age, sex, SES; 2 years exposure to communication.	Oral = TC overall psychological dev. Oral = TC self image Oral = TC impulsivity Parents judged oral youngsters +> TC
Nix, 1981	Reviews 7 studies	Summarizes "it does not appear that the use of signs and fingerspelling contribute in a positive way to a child's development and use of speech and speech reception skills . . . [on this basis] it is not included in the auditory-oral purposes of the AGB . . . who is not anti-sign, but rather pro speech."
Parasnis, 1983	38 NTID deaf/deaf delay sign/deaf/hearing	deaf/hearing +> deaf/deaf all speech deaf/hearing = deaf/deaf cognition
Geers, Moog, and Schick, 1984	168 oral/aural matched 159 TC children	O/A +> TC grammatical categories gen. O/A +> TC grammatical categories 50% TC +> O/A grammatical categories 20% MCE do not develop competence with early English syntax at a rate faster than those not using signs.
Luterman and Chasin, 1981	Deafness management quotient score 29 child. DMQ = sum hearing, SES Central intactness, and family constellation	High DMQ +> low DMQ for speech discrimination, auditory discrimination, speech articulation, above sig. Also more speech, fewer signs, more mainstreamed (not significant)
Quigley & Paul, 1984a	Summarizing Messerly and Abram (1980), Doehring, Bonnycastle, and Ling (1978), Lane and Baker (1974)	"Deaf children in incontestably oral programs develop better language and academic skills than deaf children in the general population" (p. 20)

Key: + means more, better, improves; +> means better; > means worse than next group; = means no difference between groups; − means less, worse disimproves;

* Cited in Nix, 1981. (SOURCE: From "Total communication in perspective" by H. Schlesinger, in D. Luterman (Ed.), 1986, *Deafness in Perspective*. San Diego: College Hill Press. Reprinted by permission.)

TABLE 4.2. Positive Effects of Total Communication on Deaf Children

Studies	Subjects	Results
Montgomery, 1966	59 Scottish	Manual communication did not influence speech negatively
Stuckless and Birch, 1966	105 deaf of deaf parents manual 337 deaf of hearing parents oral	Deaf/deaf = speech deaf/hearing Deaf/deaf + speechreading Deaf/deaf + reading Deaf/deaf + writing Deaf/deaf? + psychosocial development
Quigley, 1968	16 total communication 16 oral children	TC + language TC + speechreading TC + academic achievement
Vernon and Koh, 1970	32 genetically deaf manual 32 gentically deaf oral	Manual + Stanford Achievement Manual + Stanford Reading Manual + Stanford Paragraph Meaning Manual + Stanford Vocabulary Manual + written language Manual = oral speech Manual = oral speechreading Manual = oral psychosocial Development
Meadow, 1967	56 deaf of deaf 56 deaf of hearing	Deaf/Deaf + reading Deaf/Deaf + math Deaf/Deaf + overall achievement Deaf/Deaf + social adjustment Deaf/Deaf + written language Deaf/Deaf = deaf/hearing speech Deaf/Deaf = deaf/hearing speechreading
Vernon, 1972	Summarized 11 studies	Early manual communication has + effect
Schlesinger and Meadow, 1972	Studied profoundly deaf children; 2 with deaf parents 2 with hearing parents; both use signs	Bilingualism/deaf/deaf + language Bilingualism/deaf/deaf + code switch Bilingualism/deaf/deaf + oral skills Signs accelerate language acquisition Signs accelerate speech

Reference	Study	Findings
Furfey, 1974	137 adults studies for ability to communicate with hearing and deaf individuals	Post-lingual deaf or Hi/residual deaf} + communicate with hearing people
Brasel and Quigley, 1977	18 deaf students 10–19 years 4 groups: manual English intensive oral ASL average oral	Oral students often poor progress in school, later more isolated. Manual English + in 5 out of 6 syntax. Manual English + subtests of SAT. Manual English + paragraph meaning 2 years advanced over (next) oral
Moores, Weiss, and Goodwin, 1978	7 early education school evaluation for 6 years, receptive and expressive, academic achievement, cognitive functioning	Oral and manual +> oral assessment. Cognitive/academic emphasis + assessment. Parental involvement + assessment. TC = Rochester. Residual hearing not emphasized. Math not suffic. emphasized
Schlesinger, 1978	Deaf/hearing 3 Hard of hearing/hear. 1 Deaf/deaf 1	Children acquired morphemes more in accordance with perceptual salience than with frequency of morpheme in parent sign/speech input
Babb, 1979	36 children 10 yr SEE 11; half school only; others home and school	Home and school + educational measure. School only − educational measure
Bornstein, Saulnier, and Hamilton, 1980	20 unselected hearing impaired children taught signed English for 4 years	Signed English children had 3 yr acceleration compared to deaf child. Signed English child. vocabulary grew 43% that of hearing children
Maestas y Moores, 1980	Studied 7 deaf/deaf for language acquisition	Deaf/deaf = hearing/hearing milestones corroborates early codeswitching signs made on mother and on peers
Bornstein and Saulnier, 1981	Follow-up study of inflectional markers	Rate of growth slowed for deaf child. Deaf children used only half of 14 markers used by hearing children.
Norden, 1981	Longitudinal study prelingually deaf children	TC + normal adjustment. TC + harmonious development. TC + accelerated language development = normal hearing milestones. TC + access to equals, deaf children and adults +> self-esteem. TC + spontaneous development speech
Champie, 1981	Language acquisition one deaf child	Cooperation mother/teacher enables nearly normal language growth; language samples provided shows Lyssa's impressive language functions, discuss future, solve problems, use conditional

TABLE 4.2. *(continued)*

Studies	Subjects	Results
Dee, Rapin, and Ruben, 1982	Language acquisition 11 toddlers, 14–30 months	Sign learning + oral skills Sign learning + (+++ in knowledge and use of questions) Immediate acquisition of basic signs reduces parental hopelessness and impotence about communicating with hearing impaired child
Gardner and Zorfass, 1983	Language acquisition 1 severely to profoundly deaf child who started signs at 15 months	Early signs + attach meaning to sound Signing dev. first followed by speech At 3 years oral language compares to that of hearing child
Delaney, Stuckless, and Walter, 1984	10 year study-school changing from 0 to TC 116 students Pre-TC 40 Mix-TC 49 Post TC 27	Post-TC +> mix-TC +> Pre-TC Cal. Ach. T. Post-TC +> mix-TC +> Pre-TC Speechreading Post-TC +> mix-TC +> Pre-TC Mathematics Post-TC +> mix-TC +> Pre-TC Reading
Klopping, 1971	Level of language comprehension with different modality?	Comprehension total communication = 76.35% Rochester = 55% Speechreading and voice = 35.15% 33% did not understand language at any adequate level under any of the methods of communication
White and Stevenson, 1975	45 deaf students Amount of information assimilated reading, TC, manual, oral?	Reading +> Manual and TC +> Oral Bright = average = low for oral Bright +> low for TC, MC and reading
Newell, 1978	Comprehension of four short factual stories simultaneous communication = SC " interpreted = SI oral O, manual MC?	SC +> O and MC SI +> O and MC
Caccamise, Hatfield, and Brewer, 1978	Reception information NTID students which modality better? Sim. Comm. =SC " Interpret. =SI	in "oral successes" with little exposure to Signs Most students: SC +> SI +> MC speechreading with sound = fingerspelling with sound Some students MC +> SC or speechreading and sound +>SC

Study	Description	Findings
	Manual Comm. = MC English = MCE American Sign = ASL Fingerspell. = FS	or MCE +> ASL or ASL +> MCE Signs + FS + speech +> FS + speech for normal flow and transmission of information SC and MC (ASL or MCE +> English language M/SC does not hurt development oral/aural skills; may help
Basile, Martin, and Caccamise, 1978	1/3 of NTID students in need of M and SC communication!	
Ouellette and Sendelbaugh, 1982	45 Subjects with 80 db + loss given short story. Which modality better?	Written story +> MCE (not significant) Written story +> ASL (Significant)
Sullivan, 1982	Modality of communication effects of TC, Visual Aid and Pantomime on WISC-R Which greater effect on? genetic group questionable handicapped group multihandicapped group	WISC-R Genetic = 115 Total communication = 100 Visual aids = 93 Pantomime Questionably handicapped group = 109 Total communication = 98 Pantomime = 95 Visual aids Multihandicapped group = 104 Total communication = 90 Visual aids = 88 Pantomime
Grove and Rodda, 1984	118 severely/profoundly deaf. Reception of information through different modalities; which better?	Strong possibility standardization of WISC-R for deaf children is low, since administered in a variety of modes; TC used 77.2%; therefore, $(77.2 \times 100) + 22.8 \ (100\text{-}15)/100 = 96.5$ Reading +> TC +> manual +> oral Possible overload on short term memory, manual + oral may provide a more robust memory trace.

Key: + means more, better, improves; +> means better; –> means worse than next group; = means no difference between groups; – means less, worse, "disimproves" (SOURCE: From ""Total communication in perspective" by H. Schlesinger, in D. Luterman (Ed.), 1986, *Deafness in Perspective.* San Diego: College Hill Press. Reprinted by permission.)

TABLE 4.3 Total Communication for Hearing "Other" Populations

Studies	Subjects	Diagnosis	Age (Years)	Language Receptive	Language Expressive	Speech	Behavior
Schaeffer, et al., 1977	3	Autistic				TC+speech	
Wilbur, 1979	34	Autistic (5 studies)				TC+speech	−Negative behavior +Social
Konstantareas, Webster, and Oxman, 1979	4	Autistic	8–10	TC +> 0	TC +> 0		+Social +Self-care
Barrera and Sulzer-Azaroff, 1983	3	Autistic	6,7,9	TC +> 0	TC +> 0	TC+voc	−Echolalia
Acosta, 1982	4	Down's Syndrome	3–5	faster		TC+voc	+Behavioral +Integration
Lombardino, Williams, and MacDonald, 1981		Developmentally delayed				TC+voc	+Attention Motivation Dexterity Social −Negative behavior

Study	N	Population	Findings
Stremel-Campbell, Cantrell, and Hallie, 1977	9	T.M.R.	6 +speech
Vernon, Coley, and DuBois, 1980		Aphasics (4 studies)	+Linguistic rehabilitation
Ross, 1983	30	Mental retardation	TC +> 0; TC +>sign; +Memory
T. Harris, 1978		Severe handicap	+Learning; +Retention
Hobson and Duncan, 1979	9	Profound mental retardation	+Enjoyment

Key: + means more better, improve; +> means better; −> means worse than next group; − means less, worse, "disimproves"; = means no difference between groups; (SOURCE: From "Total communication in perspective" by H. Schlesinger, in D. Luterman (Ed.), 1986, *Deafness in Perspective*. San Diego: College Hill Press. Reprinted by permission.)

Signs and fingerspelling have also been helpful in teaching reading to handicapped children. Numerous clinical studies and classroom case studies have been reported that show specifically how manual language can promote the acquisition of reading skills in children with learning disabilities, mental retardation, blindness, deafness, and autism. There are lesson plans, instructional games, learning stations, and reproducible student sheets available for teachers interested in using these methods (Hafer & Wilson, 1986; Greenberg, Vernon, DuBois & McKnight, 1981).

ADULT INTEREST IN SIGN LANGUAGE

Sign language classes are popular in high schools, colleges, and universities (Wilcox, 1988). In the past, sign language was learned by hearing persons from a deaf parent or relative, a deaf co-worker, or a deaf neighbor or church member. Today many colleges and universities offer courses in sign language. Specifically, there are approximately 772 colleges and universities in the United Sates which provide courses or programs in sign language or manual communication (Cokely, 1986). The courses are taken primarily by those planning careers in teaching, social work, vocational rehabilitation, psychology, or interpreting. Many of these institutions offer advanced degrees in interpreting or sign language teaching. Harvard, New York University, American University, and others accept American Sign Language to meet the language proficiency requirement for the Ph.D. degree. Churches, YWCAs, the Red Cross, and other community service organizations also offer sign language classes.

This growing interest in sign is also seen in media coverage. It is not uncommon to see an interpreter inserted in the corner of the TV set for newscasts or religious shows. Also the presence of actress Linda Bove on "Sesame Street" and other deaf actors in soap operas, on commercials, on serials such as "Dallas," the TV drama *Love Is Never Silent,* and the movie production of *Children of a Lesser God*—all have generated public interest in learning sign language—and greatly increased its acceptance by the general public.

SIGN LANGUAGE TEACHING AND INTERPRETING

TEACHING

How is sign language instruction provided in the classroom? In the past, the teaching involved memorizing lists of signs with English word equivalents. Since 1856 there have been sign language dictionaries which present verbal descriptions of how to produce the signs, often with corresponding illustrations. Most of these signs are arranged alphabetically or grouped according to topic. Today there are at least 15 to 20 sign books from which to choose (Cokely, 1980; Frishberg, 1986).

Because of growing interest in teaching signs, the National Association of the Deaf in 1967 established a Communication Skills Program (CSP) to provide guidance to sign language teachers. Current information was made available through a series of symposia and workshops. In 1975 the CSP began a national organization of sign language teachers called the Sign Instructors Guidance Network (S.I.G.N.) to upgrade signing skills of teachers. The CSP has held annual national symposia on sign language research and teaching since 1977 (Frishberg, 1986).

Recently the teaching of sign language has been influenced by linguistic research guided by the work of William Stokoe (1960). Stokoe and his associates compiled the first dictionary of signs based on linguistic principles (Stokoe, Casterline, & Croneberg, 1965). He used a notation system of writing signs, involving a symbol of each parameter of signs, and arranged the entries according to hand shape. While his notation system is used by sign language researchers, it is not used by sign language teachers because of its complexity. Nevertheless, about 10 sign language texts have followed Stokoe's work, teaching signs through linguistic principles. Curriculi and teaching materials have been developed for ASL instruction (Baker & Cokely, 1980; Smith, 1988).

INTERPRETING

Interpreters are typically hearing persons who translate the voice of a speaker into American Sign Language or manual English for a deaf person. An interpreter may also work in reverse, translating the signs of the deaf person into voice for a hearing audience. Deaf persons may also function as intermediary interpreters assisting the hearing interpreter with clients who are deaf-blind or have minimal language skills (Frishberg, 1986). There are also oral interpreters, who mouth the words of the speaker for nonsigning deaf people.

Traditionally, most interpreters were children of deaf parents who had no formal training but acquired sign language as their first language. At a very young age they would interpret for their parents. In her novel *In This Sign,* Joanne Greenberg writes of the pressures young hearing children face when given the responsibility of interpreting at an early age in such difficult situations as with an undertaker or with a salesman.

A nonfiction account of a hearing girl who interpreted the business transactions for her deaf parents is found in Lou Ann Walker's *A Loss for Words* (Walker, 1986). Many children of deaf parents, who learned American Sign Language as their first language, will enter the field of interpreting. For example, Cokely (1981—cited in Frishberg, 1986) surveyed 160 interpreters at a national conference and found that a third of them had learned ASL from deaf parents as young children.

Colleges, universities, and community colleges have interpreter training programs; some offer certificates, others Bachelor's or Master's degrees. The programs vary greatly in quality because the field is new. Much depends on the instructor's qualifications and the availability of deaf adults in the area who can provide field experience for the students.

THE WORK OF AN INTERPRETER

Interpreters may be used in religious, vocational, educational, medical, legal, and theatrical settings, and also with people who have English language limitations or various handicaps.

Interpreters have traditionally worked for churches and other religious organizations. These have been pioneers in providing such services for deaf people. Some churches will have deaf clergy and deaf signing choirs.

Because federal legislation has mandated the integration of deaf people in the hearing world, there is an increasing need for trained interpreters in a variety of work and educational settings (Frishberg, 1986; Tucker, 1986). For example, the

Vocational Rehabilitation Act Amendment of 1965 (Public Law 89-33) authorized the employment of interpreters as part of the vocational rehabilitation expenses when a hearing-impaired client was involved. The Rehabilitation Act of 1973 prohibits discrimination against hearing-impaired people and requires accessibility in employment, education, and other health, welfare, or social services programs. This act has several sections that have strong implications about access to employment for disabled people. The 1978 amendments to the 1973 Act clarifies what accessibility means for the hearing-impaired and includes removing communication barriers by providing interpreters (DuBow et al., 1982). This landmark amendment opened many doors for deaf people while simultaneously creating a whole world of new jobs for interpreters.

Since 1975, interpreters have been needed for the younger deaf population in public elementary schools and secondary schools because of P.L. 94-142, the Education for All Handicapped Children Act of 1975. This act mainstreamed deaf students into public schools with support services such as tutoring, speech training, and interpreting. Moores (1984) quoted from the Annual Survey of Hearing-Impaired Children and Youth (1983) that educational interpreting services were being provided to more than 6,300 school-age deaf children during 1983. Since more deaf children have been mainstreamed since then, these numbers have undoubtedly increased.

Interpreting for young deaf children takes more skills than just translating what the teacher has said. It may involve some tutoring, especially at elementary and secondary levels. The interpreter often must assume multiple roles as interpreter, tutor, aide, and counselor. Since this is a relatively new area of interpreting, the responsibility of the interpreter-tutor is still being defined (Frishberg, 1986; Moores, 1984; Zawolkow & DeFiore, 1986).

Interpreting for students in rural settings may pose additional problems. For example, hearing-impaired and deaf students from rural Kentucky often have poor oral skills and use only "home signs" because they have been isolated from other deaf children. An interpreter-tutor in this region needs to be aware of such students' backgrounds and must develop strategies to work with them within public schools. In fact, to be effective, the interpreter must function much like a certified teacher of deaf children (Andrews, 1985).

Other settings for interpreters include doctors' offices, hospitals, courtroom trials, and attorneys' offices, as well as at policemen's questioning (DuBow, Goldberg, Greer, Gardner, Penn, Conlon, & Charmatz, 1984). Several states allow deaf persons to serve on juries with interpreters (Tucker, 1986). Forty-eight states have passed laws specifying that interpreters must be provided for deaf citizens in state court proceedings (Tucker, 1986).

Interpreting in the performing arts is widely done in various contexts such as TV and theatrical productions (Frishberg, 1986).

There is a specialized kind of interpreting for minority deaf populations such as those who have limited language abilities, are multiply handicapped (cerebral palsy, deaf-blindness, etc.) or use only oral methods of communication.

Deaf persons with minimal language skills are those who do not speak well, do not read or write, and are not familiar with English or with ASL. This does not mean they are not intelligent. They may have been isolated from other deaf people and thus never learned a standard communication system. They may have developed only "home signs" or gestures. Many are totally without any linguistic symbol system, oral or manual. They pose the most difficult challenge an interpreter can face. Often a deaf person will function with a hearing interpreter as an intermediary interpreter. Mime, gesture, and "acting out" scenes are used to communicate ideas.

Interpreting for deaf multi-handicapped persons requires knowledge of methods for using tactile expression and reception, controlling rate of message transmission, and other skills in dealing with specific handicaps (Frishberg, 1986). Oral interpreting, too, requires specialized skills (Frishberg, 1986).

State Commissions on Deaf exist which often provide quality assurance screening programs, evaluate interpreters, put on workshops, and act as a referral system to employ interpreters.

A national organization in this field is the Registry of Interpreters for the Deaf (RID). Founded in 1964, it has over 3,000 members, with chapters in all 50 states. Its major goals are to maintain current listings of certified interpreters, develop ethics and standards, establish evaluation procedures, promote public awareness of interpreters, formulate a code of ethics, work with national and state organizations, and make job referrals.

Inherent Difficulties

Inherent in the relationship of deaf people to interpreters is a dimension of hostile-dependence. Hostile-dependency feelings emerge when a person must depend on another for some need yet feels angry toward that person at the same time. It is difficult for any human being to be as dependent on another as a deaf person is on an interpreter. By virtue of this relationship, tremendous control and power rest with the interpreter. Inevitably, this power leads to abuse and consequent anger. There is also the tendency of the deaf person to see the interpreter as omnipotent. Then when things go wrong, the deaf person blames the interpreter, not himself or the person whose speech was interpreted.

AMERICAN SIGN LANGUAGE IN PSYCHOLOGY AND LINGUISTICS

American Sign Language has been used in psychology, linguistics, psycholinguistics, and neurolinguistics in the investigation of definitions of language, human and primate language acquisition, and human language processing. These studies have shed new light on previously held theories.

LANGUAGE THEORIES

Traditional definitions of language emphasized the importance of speech. Prior to the 1960s modern linguistics had drawn its conclusions about the nature of language exclusively from spoken language. Klima & Bellugi quote Chomsky as having said, "A language is a specific sound-meaning correspondence . . ." (Chomsky, 1967, cited in Klima & Bellugi, 1979). Chomsky later rephrased the quote to "a specific signal-meaning correspondence." This shift of language definition to include the visual-gestural language of the deaf community has significantly altered the point of view toward what is fundamental about language (Klima & Bellugi, 1979; Stokoe, 1960).

LANGUAGE ACQUISITION

For many years, because of the assumption that language could be acquired only in spoken form, it was believed that deaf children would never acquire language in a normal manner. However, studies of the acquisition of American Sign Language by deaf children of deaf parents have changed this point of view (Schlesinger & Meadow, 1972; Bonvillian et al., 1983; Newport & Meier, 1986). These studies and others show that the process of learning ASL as a first language resembles stages of acquiring spoken language by hearing infants. Further, the deaf mother–child interactions parallel hearing mother–child interactions in the linguistic nature of their rich communicative patterning. The two acquisition processes do differ in some ways, though. For example the deaf infant begins to symbolize by producing his or her first sign at about 9 months, whereas the hearing infant says the first word at about one year. One reason given is that motor development of the hands predates motor development of the speech muscles. While the content of deaf and hearing infants' words are similar (words in their environment), the deaf child does not typically acquire function words like "a," "the," or "of." Both infants, though, make use of processes such as overextension and underextension and acquire semantic and syntactic relations and combinations in similar manners. Future longitudinal studies using American Sign Language will undoubtedly contribute to the understanding of language acquisition.

Studies of American Sign Language acquired by deaf children over 5 raise questions about the existence of an optimal or critical period for language development (Vernon & Ottinger, 1986). The case in point is that many deaf children may not meet other deaf adults or gain exposure to ASL until their teens or later and yet they still are able to acquire ASL fluently. These findings cast doubts on the critical period theories, at least for a visual nonauditory language (see chapter 13).

PRIMATE STUDIES

After years of research showing that animals could not acquire a spoken vocabulary, studies have shown that primates can use signs to learn to communicate (Fouts, 1983). There is disagreement among psychologists and linguists as to whether animals are actually using a linguistic system (i.e., a language) or whether they merely have imitation abilities. Some linguists, for example, maintain that the chimps are only displaying advanced imitation skills. Regardless of these findings, it has been demonstrated on films that chimps can acquire a sign vocabulary, combine them into two-sign utterances, and use them to communicate. Besides giving some understanding of the language capabilities of chimpanzees, this research has been applied to help noncommunicating children in language intervention (Fouts, Shapiro, & O'Neil, 1978).

LANGUAGE PROCESSING

The study of sign language processing provides a way to understand the more general question of how the brain processes language. ASL has the complex organizational properties found in spoken language but with the visual-gestural modality (Bellugi, Poizner, & Klima, 1983). Hearing and speech are not necessary for the development of hemispheric specialization, as it once was believed. Generally, the left hemisphere takes care of oral language and linguistic structures whereas the right hemisphere takes care of spatial relations and motor functions. ASL has both complex language structures and complex spatial relations which, for hearing people, show a differing specialization. Because of these dual attributes, the study of the processing of ASL offers insights into the more fundamental issue of the functioning of the two brain hemispheres (Bellugi, Poizner, & Klima, 1983).

FUTURE NEEDS

American Sign Language of the deaf community has proven valuable for hearing educators, researchers, and scientists studying language behavior per se in addition to its pragmatic benefits in teaching deaf children. It is widely used in many programs for training professionals to work with deaf adults. Much of the teaching effort and material design has been for hearing adults who wish to learn ASL, not for deaf people. The rationale is, perhaps, that if more hearing adults can use it, then they will be able to communicate with deaf adults and thus make more information easily accessible to the deaf community. However, a more concentrated effort in research, teaching methods, and materials utilizing American Sign Language needs to be focused on those who need it most—deaf children and their teachers. Perhaps with the increasing knowledge of ASL linguistics among academics, this information will become more accessible and practical to educators working with deaf children.

REFERENCES

Allen, T. E., & Woodward, J. C. (1986, May). *How teachers communicate with deaf students today.* Paper presented at a seminar on sign language for deaf culture. Gallaudet Research Institute, Washington, DC.

Andrews, J. F. (1985). *Training of personnel to be interpreters for hearing-impaired children and youth in classrooms in Appalachian Kentucky.* Washington, DC: U.S. Department of Education, Office of Special Education and Rehabilitative Services.

Annual Survey of Hearing-Impaired Children and Youth. (1983). Washington, DC: Gallaudet Research Institute.

Baker, C., & Cokely, D. (1980). *American Sign Language: A teacher's resource text on grammar and culture.* Silver Spring, MD: T. J. Publishers.

Baker-Shenk, C. (1985). The facial behavior of deaf signers: Evidence of a complex language. *American Annals of the Deaf, 130*(4), 297–304.

Bellugi, U., Poizner, H., & Klima, E. S. (1983). Brain organization for language: Clues from sign aphasia. *Human Neurobiology, 2,* 155–170.

Bonvillian, J. D., Nelson, K. E., & Rhyne, J. M. (1981). Sign language and autism. *Journal of Autism and Developmental Disorders, 11*(1), 125–137.

Bonvillian, J. D., Orlansky, M. D., Novack, L. L., Folven, R. J., & Holley-Wilcox, P. (1983, June). Language, cognitive and cherological development: The first steps in language acquisition. In W. Stokoe & V. Volterra (Eds.), *Proceedings of the III. International Symposium on Sign Language Research.* Rome, Italy. Silver Spring, MD: Linstok Press.

Bornstein, A. L., Hamilton, L., Kannapell, B., Roy, H., & Saulnier, K. (1975). The signed English dictionary for preschool and elementary levels. Washington, DC, Gallaudet University Press.

Bornstein, H., & Saulnier, K. (1984). *The Signed English starter,* Washington, DC: Kendall Green Publications, Gallaudet College Press.

Bornstein, H., Saulnier, K., & Hamilton, L. (1983). *The comprehensive Signed English dictionary.* Washington, DC: Kendall Green Publications, Gallaudet College Press.

Brill, R. G. (1984). *International congresses on education of the deaf: An analytical history 1878–1980.* Washington, DC: Gallaudet College Press.

Bryen, D. N., & Joyce, D. G. (1985). Language intervention with the severely handicapped: A decade of research. *The Journal of Special Education, 19,*(1), 7–39.

Bryen, D. N., & Joyce, D. G. (1986). Sign language and the severely handicapped. *The Journal of Special Education, 20,* 183–194.

Cirrin, F. M., & Rowland, C. M. (1985). Communicative assessment of nonverbal youths with severe/profound retardation. *Mental Retardation, 23*(2), 52–62.

Cokely, D. (1980). Sign language: Teaching, interpreting and educational policy. In C. Baker and R. Battison (Eds.), *Sign language and the deaf community: Essays in honor of William C. Stokoe.* Washington, DC: Gallaudet College Press.

Cokely, D. (1981). Sign language interpreters: A demographic survey. *Sign Language Studies, 32,* 261–286.

Cokely, D. (1986). A resource list: 772 college level programs teaching sign language or manual communication. *Sign Language Studies, 50,* 78–92.

DeViveiros, C. E., & McLaughlin, T. F. (1982). Effects of manual sign on the expressive language of four hearing kindergarten children. *Sign Language Studies, 35,* 169–177.

DuBow, S., Goldberg, Geer, S., Gardner, E., Penn, A., Conlon, S., and Charmatz, M. (1984). *Legal rights of hearing-impaired people.* Washington, DC: Gallaudet University Press.

Erting, C. (1985). Sociocultural dimensions of deaf education: Belief systems and communicative interaction. *Sign Language Studies, 47,* 11–126.

Fischer, S. (1978). Sign language and creoles. In P. Siple (Ed.), *Understanding language through sign language research.* New York: Academic Press.

Fouts, R. S. (1983). Acquisition and testing of gestural signs in four young chimpanzees. *Science, 180,* 978–980.

Fouts, R. S., Shapiro, G., & O'Neil, C. (1978). Studies of linguistic behavior in apes and children. In P. Siple (Ed.), *Understanding language through sign language research.* New York: Academic Press.

Frishburg, N. (1986). *Interpreting: An introduction.* Silver Spring, MD: RID Publications.

Garcia, W. J. (Ed.) (1983). *Medical sign language.* Springfield, IL: Charles C. Thomas.

Greenburg, J. C., Vernon, M., DuBois, J., & McKnight, J. (1981). *The language arts handbook: A total communication approach.* Baltimore: University Park Press.

Griffith, P. L., & Robinson, J. H. (1980). Influence of iconicity and phonological similarity on sign learning by mentally retarded children. *American Journal of Mental Deficiency, 85*(3), 291–298.

Groce, N. (1985). *Everyone here spoke sign language.* Cambridge, MA: Harvard University Press.

Hafer, J. C., & Wilson, R. M. (1986). *Signing for reading success.* Washington, DC: Kendall Green Publications, Gallaudet College Press.

Higgins, P. C. (1980). *Outsiders in a hearing world: A sociology of deafness.* Beverly Hills, CA: Sage Publications.

Jamison, S. (1973). *Signs for computing terminology.* Silver Spring, MD: National Association of the Deaf.

Jordan, I. K., & Karchmer, M. A. (1986). Patterns of sign use among hearing impaired students. In A. Schildroth & M. Karchmer (Eds.), *Deaf children in America.* San Diego; College-Hill Press.

Jordan, K. G., Gustason, G., & Rosen, R. (1976, December). Current communication trends at programs for the deaf. *American Annals of the Deaf.* pp. 527–532.

Kannapell, B., Hamilton, L., & Bornstein, H. (1969). Signs for instructional purposes. Washington, DC: Gallaudet University Press.

Klima, E., & Bellugi, U. (1979). *The signs of language.* Cambridge, MA: Harvard University Press.

Kluwin, T. N. (1983). Discourse in deaf classrooms: The structure of teaching episodes. *Discourage Processes, 6,* 275–293.

Konstantareas, M., Hunter, D., & Sloman, L. (1985). Training a blind autistic child to communicate through signs. *Journal of Autism and Developmental Disorders, 12*(1), 1–11.

Konstantareas, M. M. (1985). Sign language as a communication prosthesis with language-impaired children. *Journal of Autism and Developmental Disorders, 12*(1), 1–11.

Lane, H. (1984). *When the mind hears.* New York: Random House.

Lane, H., & Phillip, F. (1984). *The deaf experience.* Cambridge, MA: Harvard University Press.

Meadow, K. P. (1968). Early manual communication in relation to the deaf child's intellectual, social and communication function. *American Annals of the Deaf, 113,* 29–41.

Miles, D. (1976). *Gestures: Poetry in sign language.* Northridge, CA: Joyce Motion Picture Co.

Moores, D. F. (1987). *Education of the deaf: Psychology, principles, and practices* (2nd ed.). Boston: Houghton Mifflin.

Moores, D. F. (1984). Interpreting in the public schools. *Perspectives for Teachers of the Hearing Impaired,* 13–15, Gallaudet University Symposium.

Musselwhite, C. R. (1986). Using signs as gestural cues for children with communicative impairments. *Teaching Exceptional Children, 19*(1), 32–35.

Musselwhite, C. R., & St. Louis, K. W. (1982). *Communication programming for the severely handicapped: Vocal and non-vocal strategies.* San Diego: College-Hill Press.

Nash, J. E. (1987). Who signs to whom?: The American Sign Language Community. In P. Higgins & J. Nash (Eds.), *Understanding deafness socially.* Springfield, IL: Charles C. Thomas.

Newport, E. L., & Meier, R. R. (1986). Acquisition of American Sign Language. In D. Slobin (Ed.), *The cross-linguistic study of language acquisition.* Hillsdale, NJ: Lawrence Erlbaum Associates.

Padden, C. (1980). The deaf community and the culture of deaf people. In *Sign language and the deaf community: Essays in honor of William Stokoe.* (Ed.). C. Baker and R. Battison. Silver Spring, MD: National Association of the Deaf.

Poulton, K. R., & Algozzine, B. (1980). Manual communication and mental retardation: A review of research and implications. *American Journal of Mental Deficiency, 85*(2), 124–152.

Quigley, S. P. (1968). The influence of fingerspelling on the development of language, communication and educational achievement in deaf children. Department of Special Education, University of Illinois, Champaign.

Sandager, O. K. (1985). *Sign languages around the world.* North Hollywood, CA: OK Publishing Co.

Schlesinger, H., & Meadow, K. (1972). *Sound and sign: Childhood deafness and mental health.* Berkeley: University of California Press.

Scouten, E. L. (1984). *Turning points in the education of deaf people.* Danville, IL: The Interstate Printers & Publishers.

Smith, C. (1988). Signing naturally: Notes on the development of the ASL curriculum project at Vista College. In S. Wilcox (Ed.), Academic acceptance of American Sign Language [Special issue], *Sign Language Studies, 59.*

Stokoe, W. C. (1960). *Sign language structure: An outline of visual communication systems of the American deaf.* Studies in Linguistics, Occasional Paper, Buffalo, NY.

Stokoe, W. C., Casterline, D., & Croneberg, C. (1965). *Dictionary of American Sign Language.* Washington, DC: Gallaudet College Press.

Stuckless, R., & Birch, J. W. (1966). The influence of early manual communication on linguistic development in deaf children. *American Annals of the Deaf, 3,* 452–460.

Tucker, B. P. (1986). Interpreter services: Legal rights of hearing-impaired persons. In W. Northcott, (Ed.), *Oral interpreting: Principles and practices.* Baltimore: University Park Press.

Vernon, M. (1983). A new approach to reading. *Claremont Reading Conference 47th Yearbook,* Claremont, CA.

Vernon, M., & Coley, J. D. (1978). The sign language of the deaf and reading-language development. *The Reading Teacher, 32*(3), 297–301.

Vernon, M., Coley, J., & Ottinger, P. (1979). The use of sign language in the reading-language development process. *Sign Language Studies, 22,* 89–94.

Vernon, M., & Koh, S. E. (1971). Effects of oral preschool compared to early manual communication on education and communication in deaf children. *American Annals of the Deaf, 116,* 569–574.

Vernon, M., & Ottinger, P. (1986). *Theoretical perspectives on deafness.* Working paper, Western Maryland College, Westminster.

Walker, L. A. (1986). *A loss for words: The story of deafness in a family.* New York: Harper & Row.

Wilcox, S. (1988). Academic acceptance of American Sign Language [Special issue]. *Sign Language Studies, 59.*

Wilson, R., & Hoyer, J. (1985). The use of signing as a reinforcement of sight vocabulary in the primary grades (pp. 41–43). *1985 Yearbook of the State of Maryland International Reading Association.*

Wilson, R., Teague, J., & Teague, M. (1985). The use of signing and fingerspelling to improve spelling performance with hearing children. *Reading Psychology, 4,* 267–273.

Woodward, J. C. (1978). Historical bases of American Sign Language. In R. Siple (Ed.), *Understanding language through sign language research.* New York: Academic Press.

Woodward, J. (1980). *Signs of drug use.* Silver Spring, MD: National Association of the Deaf.

Zawolkow, E. G., & DeFiore, S. (1986). Educational interpreting for elementary and secondary-level hearing-impaired students. *American Annals of the Deaf, 131*(1), 26–32.

CHAPTER 5
Other Forms
of Communication

It is luxury to be understood.   *Emerson*

The psychological effects of a hearing loss are clearest and, in some respects, most severe when the onset is early in life and when the degree of loss is profound. These effects are primarily in the area of communication. Therefore, to understand them requires a careful look at communication options deaf individuals can utilize. This chapter will examine the advantages and disadvantages of these communication options: speech; speechreading; amplification; manual systems such as Cued Speech, fingerspelling, and manual codes of English; written English; and reading.

SPEECH

INTELLIGIBILITY

For a person whose hearing deficit occurred before age 3 and whose loss is severe enough to prevent the *understanding* of speech with or without a hearing aid, it is impossible to learn to talk normally. Even after years of training, intelligible speech for conversational use is rarely acquired (Jensema, Karchmer, & Trybus, 1978). Only in extremely rare cases is it mastered by deaf people (Conrad, 1979; Freeman, Carbin, & Boese, 1980, Levine, 1980).

What is there about early onset of profound deafness that makes normal speech impossible and intelligible speech rare? Speech is not simply the imitation of isolated sounds but is a continuously changing acoustic stream produced by dynamic articulatory processes (Borden & Harris, 1984). The basic problem is that to articulate correctly, one must not only learn how to produce individual phonemes or sounds by imitation but learn how to produce them in a continuous stream of speech in contexts that are influenced and changed by their neighboring sounds. For example, say the words "kit" and "skip" and listen to how you say the sound "k." We pronounce "k" in "kit" as a voiceless stop-plosive whereas we pronounce this same sound as a voiced stop-plosive in "skip" (sgip). The phoneme "k" changes to "g" in this environment. In "kit," "k" is followed by an audible puff of air; in "skip" it is not; it sounds almost, but not quite, like a "g". This process causes us to coarticulate, or move our articulators at the same time (Borden & Harris, 1984). These speech processes—coarticulation and assimilation—are what make speech transmission a rapid and efficient system. Teaching these procedures by sight or touch to children who cannot hear is most difficult. Another example amplifies this point. Could you distinguish between the sound "g" (as in "good") from the sound "k" (as in "kit") or between the "i" (as in "hit") and the "e" (as in "bet") if you had to depend on feeling their differences kinesthetically?

Even for those who hear, the process of speech development and articulation is infinitely more difficult than is generally realized. For example, those of us who have studied a foreign language realize how difficult it was to say the words and dialogues even when we heard them perfectly. Imagine the problem of articulating them intelligibly if we had not been able to hear them. Another example that helps to illustrate the profoundly deaf person's problem in learning speech is our own difficulty with accents. Suppose a professor's accent reflects a rural Southern background. It would be far more prestigious for such a professor to have a "part Harvard—part British" accent. However, even with normal hearing to monitor his speech, the professor's accent is likely to remain "Southern." Even professionally trained actors have difficulty changing their accents when their roles require it. If it is this arduous for professional actors to control their articulation when they can hear what is being said, imagine the difficulty for the person who has never heard the sounds of speech.

Even for the normally hearing child, speech is far more difficult than we realize. It takes a child about 8 years to master fully the sounds of English (Sanders, 1972) and a French child almost 15 years to master fully the articulation of French at an adult level. Relevant to this is the fact that people who are exposed to a new language after age 8 almost never learn to speak it without an accent (Lenneberg, 1967).

The point of this extensive explanation is to give some understanding and empathy to the problem the prelingually profoundly deaf person faces. It is no wonder that none develop normal speech and that only a tiny minority develop intelligible speech. Unfortunately, almost all parents, many professionals, and the lay public assume all deaf people can learn to talk if given the chance.

PRELINGUAL DEAFNESS

With good speech and auditory training most profoundly prelingually deafened children can learn to say a limited repertory of words and phrases intelligibly (Benderly, 1980; Northcott, 1981). Some of their speech can be understood by those who are used to it—family members, close friends, and co-workers. This degree of speech competence is worthwhile. The tragedy arises from the almost universally *unrealistic expectations* for speech development. Parents are invariably told by well-intended friends about some deaf person with perfect speech skills. Inevitably, these individuals turn out to be hard-of-hearing persons or individuals who became deaf after learning to speak.

With prelingually hearing-impaired children who have enough hearing to understand some speech, the potential for speech development improves. In general, the more speech the child can hear and understand, the greater the potential for intelligible speech to develop (Conrad, 1979). Other issues enter, such as structure of the vocal mechanism, motor skills, motivation, the configuration of the audiogram, and quality of teaching. Just as there are individual aptitudes for music, mathematics, and foreign languages, there are also greatly varying aptitudes among hearing-impaired children for speech development. Just as every child who studies music cannot become a professional musician, all hearing-impaired children do not have the potential for speech.

POSTLINGUAL DEAFNESS

People who lose their hearing after acquiring speech have a much different problem, that of retaining articulatory skills already developed. In general, the older the person is when becoming deaf, the more intelligible his or her speech tends to be. For example, those deafened after age 10 usually retain fully intelligible speech, whereas those deafened at age 4 or 5 generally have speech better than congenitally deaf persons but likely not fully intelligible. In all postlingually deafened people, voice quality tends to become monotone over time, newly learned words are mispronounced, and there is a general decline in overall quality and clarity of articulation. It is important that the postlingually deafened obtain speech therapy to conserve what they have. It should be a different kind of therapy than that used with congenitally deaf children.

SOME ADDITIONAL COMMENTS

Some additional points about speech and hearing impairment need to be made. First, many brilliant, successful prelingually deaf people have little or no comprehensible speech. This is not to say that speech skills do not make success easier. They do, but their absence does not preclude success. Second, speech and language are not the same. Parrots and crows can be trained to speak intelligibly, but they do not understand the language they use. Similarly, some hearing-impaired persons who can articulate words have little or no knowledge of their meaning or the syntactical rules used to join them together. Reciprocally, some deaf persons totally unable to speak have an excellent command of language, both English and sign.

SPEECH IMPROVEMENT

An unanswered question in regard to speech development in profoundly prelingually deaf children is their rate of improvement in speech and how long this continues. For example, is it like improvement in walking, in that skills increase significantly for a few years and then remain essentially the same? This is true of many motor skills. Or does basic speech continue to improve indefinitely with appropriate help?

Although speech is taught in all programs for deaf children, there are few objective data that measure improvement or change as a function of time and instruction. One study, using a teacher-rating scale as measurement, found no significant improvement of speech intelligibility among deaf students over several years of instruction. The amount of improvement that did occur was more a function of the amount of residual hearing than of instruction (Jensema, Karchmer, & Trybus, 1978).

All deaf children should be given the opportunity to learn to speak. Progress should be assessed objectively, and as long as significant improvement occurs, instruction should be continued. Even after there has been a leveling off, some instruction is needed to maintain existing skills. The tragedy occurs either when many hours of vital school time is spent teaching speech, at the expense of other instruction, to children whose speech intelligibility has ceased to improve significantly or when persons who could benefit from speech instruction are not given it.

SPEECHREADING/LIPREADING

Periodically there will appear in the newspaper or on television a story about a deaf person who "lipreads the Queen of England from the opposite side of a Rugby field" or who "lipreads a Russian spy 100 feet away in a dimly lit restaurant." These tales are misleading. They cause the general public to perceive of speechreading (the technical term for lipreading) as being a means of receptive communication almost as effective as hearing. Such is not the case.

VISIBILITY OF SOUND FORMATION

Two-thirds of the 42 sounds (phonemes) that make up the English language either are invisible or else look just like some other sound formed on the lips (Hardy, 1970; Vernon 1972). Furthermore, among the most difficult sounds to lipread are the ones that are the most important and the most widely used, the vowels (Berger, 1972). The vowels are hard to lipread because vowel production is dependent upon several dimensions: place of major constriction within the pharyngeal-oral tube, degree of major constriction within the same tube, and the extent of major constriction at the mouth opening (Hixon, Shriberg, & Saxman, 1980). Of these, only the mouth opening dimension is easily visible to the lipreader. The remaining one-third of the 42 sounds, those visible for speechreading, must be grasped in the fleeting instant they are on the lips (Hardy, 1970; Vernon, 1972). All of this creates tremendous ambiguity for the lipreader. For example, the sentences "I love you" and "I'll have a few" are formed similarly on the lips. Needless to say, a failure to distinguish between the two statements could be disastrous.

OBSTACLES TO SPEECHREADING

The ambiguity inherent in the way the sounds of English are formed on the lips is further compounded by a multitude of other factors. Among these are the tendency of people to move their head when speaking; the presence of beards, mustaches, protruding teeth, cigarettes, other objects in the mouth; different accents; hand or newspapers covering the mouth; *ad infinitum.*

In group situations, by the time the deaf speechreader notices that one person has stopped talking, the next conversationalist may be halfway through his or her statement. In dimly lit settings, nothing can be lipread. Analogous type problems arise in school classrooms. These are compounded by teachers who talk with their backs to the class or in front of windows with glaring light that makes a shadow of their faces.

While all of these factors make speechreading hard enough for the deafened adult who already knows English, it is a nearly impossible task for a child born deaf. Such children must learn English by lipreading it. Their problem is analogous to that which you and I would face if a soundproof transparent "Flash Gordon" type globe were placed over our heads and we were then left in Africa and told to learn Swahili through lipreading. If we were also expected to learn calculus, African history, African culture, and vocational skills through speechreading in Swahili, we would then have an understanding of the problem faced by the congenitally profoundly deaf child who is dependent on speechreading as a primary means of communication in classrooms and other settings. The average deaf child understands about 5 percent of what is said through lipreading (Mindel & Vernon, 1971).

SUCCESSFUL LIPREADERS

It is ironic that as a group the best lipreaders are not deaf people who have studied it for 12 to 16 years. Research done by the Tracy Clinic (Lowell, 1957–1958) found that normally hearing college sophomores do better. There are two reasons. First, every time a hearing person talks to another hearing person, the listener is being taught to speechread by classical conditioning. In normal discourse between hearing people, two stimuli are being paired and presented simultaneously: the lip movements and the sound of the word. Thus the listener is being classically conditioned to associate these two stimuli just as the dog in Pavlov's experiments learned to salivate at the sound of the bell. This is the main reason hearing people lipread without being formally taught. No such conditioning occurs with the deaf persons: They see only the mouth movement and do not have the other stimulus (the sound of the spoken word) with which to associate the lip movement. Its absence obviously makes lipreading tremendously more difficult for the deaf person to learn.

The second reason that college sophomores as a group are better lipreaders is the fact that lip movements for about two-thirds of English sounds are invisible or homophonous, that is, they are formed in the speech mechanism where the lipreader cannot see them or else they look like some other sound. The speechreader then, has to guess at what the "missing words" are. It is easier for those fluent in English (college sophomores) to fill in these blanks than for persons who as a group lack good English language skills (congenitally profoundly deaf persons).

INADEQUACY OF SPEECHREADING

The end result for prelingually profoundly deaf people is that *speechreading is an inadequate form of communication.* It is of some use when the deaf person knows the context and the conversation is simple. For example, when one is passing a co-worker in the hall on the way to work, "Good morning" is the expected salutation. Thus it is easy to lipread. Similarly, in school programs for deaf children the youngsters have learned from experience that visitors usually ask one of three questions: "What is your name?" "How old are you?" or "Where are you from?" The speechreading task is to guess or distinguish which one of these questions was asked and respond accordingly.

It is when communication becomes more complex than these rudimentary exchanges that lipreading tends to be inadequate. A failure by the general public and by many professionals to realize this fact has created severe problems for deaf people. The following case illustrates the point.

> An obstetrician, treating a deaf couple during the wife's pregnancy, realized that the fetus faced possible blood problems due to complications of Rh factor. However, the infant was carried to term and had a natural childbirth. The pediatrician who took over was alerted to the problem. He told the mother orally, prior to discharging her and her baby from the hospital, that if the child got pale, turned yellow, or failed to eat, to be sure to bring her to him immediately. Although these complex directions were impossible to speechread, the deaf mother did not want to appear stupid or to irritate the busy pediatrician, so she nodded and smiled despite not understanding him. Soon after, the infant became lethargic, ate poorly, and eventually turned yellow. Finally, after a week the mother took the baby to the doctor, but by then

the bilirubin levels were so high that kernicturus had set in. The child was left severely cerebral palsied and mentally retarded. Now 28 years old, she has to be strapped in a wheelchair and is essentially capable of only the basic life functions of eating, breathing, and eliminating waste.

Every deaf person has tales to tell of lost jobs, altercations, school failures, business losses, and other serious problems resulting from the confusion created by dependence upon speechreading. The fact that over half of the sounds of English look like some other sound when formed on the lips is obviously at the heart of these misfortunes.

COPING BEHAVIORS

There is another dimension to the problem. Deaf people are like anybody else in that they do not wish to appear stupid or to be the object of other people's anger. If they repeatedly say "I do not understand" or "Please repeat that," hearing people find it frustrating. Because they think lipreading is easy, their only conclusion from the deaf person's failure to understand is that he is either too stupid or too indifferent to follow what is said. In either case, the speaker becomes frustrated and angry and perceives the deaf individual as incompetent.

To avoid this reaction, deaf people become experts at smiling and nodding in an understanding way, even when they have grasped nothing of what was said. More sophisticated deaf persons become masters of Rogerian therapeutic techniques, giving "hmmm's" and other neutral responses that not only falsely convey understanding but also encourage the speaker to continue talking.

For most deaf people, being put in the position of having to depend on speechreading is a no-win situation. They either have to ask for continuous repetition and face anger or depreciation, or they have to pretend to understand when they do not. Some deaf people cope by insisting that the hearing person write everything down, but this is obviously not totally satisfactory. It takes time, many people cannot write well, and others just refuse to take the time.

VARYING LIPREADING ABILITIES

As is the case with speech, skill in speechreading is not directly related to intelligence (Berger, 1972). Some exceptionally bright deaf people are poor lipreaders. Individuals vary greatly in their aptitude for speechreading. Factors such as visual acuity, age, gender, and personality structure play a role (Berger, 1972).

Speechreading is of greatest value to those who have enough residual hearing to hear and understand some speech sounds (O'Neill & Oyer, 1981). In fact, when an individual can supplement speechreading with significant amounts of residual hearing, the total amount understood increases dramatically (Berger, 1972; Jeffers & Berley, 1971). However, when auditory losses are profound, residual hearing is relatively useless as a supplement to speechreading (Frisina, 1963).

The group that finds speechreading the most frustrating and disappointing are those with sudden late onset deafness and those who become deaf gradually, starting in their later years (Kaplan, 1985; Sayre, 1980). For them, the visual, cognitive, and other changes of aging make it extremely difficult to learn to speechread. For example, the bifocal lens enables a person to see at reading distance and far away but does not give a good correction for the 3- to 6-feet distances at which most speechreading takes place. Lipreading also requires quick responses. The lip movement is present for only fleeting moments. It must be perceived and synthesized with subsequent cues at a rapid rate if speech is to be understood. This quickness of reaction is not present in most elderly persons.

AMPLIFICATION

Hearing aids have improved significantly over the last 10 to 15 years. Today they can help many hearing-impaired people understand speech and function adequately in an aural environment. Such advances represent a major service to hundreds of thousands of hearing aid users.

Difficulties arise when hearing aids are perceived as panaceas for deafness. There are many deaf people who get no benefit from amplification and others who only hear loud noise but understand no speech. Some general qualifications need to be made regarding hearing aids.

First, wearing a hearing aid is not just like wearing glasses. Glasses can correct imperfections in the lens of the eye and often deliver a perfect image to the retina. Hearing aids do not do this for the person with sensorineural deafness. They make sounds louder, but not necessarily clearer. If the auditory nerve is not functioning, regardless of how loud the sound is amplified, the hearing aid does no good. By analogy, glasses that magnify an image to a severed retina do nothing to help blind people see. When the auditory mechanism is damaged, the amplified sound of the hearing aid is usually distorted. Thus the brain gets an unclear message. As a result, for many deaf people, aids are not helpful for understanding language. The public is sometimes confused at this point; they assume that the presence of the aid means that the wearer can, with some effort, understand speech.

Hearing aids may also amplify background noises disproportionately. For example, an air conditioner that we hardly notice often sounds like a roaring ocean to a person wearing a hearing aid.

There is a potential danger from amplification, especially in infants and young children. If the level of sound is increased too much, it will damage the auditory mechanism (Macrae, 1968; Madell, 1978). This is a rarely mentioned but real danger of hearing aids.

Some deaf people wear hearing aids not because the devices enable them to hear, but because they alert others to their hearing problem. Once alerted, people sometimes speak more distinctly. By contrast, there are many who could benefit from aids but who refuse to wear them because of shame, vanity, ignorance, discomfort, or general social sensitivity. They associate hearing aids with old people and crude humor. They want no part of either.

Hearing devices are now being surgically implanted in the cochlear. Thus far these devices do not yield as good a perception of speech as hearing aids (Owens & Telleen, 1981). Cochlear implants are currently an experimental procedure, not a realistic alternative for most prelingually deaf people (Owens & Telleen, 1981).

MANUAL SYSTEMS AND CODES

In chapter 4 we discussed at length the characteristics of American Sign Language and its use with deaf people. The use of ASL is the major identifying characteristic of the deaf community (see also chapter 1).

Instead of using the sign language of the deaf community, educators have invented manual systems or codes and have combined them with spoken language. Therefore, a variety of sign languages and systems are currently used in programs for deaf children. Some of these use elements of ASL but in drastically altered ways. It is important to note that these systems are *not* languages in themselves but are systems devised to represent English visibly to deaf persons. The following sections discuss the advantages and disadvantages of each system and also contrast them with American Sign Language.

Cued Speech

Cued Speech is a manual system that uses hand cues to make English sounds or phonemes visible (Cornett, 1967). In English, Cued Speech uses eight handshapes and four hand locations near the face to supplement the lip, teeth, and tongue movements in order to eliminate the ambiguities of speechreading. For example, in the sentence, "Let's go," the phonemes that are not easily distinguished on the lips now become visible with the manual cues. (See Figure 5.1.)

This system is cumbersome for several reasons. First of all, it depends on lipreading. If you cannot lipread, then the cues have no meaning. Secondly, the person receiving the cues must face the speaker. As with the oral-only method, group discussions are virtually impossible. Another problem is that it is hard to synchronize the hand movements with the lip movements for each homophonous sound. The user must process information, make complex associations, and finally interpret them to understand what is said. Finally, learning Cued Speech is difficult enough for those who have already mastered English. For young deaf children attempting to acquire English, it can be close to impossible. Cued Speech can be advantageous as an aid in teaching articulation, or to facilitate lipreading. It is inappropriate as a manual supplement to speech in a program that uses signs and speech.

Other countries have their own variations of Cued Speech. For example, the Bagheban system does for Farsee what Cued Speech does for English.

Fingerspelling

Each of the 26 letters of the alphabet can be formed on the hand. Just as in writing, the letters can then be combined into words and sentences (see Figure 5.2). The result is a complete communication system. When combined with speech, it is known as the Rochester method in the United States and as neo-oralism in Russia (Moores, 1987).

Fingerspelling has several major benefits. First, it is isomorphic with written English, that is, a sentence fingerspelled on the hand is identical to its counterpart written on paper. Thus the deaf child who learns to communicate exclusively by fingerspelling is getting direct exposure to English syntax and vocabulary. This relationship between English and fingerspelling makes the method especially useful for persons who have later onset hearing losses.

Another advantage of fingerspelling is that each letter of the alphabet is visually clear and is distinct from all others. There is not the ambiguity pervasive in speechreading. Obviously, this is a key benefit because ambiguity and lack of clarity are overwhelming impediments to communication.

The ease with which fingerspelling can be learned adds to its appeal. The average person can master the hand alphabet in about 20 minutes. They can then communicate with a deaf person, but the process is initially extremely slow. It takes months and sometimes years of frequent exposure to fingerspelling to be able to read it and use it expressively at a fast rate. Advocates of fingerspelling claim that it can be used at between 100 and 200 words per minute, about the rate of normal speech (Scouten, 1942). Our clinical view is that 80 to 90 words per minute is more realistic for most experienced fingerspellers.

The effective reading of fingerspelling and regular print have one important factor in common. Neither involves the reading of each individual letter but instead requires the perception of groups of letters and words as they form patterns or "Gestalts." Just as the beginning reader in the first grade initially has to go letter by letter to grasp the printed words, the beginning reader of fingerspelling must also

FIGURE 5.1.   Cued speech sentence, "Let's go."

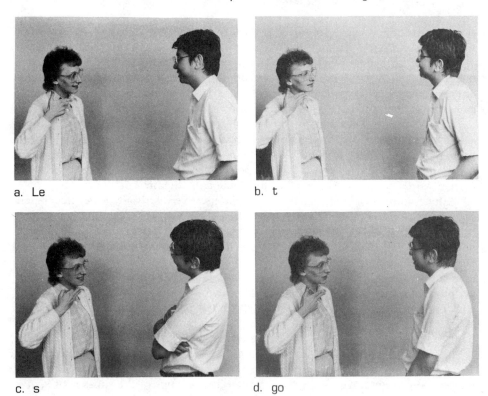

a. Le   b. t

c. s   d. go

NATIONAL ASSOCIATION OF THE DEAF

The Manual Alphabet
(as seen by the receiver)

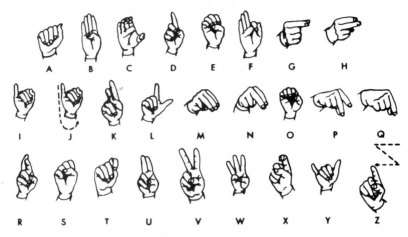

FIGURE 5.2.   The manual alphabet, in which each printed letter is represented by a separate hand position [Source: O'Rourke, T. (ed.). (1973). *A basic course in manual communication.* Silver Spring, Md.: National Association of the Deaf. Reprinted by permission.

start at this tedious pace. However, groups of letters (e.g., *ion, ing, ed, nd*), then words (e.g., *and, for, if*), and finally entire phrases are soon perceived as units.

Many hearing people who work, live next to, or have deaf relatives will learn to fingerspell. Often they do it slowly, and they usually have particular trouble understanding what is spelled to them. Despite these problems, fingerspelling can be a highly useful method of communication between deaf and hearing people. It is not unreasonable for the deaf person to expect hearing relatives, co-workers, neighbors, and others with whom interaction is frequent to take 20 minutes to learn to fingerspell. It is especially helpful as a supplement to lipreading, with the hearing person fingerspelling key words the deaf person may miss or the deaf person spelling certain words he or she is unable to pronounce intelligibly.

Along with its benefits, there are communicative disadvantages of fingerspelling. First, if the deaf person lacks competence in English, as many do, it is relatively useless. The situation is analogous to someone writing in Russian to an American who knows only English. For the deaf infant during the critical stages of language development, it is totally unsatisfactory.

The slowness of fingerspelling for most people is another disadvantage. Few people, if any, can do and read fingerspelling at conversational speeds. For those few who can, it is a tremendous strain which cannot be sustained for long. For most people, fingerspelling significantly slows down communication. This slow rate can be frustrating and may remove from the process much of its spontaneity and zest.

Finally, fingerspelling lacks the affect associated with sign language and speech. The voice qualities and facial expression of speech and the body language and facial expression of sign language carry with them the feelings of the speaker or signer. These rich dimensions of communication are diminished in fingerspelling.

Manual Codes of English

There are several manual codes of English, sometimes referred to as MCE. Examples of these contrived systems are Seeing Essential English or SEE1 (Anthony, 1971), Signing Exact English or SEE2 (Gustason, Pfetzing, & Zawalkow, 1972) and the Linguistics of Visual English or L.O.V.E. (Wampler, 1972). Another manual system is called Signed English (Bornstein, Hamilton, Kannapell, Roy, & Saulnier, 1975). The purpose of these manual codes is to give the deaf child a visible exposure to the rules of English word formation and grammar.

The photographs in Figure 5.3 through 5.6, (pages 107–111) illustrate the differences of these systems to each other and to American Sign Language. The students are demonstrating the English sentence, "Are you a good student?" in ASL, in the SEE system, and in Signed English.

These manual codes or systems are not natural languages. They are artificial systems which do several things with ASL and English. First, they borrow lexical items from ASL. For example, the signs *you* and *good* are borrowed ASL signs (see Figures 5.4, 5.5, and 5.6). Second, manual systems may also alter existing signs. For example, notice in Figure 5.3 that the sign for *yes* (typically made with a closed fist) has been altered to begin with the handshape "y." Many other signs in these systems follow this "borrowing" rule. A third difference is that manual systems invent additional signs for English morphemes, articles, and other grammatical markers which are not found in ASL. For example, Figures 5.5 and 5.6 illustrate that signs have been invented for the verb *are* and the article *a*. Signed English has 14 invented grammatical markers, and the SEE systems have over 50 invented signs for affixes. Notice again (Figure 5.5) that the suffix *-ent* has its own invented sign. Fourth, the manual systems will order their signs in English word order. Again, look at Figures 5.4–5.6 and contrast the syntax of each sentence.

The proponents of Signed English emphasize that it differs from the other manual codes or SEE systems in that it alone follows the "meanings" of ASL lexical signs. That is, the user of manual codes will follow spelling alone and disregard the

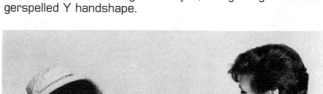

FIGURE 5.3. The sign for "yes," beginning with fingerspelled Y handshape.

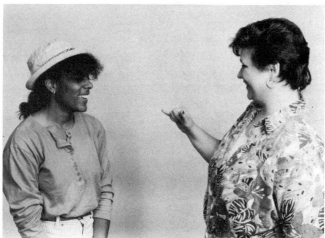

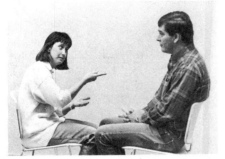

a. You

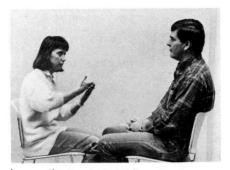

b. good

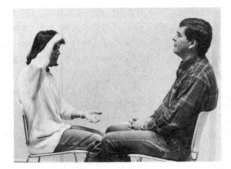

c. learn

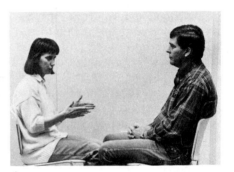

d. person

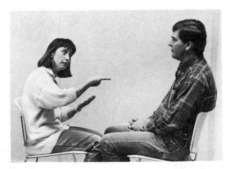

e. you

FIGURE 5.4. The sentence, "Are you a good student?" In American Sign Language (ASL)

FIGURE 5.5. The sentence, "Are you a good student?" in Signed Exact English (SEE)

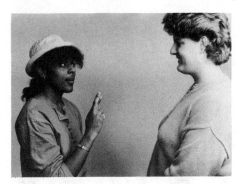

a. Are

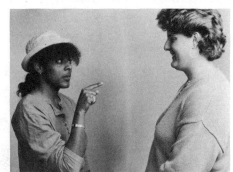

b. you

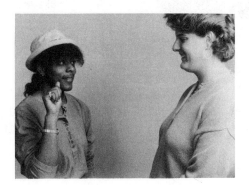

c. a

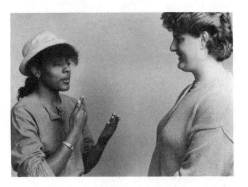

d. good

(continued)

FIGURE 5.5. (*continued*)

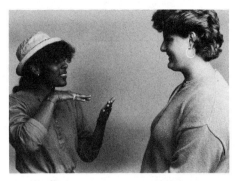

e. stud-

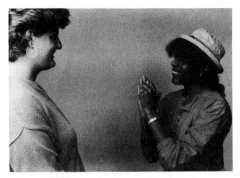

f. -ent

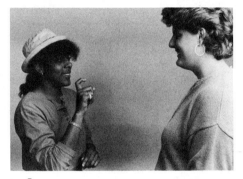

g. ?

FIGURE 5.6. The sentence, "Are you a good student?" in Signed English

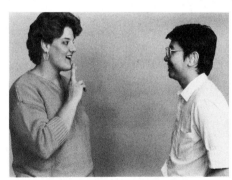

a. Are

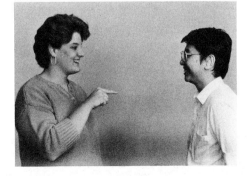

b. you

FIGURE 5.6. (*continued*)

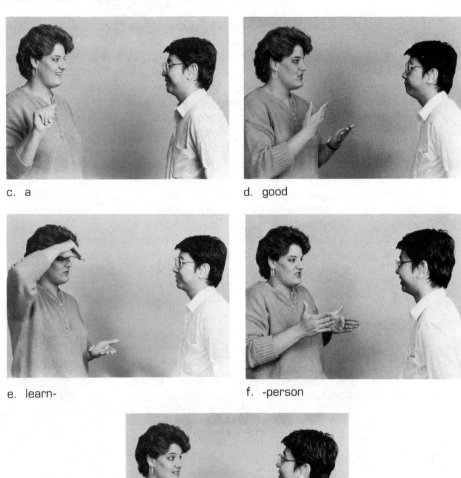

c. a

d. good

e. learn-

f. -person

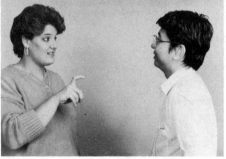

g. ?

fact that some words have multiple meanings. For example, in the phrase "run up a bill" and "run a race," both signs for *run* would be made the same in the SEE systems; in contrast, Signed English will follow the ASL lexical sign for each meaning of the phrases.

MANUAL CODES VERSUS ASL

As was mentioned above, the major advantage of all these manual codes and systems is that they make the grammatical forms of English visible to the deaf child. On the negative side, they are considered by many linguists and educators to be slow, cumbersome, and difficult to learn. They also lack the expressiveness found in American Sign Language.

Manual codes of English differ from both English and American Sign Language in significant ways (Baker, 1978; Baker & Cokely, 1980; Reagan, 1985; Vernon, 1987; Wilbur, 1979). As was mentioned, American Sign Language is a natural language whereas sign codes are only systems by which a particular spoken language can be presented visually instead of auditorally. Manual signs in ASL stand for a concept or an idea, while in the sign codes the signs stand for the words of the spoken language they are to represent. In these codes, signs are really more comparable to the written form of a spoken language than to a language in itself.

Signs in ASL took many years to evolve and are visually and gesturally easy to make. By contrast, manual codes invent signs with arbitrary hand positions and movements which are difficult to read and to form on the hands. Whereas ASL uses hands, fingers, arms, the head, facial muscles, eyes, and body movements to express lexical items and grammatical operations (Baker-Shenk, 1985), sign codes omit these nonmanual cues, thus disrupting the morphological and grammatical processes of both languages. Not only are these manual codes awkward and cumbersome for the user but, by altering the linguistic integrity of each system, the processes of acquisition and development inherent in all natural language are violated.

Total Communication

Using both signs and speech is referred to as *total communication.* This term also incorporates a theory that supports the use of all modes—visual, gestural and auditory, and written—to be made available to deaf children (Denton, 1970). Total communication has also been referred to as *bimodal* or *simultaneous communication* (Sim-Com) (i.e., when communicating with a deaf child you talk and use signs at the same time).

Educational programs will differ on the selection of a manual system to combine with speech. For example, some schools will use speech with a Pidgin Sign English, a blend of ASL and English (see chapter 4). Other programs will use a Signed English with speech or a manual code (the SEE systems). All of these systems incorporate fingerspelling. While bimodal input is widely accepted, a controversy exists in the field as to which sign language or sign system is the most effective (Vernon, 1987).

The advantage of total communication is that it opens all avenues and modes of communication for the deaf child. The child is not forced to rely on only one mode. Further, research studies have repeatedly demonstrated the beneficial effects of total communication in all areas of deaf children's development—psychosocial, linguistic, and academic achievement. (See Table 4.2.)

On the other hand, there are also some difficulties inherent in combining either ASL or an English manual system with speech in a system of communication for deaf children (Sim-Com). First, the linguistic integrity of each system is dramatically altered. English is an aural-oral language whereas Sign Language is visual-gestural in form, and there are structures in each language that cannot be adequately and completely represented in the other (Baker & Cokely, 1980). Second, teachers, parents, and children tend to use an abbreviated telegraphic or fragmented version of English in the manual code (Kluwin, 1983; Bornstein & Saulnier, 1981; Bornstein,

Saulnier, & Hamilton, 1980). The reason cited for this is that Sim-Com is cognitively demanding. It causes signers to slow down their speech and leave out many things in their signs which they are saying orally (Erting, 1985; Kluwin, 1983; Baker, 1978). Concepts, grammatical markers, and articles tend to be deleted, giving deaf children an inaccurate, incomplete representation of English (Baker, 1978; Marmour & Pettito, 1979; Reich & Bick, 1977). However, it is not as inaccurate a version of English as is that given to the deaf person dependent on lipreading alone. Future research is needed to investigate the acquisition and development of English with different populations of deaf children using the different manual systems.

WRITTEN LANGUAGE

Writing notes and letters is another avenue for communication. Unfortunately, the consequence of early profound hearing loss most difficult for professionals and the lay public to understand is its effect on English language skills. Most deaf and severely hard-of-hearing persons whose auditory loss was prelingual lack fluency in English. The language sample below illustrates the problem. It is representative of the competency in English of the lower 30 percent of persons born deaf who are 16 or older.

Deafness
My Name is Norman Sadness

I'm sorry, regret forgive me. I am answer, he said we have no money, break, no church. Patience bear endure suffer I've been very business, busy leave depart refuse, won't Mother is not well, Lydia have possess money secret hid book bank. Pocket handbags, Norman I know, watch look at, Mother he said forgive $1.60 dollar, his Norman says guess, miss I'm not always good. $1.60 dollar everyday Daily Not good $1.60 dollar, week, weekly. That's a lie. Mother Lydia have possess money pocket handbags. His Norman sadness no money no work.

The language sample below is representative of the written language competence of the average (25th to 75th percentile) prelingually deafened adult.

Good Morning

That's all right. I understand. I am answer has stopped drinking. How my life has changed! My health and mind is so much better, I also was bad drinker, but I haven't taken a drop since and haven't wanted any. thanks to God! Prayer stops drink. I want to tell you about the great help I received from your prayers, I had been drinking pretty heavily so I asked you to pray with me, so I could stop. Today I hate alcohol and I can't look at it. We have nothing to do he doesn't matter. God bless you all. Thank O.K.

To understand why this difficulty with English exists, let's return to an analogy used earlier. Let's assume that we had a transparent sound-proof "Flash Gordon" type glass globe placed over our head and we were flown to Moscow. Assume that we were told to learn Russian but that we could not use English as a frame of reference; for example, we could not use an English-to-Russian dictionary. After 20 years in Moscow under these circumstances, even with major effort, we would know very little Russian. We would have learned basic nouns, especially if they stood for concrete objects which could be shown in pictures. However, our mastery of Russian syntax would be minimal. We would be forced to learn a language we did not know primarily by trying to lipread it. Our teacher would write words in Russian for which there were pictures (dog, cat, milk, house) but would we learn terms such as love, theory, concept, imagine? Syntactical constructions such as the perfect tense, irregular verb conjunctions, the passive voice, idioms, and intransitive verbs would be tremendously difficult or impossible to master. Our exposure to Russian through lipreading would be minimal because it would require that we be specifically watching with full attention to the lip movements of a person when they were speaking.

This analogy helps to clarify the prelingually deafened person's problem mastering English. Instead of hearing it on television, from parents, from friends, from radio, *ad infinitum* almost continually during 12 to 18 waking hours a day, the deaf child hears absolutely no English. He sees it for fleeting moments on the lips but, not knowing English, he understands little if any of these mouth movements. At school he is shown pictures matched with the appropriate words to describe them (e.g., the picture of a tree and the word "tree"), and other lessons are provided. Still, observation of traditional classrooms shows that actual exposure to comprehensible English averages less than 30 minutes a day. Furthermore, other formal instruction does not begin until optimal years for learning as passed.

The understandable result is that few prelingually deaf people master English and many are unable to use it well enough to read and write effectively (Jensema & Trybus, 1978; Quigley & Paul, 1984). The problem is pervasive among deaf people. Sadly, their poor English is often misconstrued as a reflection of low intelligence (Vernon, 1976). Actually, it is a manifestation of lack of exposure to English because of not hearing it.

READING

Author Joanne Greenburg wrote a novel, *In This Sign,* a most vividly cogent and powerful statement on the human condition of deafness (see reference in chapter 1). It clearly captures and describes the difficulty deaf people have with English. Despite this, when Mrs. Greenberg lectures, people continually ask her why deaf people do not read more.

Most deaf people do not read much because they cannot. Looking at the two language samples in the above section makes this fact understandable. Lacking in English vocabulary and syntax makes reading an extremely laborious and slow process for the average deaf person. Such an individual faces a problem similar to that of a student who, after studying one or two years of college French, tries to read a French novel.

Stating the problem statistically, 30 percent of deaf students leave school functionally illiterate: at grade 2.8 or below on educational achievement tests. Sixty percent read at grade level 5.3 or below (Conrad, 1979; DiFrancesca, 1972; Furth,

1966; Hammermeister, 1971; Trybus & Karchmer, 1977; Wrightstone, Aronow, & Moskowitz, 1963). Only 5 percent achieve at 10th grade or above (Jensema & Trybus, 1978; Office of Demographic Studies, 1971).

Looked at it somewhat differently, the average deaf child gains eight months in reading achievement from age 10 until 16 (Vernon, 1972). By contrast, the average hearing student gains six years during the same time span.

The situation with prelingually hard-of-hearing persons is not as severe. However, because of the degree of language and reading problems of these individuals, a high percentage of them are closer in reading and written skills to those born deaf than to the normally hearing (Davis, 1977).

In sum, these data on reading mean that for most deaf people, reading is a severely limited means of getting knowledge. For over one-third, it is essentially an unavailable tool. The ramifications are awesome. For the prelingually hard-of-hearing, the problems tend to also be significant, but to a lesser degree. We will elaborate on the issue of literacy in the deaf population in chapter 11.

Overall, it is clear that the disability of early onset hearing impairment significantly affects communication. This limitation, in turn, affects the behavior of deaf persons in other areas of life. Careers, marriages, friends, education, self-concept, and almost all of the person's psychology is in some significant way impacted by deafness.

REFERENCES

Anthony, D. (1971). Seeing essential English (Vols. 1 and 2). Anaheim, CA: Educational Service Division, Anaheim Union School District.

Baker, C. (1978, October). How does "Sim-Com" fit into a bilingual approach to education. In F. Caccamise and D. Hicks (Eds.), *Proceedings of the Second National Symposium on Sign Language Research and Teaching,* Coronado, CA.

Baker, C., & Cokely, D. (1980). *American Sigh Language: A teacher's resource text on grammar and culture.* Silver Spring, MD: T. J. Publishers.

Baker-Shenk, C. (1985). The facial behavior of deaf signers: Evidence of a complex language. *American Annals of the Deaf, 130*(4), 297–304.

Benderly, B. L. (1980). *Dancing without music: The deaf in America.* Garden City, NY: Anchor Press/Doubleday.

Berger, K. W. (1972). *Speechreading: Principles and methods.* Baltimore: National Education Press.

Borden, G. J., & Harris, K. S. (1984). *Speech science primer: Physiology, acoustics, and perception of speech* (2nd ed.) (p. 126). Baltimore: Williams and Wilkins Publishing.

Bornstein, H., Saulnier, K., & Hamilton, L. (1980). Signed English: A first evaluation. *American Annals of the Deaf, 125,* 467–481.

Bornstein, H., & Saulnier, K. (1981). Signed English: A brief follow-up to the first evaluation. *American Annals of the Deaf, 126,* 69–72.

Bornstein, A. L., Hamilton, L., Kannapell, B., Roy, H., & Saulnier, K. (1975). The Signed English dictionary for preschool and elementary levels. Washington, DC, Gallaudet University Press.

Conrad, R. (1974). *The deaf school child.* London: Harper & Row.

Cornett, R. O. (1967). Cued speech. *American Annals of the Deaf, 112,* 3–13.

Davis, J. (1977). *Our forgotten children: Hard-of-hearing pupils in the schools.* Minneapolis: Audio Visual Library Service.

Denton, D. M. (1970). Remarks in support of a system of total communication for deaf children. In *Communication Symposium*. Frederick: Maryland School for the Deaf.

DiFrancesca, S. (1972). Academic achievement test results of a national testing program for hearing impaired students, United States, Spring 1971 (Series D, No. 9). Washington, DC: Gallaudet College, Office of Demographic Studies.

Erting, C. (1985). Sociocultural dimensions of deaf education: Belief systems and communicative interaction. *Sign Language Studies, 47,* 11–126.

Freeman, R. D., Cargin, C. F., & Boese, R. J. (1980). *Can't your child hear?* Baltimore: University Park Press.

Frisina, D. R. (1963). Speechreading. *Proceedings of the International Congress on the Education of the Deaf* (pp. 191–207).

Furth, H. (1966). A comparison of reading test norms of deaf and hearing children. *American Annals of the Deaf, 3,* 461–462.

Gustason, C., Pfetzing, D., & Zowalkow, E. (1972). *Signing exact English.* Silver Spring, MD: Modern Signs Press.

Hammermeister, F. (1971). Reading achievement in deaf adults. *American Annals of the Deaf, 116,* 25–28.

Hardy, M. (1970). Speechreading. In H. Davis & S. R. Silverman (Eds.), *Hearing and Deafness* (pp. 335–345). New York: Holt, Rinehart & Winston.

Hixon, T., Shriberg, D., & Saxman, H. (Ed.). (1980). *Introduction to communication disorders* (p. 80). Englewood Cliffs, NJ: Prentice-Hall.

Jeffers, J., & Barley, J. (1980). *Speechreading (Lipreading).* Springfield, IL: Charles C Thomas, 1971.

Jensema, C. J., Karchmer, M. A., & Trybus, R. J. (1978). The raged speech intelligibility of hearing impaired children: Basic relationships and a detail analysis (Series R, No. 6). Washington, DC: Gallaudet College, Office of Demographic Studies.

Jensema, C. J., & Trybus, R. J. (1978). Communication patterns and educational achievement of hearing impaired students. Washington, DC: Office of Demographic Studies.

Kaplan, H. (1985). Benefits and limitations of amplification and speechreading for the elderly. In H. Orlans (Ed.), *Adjustment to adult hearing loss* (pp. 85–98). San Diego: College Hill Press.

Kluwin, T. N. (1983). Discourse in deaf classrooms: The structure of teaching episodes. *Discourse Processes, 6,* 275–293.

Lenneberg, E. H. (1967). *Biological foundations of language.* New York: John Wiley & Sons.

Levine, E. S. (1980). *The ecology of early deafness.* New York: Columbia University Press.

Lowell, E. L. (1957–1958). John Tracy clinic research papers III, V, VI, & VII. Los Angeles: The John Tracy Clinic.

Macrae, J. H. (1968). Deterioration of the residual hearing of children with sensorineural deafness. *Acta Oto-Laryngologica, 66,* 33–39.

Madell, J. R. (1978). Amplification for hearing impaired children: Basic considerations. *Journal of Communication Disorders, 11,* 125–135.

Marmour, G., & Pettito, L. (1979). Simultaneous communication in the classroom: How well is English grammar represented? *Sign Language Studies, 23,* 99–136.

Mindel, E. D., & Vernon, M. (1971). *They grow in silence,* Silver Spring, MD: National Association for Deaf Press.

Moores, D. F. (1987). *Education of the deaf: Psychology, principles, and practices* (2nd ed.). Boston: Houghton Mifflin.

Northcott, W. H. (1981). Freedom through speech; Every child's right. *Volta Review, 83,* 162–181.

Office of Demographic Studies. (1971). Academic Achievement Test Results of a National Testing Program for Hearing Impaired Students in the United States. Washington, DC: Gallaudet College.

O'Neill, J. J., & Oyer, H.J. (1981). *Visual communication for the hard of hearing.* Englewood Cliffs, NJ: Prentice-Hall.

Owens, E., & Telleen, C. C. (1981). Speech perception with hearing aids and cochlear implants. *Archives of Otolaryngology, 107,* 160–163.

Quigley, S. P., & Paul, P. (1984). *Language and deafness.* San Diego: College Hill Press.

Reagan, T. (1985). The deaf as a linguistic minority: Educational consideration. *Harvard Educational Review, 55* (3), 265–277.

Reich, P., & Bick, M. (1977). How visible is visible English? *Sign Language Studies, 14,* 59–72.

Sanders, E. (1972). When are speech sounds learned? *Journal of Speech and Hearing Research, 37,* 55–63.

Sayre, J. R. (1980). *Handbook for the hearing impaired older adult.* Danville, IL: Interstate Printers & Publishers.

Scouten, E. L. (1942). *A re-evaluation of the Rochester method* (pamphlet p. 52). Rochester, NY: Alumni Association of Rochester School for the Deaf.

Trybus, R., & Karchmer, M. (1977). School achievement scores of hearing impaired children: National data on achievement status and growth patterns. *American Annals of the Deaf Directory of Programs and Services, 122,* 62–69.

Vernon, M. (1972). Mind over mouth: A rationale for total communication. *Volta Review, 74,* 529–540.

Vernon, M. (1976). Psychologic evaluation of hearing impaired children. In L. Lloyd (Ed.), *Communication, assessment, and intervention strategies* (pp. 195–223). Baltimore: University Park Press.

Vernon, M. (1987). Controversy in Sign Language *ACEHI Journal, 12,* 155–164.

Wampler, D. (1972). Linguistics of Visual English. Santa Rosa, CA: Early childhood education Department, Aurally Handicapped Program, Santa Rosa City Schools.

Wilbur, R. B. (1979). *American Sign Language and sign systems.* Baltimore: University Park Press.

Wrightstone, J., Aronow, M., & Moskowitz, S. (1963). Developing reading test norms for deaf children. *American Annals of the Deaf, 108,* 311–316.

SECTION II SUMMARY

Chapter 4 traced the development of American Sign Language both linguistically and historically. It showed how ASL was influenced by signs used in America in addition to the French influence brought from Paris by Laurent Clerc. The linguistic form and content of ASL were examined, and its significant differences from English or any other spoken languages were noted. The chapter described how sign language is used in schools for deaf children, schools for hearing children, and clinics and programs for exceptional populations. It showed how ASL evolved from originally being a language passed down from deaf parents to their hearing and deaf offspring, to the point where formal classes in sign language are now available in high schools and universities. Finally, it discussed how researchers in linguistics and psychology are using sign language to challenge current theoretical frameworks.

Chapter 5 discussed the other forms of communication that are options for deaf persons, such as speech; speechreading; amplification; manual codes or systems such as Cued Speech, fingerspelling, the SEE systems, and Signed English; writing; and reading. It emphasized that the use of signs and speech (total communication or bimodal communication) is generally accepted in most programs for deaf students because research has demonstrated its benefits for them. It pointed out the intrinsic difficulties from combining the aural-oral and the visual-gestural modalities. Finally, the advantages and disadvantages of each of the different forms were discussed, along with the attitudes of the deaf community toward these forms of communication.

REVIEW QUESTIONS

1. American Sign Language is different from spoken English in several ways. Explain.
2. How has literature such as novels, nonfiction, plays, and poetry captured the attitudes and feelings of deaf people toward American Sign Language?
3. Why is lipreading difficult for deaf persons?
4. What are the advantages and disadvantages of combining speech and sign into one communication system?

SECTION III

The Psychology of Deafness

OVERVIEW

Chapter 6 first shows how families' reactions to deafness have a permanent psychological effect on the deaf child and influence the entire emotional structure of the family. It describes the grief process parents typically go through and the coping mechanisms they adopt. The victims' reactions to deafness are dealt with in chapters 7 and 8, which cover adjustment patterns. These range from unique behavioral patterns to psychotic and nonpsychotic disturbances. There are significant differences between hearing and deaf people among the types of nonpsychotic or behavioral disorders less severe than psychosis. Many of these milder disorders are caused not by deafness, but by communication problems and societal rejection. Most psychotic disorders, on the other hand, are distributed in the deaf population in essentially the same proportion as among the hearing. It is suggested in this section that knowledge about behavioral patterns can be used to set up model services and methods of psychotherapy.

Chapter 9 shows that a psychology of deafness must take into account the attitudes of hearing people toward deaf people, because the stigma of deafness tends to permeate the deaf child's relationship with family, with educational environment, with employers, and with fellow workers. The chapter focuses on the dynamics that underlie the "authoritarian personality"—a negative personality type that is frequently found in those who have positions over deaf people. Finally, healthier attitudes towards the deaf population are suggested that help rather than hinder their education and rehabilitation.

CHAPTER 6
Psychodynamics Surrounding the Diagnosis of Deafness

The best brought-up children are those who have seen their parents as they are. Hypocrisy is not the parents' first duty.

Shaw

Intense emotional shock is the inevitable reaction of parents to the discovery that their child is deaf. The extreme depth of feeling at this traumatic time has a permanent psychological effect on the deaf child and influences the entire emotional structure of the family.

The physician, audiologist, or other professional who makes the diagnosis also has a strong, although less readily apparent, emotional reaction. Irreversible deafness represents frustration and failure to an otolaryngologist or audiologist who devotes his or her professional life to the prevention or amelioration of hearing loss (Mindel & Vernon, 1971).

In view of both the intense nature of the reactions to the discovery of deafness, and the permanent ramifications involved, a careful examination of the dynamics that underlie these responses is essential. Thus their development will be traced from the time of conception through the later life of the deaf child and his or her family.

PREGNANCY

Few pregnancies occur at the ideal time. Some are received with great joy; a significant number are unwelcome (Hubert, 1974). About 67 percent of pregnancies in married couples are unplanned and 50 percent are not wanted. This uncomfortable reality is studiously avoided in professional literature and lay discussion. However, the profoundness and complexity of feelings associated with pregnancy must be faced. They have great impact upon the later reactions of parents when their child's deafness is diagnosed.

Parental emotions during pregnancy are generally mixed. On the one hand, there is the joy associated with the great hopes and expectations envisioned for the unborn child. The expected offspring is often perceived as the agent for the fulfillment of the parents' own frustrated ambitions, an escape from disappointment, a proof of the success of the marriage, or the realization of the adult roles played by the parents.

Along with these happy expectations are negative reactions, especially in the many families where the pregnancy is unplanned. Often one spouse blames the other for the unexpected conception. Wishful fantasies that the pregnancy will terminate are not uncommon and may be associated with both conscious and unconscious efforts to interrupt the pregnancy. For example, the wife may carry heavy laundry, drink excessively, or indulge in other physical activity known to be inappropriate during gestation. Actual abortion attempts with hot salt baths, quinine, or probing of the uterus are reported in in-depth psychological interviews with mothers of newborn children.

This kind of behavior and the underlying anger toward the responsibility and physical changes represented by the conception of a child, need to be understood, along with the joys and hopes that characterize expected parenthood. Our society tends to regard the anger as abnormal, when actually such feelings are almost universal over the nine-month course of pregnancy. By contrast, positive reactions are idealized and romanticized far beyond reality. Parents, indoctrinated by versions of how euphoric they "should" feel, become guilt-ridden or sense they are abnormal when their own responses are different.

The result is that when an infant is born defective, the negative thoughts and behavior that occurred during the pregnancy are brought back in the form of conscious and unconscious feelings about the infant and the marriage itself. The child's defect is often seen as an actualization of hostile feelings held during pregnancy. Not infrequently, the defect is thought to be an actual result of real or imagined efforts to terminate the pregnancy. Guilt and a sense that the deafness is punishment for their "sinful" attitudes or poor prenatal care combine with genuine grief over the tragedy to influence pervasively parental reactions to the discovery of deafness.

FROM BIRTH TO THE DISCOVERY OF DEAFNESS

It is surprising to most people that children's deafness is rarely discovered until they are between 1 and 3 years old. The time of diagnosis varies as a function of such factors as the degree of the hearing loss, the alertness of the physician, the presence of a genetic history of deafness, the occurrence of a prenatal disease such as rubella which is known to cause deafness, or the number of other children in the family. (For example, the mother of an only child lacks a basis for comparison and is less likely to detect any difference in her child's development that might suggest deafness.) Deaf parents, on the other hand, are personally aware of the behavior indicative of deafness and may make the diagnosis as early as four months.

One reason for the delay in diagnosis is that deafness is rarely total. Almost all infants can hear a foghorn, a gunshot, pots banging, thunder, or other grossly loud sounds. They also respond to the vibrations a mother makes walking across the nursery floor, or the shadow she casts as she crosses the doorway. Consequently, parents usually see their child respond to some sort of noise or related cue and do not suspect deafness.

Even though deafness is not readily apparent during infancy, parents generally sense something is wrong. They feel a vague, peremptory uneasiness. In retrospect, many parents make such comments as, "She slept right through the vacuuming," "He took no notice when I spoke," "Mary never paid attention," "Sounds never startled Jeff," all of which reflect an awareness that their child's behavior was different. Parents who relate these observations to deafness facilitate an early diagnosis. Many parents, however, ignore or deny such implications, interpreting them as signs of the child's placidity or stubbornness. Outsiders are frequently the first to identify the deafness and may bring it to the parents' attention. Even then there is a reluctance to take the possibility seriously. This kind of delayed awareness of deafness can be the first manifestation of unconscious denial, a symptom we will see much more of later.

There is, in the deaf child, a marked absence of responsiveness to sounds in general, to the mother's voice, and thus to many aspects of the intimate mother-child relationship. This absence is felt by her, at least on the intuitive or preconscious level. It affects the mother-child interaction by robbing the relationship of some of its warmth and affective interchange. Further, at a linguistics level, it disrupts the reciprocal interaction so important for the development of pragmatic behaviors (Irwin, 1982).

With the passage of time, the parents' anxiety about the undiagnosed deafness increases and their hopes are dimmed because of lack of responsiveness and a developmental slowness. Initial concerns tend to be, "Is our child backward?" "He doesn't talk—do you think he is retarded?" "Why is he so hard to manage?" or "Why doesn't he pay attention?" instead of "Is he deaf?" One parent, usually the mother, will often try to protect the other by concealing the suspected deafness.

The following experiences of Mary Jane Rhodes, mother of a deaf child and advocate of better services for deaf people, cogently illustrates what parents go through in discovering that their child is deaf.

> "My son Ronnie was jumping and yelling as he looked out the window with his back toward me. I called him but he didn't hear. When I reached his bed I was shouting and still he didn't respond. When he saw me, he held out his arms. I realized that my perfect, beautiful, happy, and healthy baby was deaf. He was alert since he used his eyes to see what he could not hear. He could not hear his own voice so he yelled instead of cooing. He slept on when the telephone rang or the radio played.
>
> "Neither our pediatrician nor family doctor nor the ear, nose, and throat doctor had any understanding of deafness or could give me any counseling. We had to wait three months for an audiologist appointment which was 170 miles away.
>
> "Advice from well-meaning relatives and friends was confusing. Some thought he was just late responding to sound or that he was a genius late in talking. I devised methods to test his hearing like sneaking up and popping paper bags and shouting, or turning the radio on loud. Ronnie would respond just enough to confuse me.
>
> "I can't remember much of the audiologist interview except that he told us, 'Your son is deaf. He has a nerve loss and no operation or hearing aid will make him hear. With proper training he can be taught speech and speechreading. Deafness is an educational handicap so he must be enrolled in the state school for the deaf.' Because Ronnie was only 2 years old, this was unacceptable to me. I was shocked and saddened but got some comfort as I had met an expert who understood my handicap.
>
> "My husband and I were totally unprepared. I had never known a deaf person. As a young girl, upon seeing deaf people on the streets, I remember asking my mother what these people were doing. She had answered, 'They are deaf and dumb, stop staring at them.' Would my son too become an object of people's curiosity?"

Mrs. Rhodes' reactions and experiences arouse empathy and provide a perspective of what parents experience when they discover that their child is deaf. The almost unbelievable problems they face in attempting to get a diagnosis need to be carefully examined.

SEEKING DIAGNOSIS

FAILURE TO MAKE DIAGNOSIS

The first step, that of parents' sensing that something is wrong with their child, is eventually followed by a visit to a physician. The frequent delay in this follow-up may be an attempt to avoid unpleasantness, that is, to avoid reality. Regardless, when the decision to see the doctor is finally made, questions such as why the child does not talk, whether he is slow, or whether he is deaf are generally foremost in the parents' mind.

Unfortunately, most of these expressions to the physician are also rather common manifestations of the anxieties of mothers of normal children. Therefore, they are usually passed off by the physician with clichés such as, "He will grow out of it," "Everything is fine, now don't you worry," "Give him time," "You are just an overanxious mother." While these responses may temporarily allay concern, albeit falsely, they soon arouse increasing frustration, confusion, and anxiety in the family. The parents realize that something is drastically wrong, yet their communication with the doctor about this concern is essentially ignored and they are often given untrue information.

Physicians who stamp their feet behind the child's back, drop books on the floor, or perform other crude tests that vibrate the entire room are a cause of special concern. Naturally, the child responds to the vibrations even when he hears nothing. The result is a false impression that the child can hear.

This failure to make the diagnosis has two serious impacts. First, it delays habilitation past the period which some believe is crucial in the psychological and educational development of the child. Second, the confusion, anxiety, fear, anger, and guilt feelings aroused in the parents cannot be constructively channeled toward the resolution of the child's problem because the family does not know what the problem is, much less how to cope with it. Consequently, these feelings may be expressed in pathologically destructive ways.

MISDIAGNOSIS

While a failure to detect deafness is bad enough, far worse are the misdiagnoses experienced by one-third of the parents of deaf children (Grinker, 1969; Sullivan & Vernon, 1979). Misdiagnosis grows out of the complex problem of making a differentiation between retardation, brain damage, aphasia, delayed speech, autism, childhood schizophrenia, and deafness. For example, in the first author's practice, over 50 persons in various institutions for the mentally retarded have been found who were of average or above intelligence (Sullivan & Vernon, 1979; Vernon & Kilcullen, 1972).

One of these was the daughter of an ophthalmologist; starting at age 2, she spent six years in a hospital for the retarded. When correctly tested, she was found to have an IQ of 113. Despite her tragic early institutionalization, she was able, when placed in an educational program for deaf children, to graduate from high school, junior college, and an art institute. In another case in the same hospital, the son of a Naval officer spent three years there. Later he was transferred to a school for the deaf and eventually he entered a university. A deaf graduate student at Western Maryland College has a similar history of early hospitalization as a mental retardate. Unfortunately, such extreme cases of misdiagnosis are not rare.

The grossest of these errors usually occur in deaf children who also have cerebral palsy, have vestibular pathology, or are in some other way multiply handicapped. While this type of complication may make the errors more understandable, it also makes them more destructive because they compound the difficulties of a child already multiply handicapped. For example, the deaf graduate student cited above had a mild case of cerebral palsy. Yet he had an IQ of 131, which should have precluded any confusion about retardation.

It is wrong to imply that all or even most cases of misdiagnosis or failure to make an early diagnosis of deafness occur with multiply-handicapped deaf children. Remember that approximately one-third of all parents of deaf children are initially given a diagnosis other than deafness (Sullivan & Vernon, 1979; and Vernon & Kilcullen, 1972). Although physicians are often at fault, some of the most extreme errors are made by psychologists who give verbal IQ tests to nonverbal children— an unpardonable mistake. The three cases cited above were all hospitalized as a result of this type of error in psychological evaluation.

A major point to make from the issue of misdiagnosis is that delayed speech or apparent failure to respond to sound should never be ignored, nor should it be "diagnosed" as autism, retardation, or anything else until hearing has been thoroughly tested audiologically.

DIAGNOSIS

By the time deafness is finally diagnosed, the child is usually in his or her second or third year. For some parents the finding of deafness results in an initial feeling of relief because they had been led to believe that the child was brain damaged, aphasic, mentally retarded, or suffering from some other problem considered more devastating than deafness.

To most parents, the discovery of deafness is a devastating emotional shock, the full depth of which is rarely sensed by the professional making the diagnosis. The anguished statement of a mother, "After being told Jimmy was deaf I do not remember a thing the doctor said," illustrates the powerful impact of the diagnosis. Mrs.Rhodes' case history shows that even when the deafness has been identified at home, the finality of the professional's verification is a blow of such intensity that little of what is said immediately thereafter is remembered. This is an important point because the diagnostician often goes into detail about long-range rehabilitation while all the parents can assimilate at the moment is what they can do immediately.

COPING WITH IRREVERSIBLE PHYSICAL DISABILITY

One can be helped to understand parents' reactions at learning about their child's deafness by research that has been conducted on families who have children with other serious irreversible disabilities. This research yields several general principles crucial to the professional whose duties involve making and communicating to parents the diagnosis of their child's deafness (Gardner, 1969; McKegney & Lange, 1971; Stein, Murdaugh, & MacLeod, 1969).

FULL REALIZATION

The first of these principles is that constructive and effective coping with permanent disability begins only after the patient and family are fully aware of the irreversibility of the condition and of the full range of its effects (Mindel & Vernon, 1971; Vash, 1981). Patients and families do not adjust to the reality of deafness or the resulting new life-circumstance if hope is extended for a possible cure or if indication is given that the ramifications of the disability can be directly overcome (i.e., speech and speechreading will eliminate the communication problems of deafness). The principle is well illustrated in blindness. As long as a blind person continues to expect his sight to return, he sits, waits, and does nothing (Cholden, 1958). Rehabilitation never begins. Once the permanence of the loss of sight is accepted, the blind patient usually seeks an earnest, constructive means of coping with the disability; for example, he learns braille, enrolls in a travel training course, and utilizes talking books (Kirtley, 1975).

Effective adaptations become possible in the families of deaf children only when the parents are helped to realize what changes are entailed in the family life-circumstance by their adjustment to deafness. The generalization that rehabilitation will not begin until the irreversibility and full implications of the handicap are communicated to the patient holds true across disability groups and is a fundamental premise upon which constructive education and rehabilitation programs must be based. It places tremendous responsibility upon the person who informs parents that their child is deaf, a responsibility that has historically been handled in a way diametrically opposite the manner in which it should be handled.

COPING MECHANISMS

The second principle derived from research on responses to irreversible disability is that certain defenses or coping procedures are almost universal (Mindel & Vernon, 1971; Vash, 1981). The initial feelings of severe shock may last for weeks or even years. They are of such intensity as to require that the parents of handicapped children "defend" or protect themselves; otherwise psychological survival would be impossible. These defenses, more accurately referred to as *coping mechanisms,* take several forms.

Denial

Denial is a universal initial response to severe trauma and by far the most important of all reactions to deafness. It is a way by which one initially protects oneself, maintains hope, emphasizes the favorable, and minimizes the unfavorable during any time of trauma, including the finding that a child is deaf. To understand the process, let us examine how it functions in several disease and life situations.

Parents of leukemic children, when first informed that their child has the dread disease, experience a more devastating shock than they can confront immediately (Grinker, 1969; Vernon, 1971). Hence the initial response is to deny the illness. The denial may go on for a few days, a week, or many years. This initial denial gives the parents a chance to mobilize their energies and pull themselves together. Without this early fending off of the shock, more serious problems would probably arise.

Denial has been used on occasion by everyone. The loss of a parent is an example. When first informed of such a tragedy, the almost reflexive response is, "This cannot be true." Following the initial denial, most persons accept the tragedy and go through a period of mourning during which the death is integrated as a reality and adjustments are made to accommodate the loss.

Denial is further illustrated by patients requiring kidney dialysis, the treatment by a machine that takes over the function of their damaged kidneys (McKegney & Lange, 1971). Often the first response of patients who are informed of their need for this sort of treatment is, "This can't happen to me." The patients frequently deny the fact that their life will be dominated by chronic infections, hypertension, skin changes, peripheral neuropathy, organic brain dysfunction, anemia, secondary hyperparathyroidism, and the other problems which they see in fellow patients undergoing dialysis.

Another example of denial is the woman who ignores a lump on her breast (Vernon, 1971). Frequently there is a delay of some six months before she goes to the doctor, but eventually the psychologically stable woman deals with the problem by seeking appropriate medical treatment.

The point of these illustrations is that denial is a normal initial reaction to an emotional shock. It is even a healthy response, but it has to be followed by an acknowledgment of the reality of the disability and a period of mourning. When a parent dies, when a child is found to have a terminal illness, mourning and grief are a painful but integral part of what must occur. Failure to feel and express these painful experiences openly has serious, pathological consequences (Schultz, 1978). For example, most of us know someone who lost a husband or a parent and yet showed no visible grief. The person carried on as though nothing had happened. When a denial reaction of this kind takes place, rather than a period of intense mourning and grief, the result is chronic repressed grief that is not consciously acknowledged and resolved. Such repression of grief is psychologically immobilizing and prevents a constructive handling of the problem. So important is the expression of grief that a primary complaint of concentration camp victims was that they "were not permitted to mourn their dead" (Siller, 1969).

With deafness, the less intimate the relationship to the deaf child, the greater the tendency to deny. Thus, close relatives deny more than parents. The mother who tends to be with the child all day is generally less denying than the father. In fact, fathers often escape from the environment of deafness and its implications by spending more time away from the home. Such behavior makes denial easier and contributes directly to the father's failure to face the implications of deafness in his child, and thus he avoids fulfilling a basic paternal responsibility. The end result is often serious marital conflict (Vernon, 1971).

Women tend to be more accepting of disability in other human beings than men (English, 1971). Part of this acceptance grows out of the culturally induced psychological need in men to be "strong" and to deny "weakness." A deaf person, especially one's own son, may symbolize to the male the weakness he struggles desperately to overcome and deny. Thus, authoritarian mechanisms are triggered (see chapter 9). In addition, the mother's continual contact with the child lessens her tendency to deny the deafness.

Guilt

The following transcription from a group psychotherapy session illustrates the relationship of guilt to the discovery of a child's deafness:

> The problem wasn't that he was deaf that bothered me. The problem was that I did it. Something I did while I was pregnant caused this brain defect, or maybe he had an ear infection when he was very small and I didn't realize it. I have horrible thoughts about what a terrible mother I am. I'd forgotten how I felt. I needed something to handle the guilt.

Guilt is an inevitable part of every parent's reaction to having a deaf child. "What did I do?" or "What is wrong with me?" are predominant sentiments voiced by these parents (Grinker, 1969).

It is normal for the parent who gives birth to a defective child to feel she caused the handicap. Compounding the problem are the aforementioned hostile fantasies parents may have had about the fetus and any attempts at abortion that may have occurred (Gardner, 1969). Fundamentalist beliefs about "the sins of the father being visited upon the sons" may contribute even further to the guilt felt by those with such religious convictions.

Thus, almost all parents having deaf children experience varying degrees of guilt. Guilt has such pervasive pathological effects on human behavior that its presence must be recognized and resolved if family and personal pathology is to be avoided.

Seeking of Many Opinions or Cures

It is appropriate to obtain more than one diagnosis from qualified specialists to verify a child's deafness and the prognosis for the restoration of hearing. However, "doctor shopping," consultation with an endless series of clinics, professionals, and quacks over an extended period of years, is a frantic effort to deny reality. The widespread prevalence of "healing cloths," "finger surgery" for nerve deafness, acupuncture, "miracle" electronic devices, and a host of similar frauds perpetrated upon deaf children and their parents bears tragic testimony to the vulnerability of these families to such quackery (Vernon, 1971). It has been established that parents of deaf children "doctor shop" more and are more susceptible to the false hopes generated by rumors and magazine articles than are families of other handicapped youth. (Hefferman, 1955).

The ultimate tragedy is that in addition to wasting the limited family financial and emotional resources, the continued false expectation for cures impedes constructive activities that could help in adjusting to deafness.

Feelings of Impotence

The parents of a deaf child want more than anything else to be able to help. Yet they do not know what to do. Rarely have they had extensive direct exposure to deafness prior to their child's birth. The tremendous anxiety they feel leaves them open to practically any suggestion whose implementation will enable them to mobilize this anxiety into channels they are led to believe will be beneficial. Unfortunately, during this period of susceptibility, parents are commonly given counseling that leads them into inappropriate and unrealistic aspirations and into endeavors that end in frustration. Were they not so desperately desirous of helping their child, they would not be so vulnerable.

Questioning the Reason for the Deafness

Understandably, most parents want to know why their child is deaf. They feel some responsibility and blame related, in some cases, to their past ambivalence about pregnancy, parenthood, and the child (Vernon, 1971). To some extent, searching for a reason is a defense against the concept that the child was meaninglessly struck by chance, a defense against the notion that in the lottery of life, probability should decree that their infant was to be among the 6 in 10,000 school-age children who are deaf.

At a conscious level all parents seem to want to know the cause of deafness. However, sometimes the actual discovery is too threatening to pursue, as is indicated in the following statement of a mother during psychotherapy:

> I think I blame myself for E. J.'s deafness and he blames himself. I'm sure that's what it is. It's something we don't discuss. Now it's too close to the heart of things. And it's too close to what the marriage is and to what everything else is and therefore it is not discussable. I've never discussed it—it shakes him up. And it's not . . . well, because there isn't any blame to be placed. I've gotten to that point now. It isn't his fault and it isn't mine. It's simply that we have two deaf children. And I can't look and say, "It's your fault because you did it," because I can't guarantee it.

Isolation of Affect

Initially, the deafness may be accepted as factual at an intellectual level, but not emotionally. In some cases, such acceptance is evidenced by excessive interest in the medical and technical minutiae of deafness and its treatment without any recognition or expression of the repressed feelings of trauma and loss that are present at an unconscious level. As was indicated earlier, when the discovery of deafness does not result in a period of depression, it is a matter of concern. A denial of these feelings of deep sadness is a failure psychologically to face reality. It results in chronic repressed grief.

Turning to Religion

Religion can be a source of understanding and support, especially when devoutness is part of deep, longstanding religious beliefs. However, it can also be an unhealthy reaction involving efforts to seek a miracle cure and an escape from reality, rather than a realistic adjustment to deafness.

Blaming the Doctor

It is common to attribute to physicians powers beyond those of medicine (Mindel & Vernon, 1971). Then when something goes wrong, such as the appearance of an auditory lesion, the doctor tends to be held responsible. He then becomes the object of displaced anger, bitterness, disappointment, despair, and helpless frustration. Obviously this reaction is unfair to the doctor and serves no constructive purpose other than as a release of pent-up feelings.

However, in the one-third of the cases of childhood deafness where there was an initial misdiagnosis and in the numerous other instances where there has been insensitivity to parental feelings and an ignorance about deafness, parent anger with the physician or other professional is an understandable and justifiable reaction.

Blaming the Other Parent

All married people at one time or another blame each other for disappointments in their relationship. The birth of a deaf child is no exception. Often blame takes the form of bringing up the name of a relative who may have had a hearing loss, implying that the cause is a genetic trait passed on from "that hard-of-hearing cousin of yours," or some more general statement about the inferiority of one spouse's family. In more extreme cases, blame may be expressed with the vehemence illustrated by the following quotations from psychotherapy sessions:

> FIRST MOTHER (quoting her husband): "I never wanted this baby. I told you to get an abortion. It's all your fault for having her.
>
> SECOND MOTHER: I never felt—maybe it was his fault—that he did it. Really, it was me, because I felt that, well, I flew in an airplane when I was pregnant. I did this, look what I've done. I've condemned my child to life of not hearing . . . It's all me. Later we found out that it's a recessive gene that both of us carry, so really, it's the fault of neither of us.
>
> THIRD MOTHER: Look, he was our firstborn son. I wasn't going to stare my husband right in the eye and say, "Look, your kid's deaf." I wasn't about to. He discovered it all by himself; he went into the bedroom and E. J. was standing looking out the window and he called to him and he called to him and he screamed and E. J. never turned around. Jeff came back in and he said, "I know what's wrong." But I had to do it that way.

Increased Motor Activity

The anxiety that accompanies finding that one has a deaf child is often expressed by excessive smoking, overeating, walking, insomnia, and other physical efforts to reduce tension. Within reason, a number of these reactions are normal ways to cope with the anxiety initially (Visotsky, Hamburg, Goss, & Lebovits, 1961).

Fears for the Future

Soon after the fact of deafness is accepted, some parents begin to wonder about the future. Their concerns are reflected in questions such as "Can deaf people work," "Do they marry?" "What will happen to the child when we are gone?" "Are the deaf retarded?" and "What about education?" These are legitimate questions about which there is relevant information (see chapter 1). However, physicians, audiologists, and professionals in the field of deafness are rarely qualified to respond to them accurately (Mindel & Vernon, 1971).

Other parents are so concerned with "will he speak" or "will he go to regular public school" that they fail to project the future at all. In these cases important issues and the total child are blocked out as part of an obsession to deny the implications of the hearing loss.

Complete Overt Rejection

With extremely narcissistic, insecure persons, a deaf child represents such a severe injury to the ego that the child cannot be tolerated. For example, one father whose adopted boy was found to be deaf at age 3 insisted that his wife give up the son even though he had accepted the child until the diagnosis. His wife's final refusal was a major factor in a divorce shortly thereafter.

Pregnancy

Many couples are somewhat hesitant to conceive additional children until they find the cause of their child's hearing loss. However, a significant number conceive again almost immediately after discovering their child's deafness (Hefferman, 1955). Depending on the individual situation, this may be an effort "to prove there is nothing wrong with us," to ensure a nonhandicapped offspring, or to meet other, more subtle psychological needs, both healthy and pathological.

Reading Medical Literature

Some parents direct their intense desires to do something for their child toward the avid reading of medical and other professional literature. Doing this can be constructive; it enables the parents to understand the problem and its implications. In a few cases, however, the reading involves quack literature on so-called miracle cures of deafness or in other ways represents an effort to deny or evade the deafness, the child, and his needs.

Reaction Formation

Occasionally, the discovery of deafness results in statements such as, "I'm glad he is deaf," or "We are lucky to have a deaf child," or something to the effect that deafness was a heavenly blessing. Well-meaning relatives and friends frequently offer this line of thinking. Some of the more radical interpretations of "the Deaf Pride Movement" are similar reflections of reaction formation.

Deafness is the loss of an important sensory modality. It is most constructively faced through a realistic awareness of this fact and an appropriate reaction. Pollyanna-like, euphoric perceptions are a form of whistling in the dark which thinly veil true feelings and stand in the way of rehabilitation.

Grief and Depression

Grief and depression are healthy, normal responses to the reality of deafness. Initially, a mother may say, "I cannot look at my child without crying." It is only when depression continues as a chronic reaction or reaches a psychotic degree of intensity that it becomes pathological.

OVERVIEW OF PARENTAL REACTIONS TO THE DIAGNOSIS OF DEAFNESS

The reactions of parents to the discovery that their child is deaf have much in common with the reactions of all human beings to the psychological trauma of facing any serious irreversible disease or other life tragedy. There is initial shock and disbelief. Denial insulates against the emotional impact of the situation but is soon followed by a developing awareness of loss. Grief and depression are experienced. Then comes the phase of mourning which is preparation for the eventual facing of reality and adaptively coping with the life circumstances.

The problem in deafness is that many parents never progress through these stages. Others do so at a time so late in their child's life that permanent social, psychological, and educational damage is done. Some never get past the stage of "How could this happen to me?" to the realization that it did not happen to them, but to their child. The fault rests, in large part, with inappropriate counseling, educational, and rehabilitative procedures.

THE PROFESSIONAL'S REACTION
TO THE DIAGNOSIS OF DEAFNESS

It was briefly mentioned at the beginning of this chapter that the professional person making the diagnosis of irreversible deafness has a strong emotional reaction to this trauma. While it is not as intense as the parents' feelings, it cannot be minimized if the total process occurring at the time of diagnosis is to be understood (Mindel & Vernon, 1971).

FACTORS LEADING TO MISINFORMATION AND DENIAL

First, it is usually a physician or an audiologist who makes the diagnosis. These professionals have extensive knowledge of the auditory mechanism. Unfortunately, this is generally all they know about deafness (Nagel, 1962; Vernon, 1980). Parents, not realizing this limitation, expect advice on social, educational, and psychological issues related to hearing loss. Surprisingly, a degree in medicine or audiology (even the specialty of otolaryngology) requires no clinical contact with profoundly deaf children and adults (Mindel & Vernon, 1971). Very few of these specialists know sign language or have any knowledge of how deaf people cope outside a clinic; yet such experience is obviously mandatory if a person is to counsel parents effectively about the implications of deafness. There is more to deafness than the ear. Professionals are long overdue in recognizing this fact.

Another factor to be considered is the psychological significance of deafness to the professional. A person whose entire career is committed to the restoration and facilitation of hearing tends to be understandably threatened by irreversible deafness, because it symbolizes failure in his or her professional endeavor. In many cases, the choice of otolaryngology or audiology as a career field reflects the tremendous value one places on hearing.

Given these psychological needs and values, plus a lack of information about the psycho-socio-educational implications of deafness, the professional generally fails parents at their time of greatest need. He does not have the facts or experience needed to help parents regarding the behavioral consequences of deafness, nor does he want to face fully the failure that irreversible deafness represents to him. Thus he is rarely qualified to cope with the parents' feelings at this time of crisis.

In failing to communicate to parents the full meaning of deafness, he simultaneously participates in a denial and tends to provide the inappropriate information.

Most commonly, he does this by extending false hopes to parents out of misguided kindness and lack of knowledge. Unrealistic expectations for hearing aids and oral communication are offered instead of a frank, honest sharing of feelings and objective information.

AUTHORITARIANISM

In addition to facilitating denial, the professional may be triggered into attitudes of authoritarianism or omnipotence by the feelings deafness arouses in him (see chapter 9). Therefore, instead of giving parents assistance and self-enhancement, he may berate and demean them. Some of these dynamics are illustrated in the following mother's statement:

> I would say that the experts cannot accept hearing loss. They are always accusing parents of not being able to accept hearing loss. The experts—if they can take a child and make him look normal, then this is their glory. This is their thrill to be able to make a child seem normal.

Such parental judgments of professionals may seem harsh. However, they are based on clinical and research findings on deafness and taken from the experiences of hundreds of parents during years of clinical practice (Grinker, 1969; Mindel & Vernon, 1971; Vernon, 1971).

SERVICE DELIVERY

In no way are the comments above intended to malign the many physicians and audiologists who, by virtue of their own deep professional commitment, have developed an understanding of deafness necessary for the enlightenment of and counseling with parents. Nor are they intended to blame other professionals for deficiencies in their training or for lack of insight for which they are not fully responsible. In the final analysis, it is the medical schools and universities preparing professionals who work with deaf people that must assume the major share of blame.

The point to be made is that the delivery of the total services parents needs at the time they discover their child's deafness is grossly deficient. As a result, permanent psychological damage is done to them and to their deaf child. Full rehabilitative services are needed that meet the medical, psychological, and audiological aspects of the problem faced by the parents and child. These services cannot be obtained unless clinics, hospitals, and relevant professions provide them in a coordinated package instead of depending upon parents to piece needed services together on their own.

COUNSELING AND SELF-HELP GROUPS

It has been shown by actual experience in deafness as well as by research in other areas of rehabilitation that self-help groups represent the most effective therapeutic approach (Vernon, 1970; Vash, 1981). For example, Synanon, an organized rehabilitation program for drug addicts utilizing ex-addicts as therapists, was initially far more successful at curing persons with this problem than expensive, long-term individual psychiatric therapy. Alcoholics Anonymous and disabled veterans' counseling groups in hospitals also demonstrate the basic principle that people who share a common problem are often the ones who can help each other most effectively.

Parents, when they first learn that their child is deaf, should have available group counseling with others who also have deaf children. The need and benefits of discussing feelings in this kind of shared environment are crucial to constructive coping with a deaf child.

Yet when parent groups are formed, two important errors are commonly made. First, most of the participants are parents of young, recently diagnosed deaf children. These parents lack the experience and knowledge that parents of older deaf children would have. This is somewhat like Alcoholics Anonymous grouping all new alcoholics together and excluding those who had already gone through rehabilitation. It is unfortunate that much group work with parents of deaf children has involved this blatant error. The mistake is especially common with those advocating an oral only approach. Parents of older deaf children and deaf adults tend to be more aware of the reality of deafness and the limitations of oralism. Thus, instead of including these parents as regular participants in the groups, the usual procedure is to invite only a select few who can be depended upon to give favorable "testimonials" for oralism.

A second mistake often made by parent groups grows out of the same basic motivation, of opposition to total communication (use of signs and speech). The intent is to prevent parental awareness of choices other than oralism only. This error is to exclude deaf parents of deaf children. For many years most of the "citadels" of oralism which provide parent counseling either specifically excluded deaf parents or else saw that they quickly lost interest by failing to provide sign language interpretation.

The value of the contributions that deaf parents of a deaf child, or even deaf adults without deaf children, could make to such groups would seem too obvious to need explanation. It is they who know better than anyone what deafness is and what adjustments are necessary in order best to cope with it, yet such adults are usually excluded. An exception occurred some years ago at the California School for the Deaf. For years the school had offered institutes for parents and their deaf preschool age children. The standard procedure was to bring in numerous high-powered authorities and teachers who lectured about what parents should do. One year, by chance, two in the parent group were deaf. The hearing parents saw the communication possibilities, the amazing range of knowledge, and the full interaction that occurred between the deaf parents and their deaf children. The stark contrast between this gratifying type of interaction and the limited possibilities they were experiencing with oralism led them quickly to realize the value of total communication. Supplementing this discovery were the long conversations that occurred in the evenings between the deaf and hearing parents, discussions that were far more informative about what it means to be deaf than were the didactic lectures of the institute faculty.

It is obvious that this sort of group interaction between hearing and deaf parents provides the participants with more useful information and with a greater range of emotional expression than any other form of counseling.

Parents of a young deaf child have two crucial needs which can and should be met by counseling. One is the requisition of information about the implications and meanings of deafness, not just from an audiologist, otologist, or other professional, but from those who have gone through the experience of rearing a deaf child and from those who have themselves been deaf most of their lives. The second need of parents is to be able to express and work through their grief, fear, depression, anger, and other feelings connected with having a deaf child.

To meet these needs through counseling, it is desirable to have a sensitive person trained in group work, parents of deaf children of widely varying ages, and deaf adults either with or without deaf children. This combination offers the best of self-help approaches with the skills of conventional group therapy and counseling.

In large metropolitan clinics and preschools, establishment of such groups is no problem. For rural areas or small towns, the best solution is to have parent institutes held at residential schools for the deaf or at colleges where living accommodations, parent group counseling, and tutoring for the children can be provided. Where this is not possible, the best alternative is for the clinic or professional to put the family of a newly diagnosed deaf child in contact with a family that is experienced raising a deaf youngster.

Effective counseling, begun as soon as deafness is discovered, can save parents and deaf children years or even decades of groping and error. The dividends in human terms are immense, as are the suffering and waste when counseling is not available. Such counseling represents the best of preventive medicine and rehabilitation.

REFERENCES

Chodoff, P., Friedman, S. B., & Hamburg, D. (1964). Stress, defenses, and coping behavior: Observations in parents of children with malignant disease. *American Journal of Psychiatry, 120,* 743–749.

Cholden, L. S. (1958). *A psychiatrist works with blindness.* New York: American Foundation for the Blind.

English, R. (1971). Correlates of stigma towards physically disabled persons. *Rehabilitation Research and Practice Review, 2,* 1–17.

Gardner, R. A. (1969). The guilt reaction of parents of children with severe physical disease. *American Journal of Psychiatry, 125,* 636–644.

Grinker, R. R., Sr., (Ed.). (1969). *Psychiatric diagnosis, therapy, and research on the psychotic deaf.* Final Report, Grant No. R.D. 2407 S. Social Rehabilitation Service, Department of Health, Education and Welfare. (Available from Dr. Grinker, Michael Reese Hospital 2959 S. Ellis Ave., Chicago, IL. 60612).

Hefferman, A. (1955). A psychiatric study of fifty children referred to hospital for suspected deafness. In G. Caplan (Ed.), *Emotional problems of childhood* (pp. 269–292). New York: Basic Books.

Hubert, J. (1974). Belief and reality: Social factors in pregnancy and childbirth. In M. P. M. Richards (Ed.), *The integration of a child into a social world.* London: Cambridge University Press.

Irwin, J. (1982). *Pragmatics: The role in language development.* LaVerne, CA: Fox Point Publishing.

Kirtley, D. K. (1975). *The psychology of blindness* (pp. 137–155). Chicago: Nelson-Hall.

McKegney, F. P., & Lange, P. (1971). The decision to no longer live on chronic hemodialysis. *American Journal of Psychiatry, 128,* 47–53.

Meadow, K. P. (1968). Parental response to the medical ambiguities of congenital deafness. *Journal of Health and Social Behavior, 9,* 299–309.

Mindel, E.D., & Vernon, M. (1971). *They grow in silence.* Silver Spring, MD: National Association of the Deaf (814 Thayer St., Silver Spring, MD).

Nagel, R. F. .(1962). Audiology and the education of the deaf. *Journal of Hearing and Speech Disorders, 27,* 188–190.

Schlesinger, H. E., & Meadow, K. P. (1971). Deafness and mental health: A developmental approach. Project #14-P-55270/9-03 (RD 2835-5). San Francisco: Langley Porter Neuropsychiatric Institute, Department of Health, Education and Welfare.

Schultz, R. (1978). *The psychology of death, dying and bereavement.* Reading, MA: Addison-Wesley.

Siller, J. (1969). Psychological concomitants of amputation in children. *Child Development, 31,* 109–120a.

Stein, E. H., Murdaugh, J., & MacLeod, J. A. (1969). Brief psychotherapy of psychiatric reactions to physical illness. *American Journal of Psychiatry, 125,* 76–83.

Sullivan, P., & Vernon, M. (1979). Psychological assessment of hearing impaired children. *School Psychology Digest, 8,* 271–290.

Vash, C. (1981). *The psychology of disability.* New York: Springer Publishing Co.

Vernon, M. (1970). The role of deaf teachers in the education of deaf children. *Deaf American, 23,* 17–20.

Vernon, M. (1971). Psychodynamics surrounding the diagnosis of deafness. Paper published by Crippled Childrens Services, Centennial Office Building, St. Paul, MN.

Vernon, M. (1980). Handicapping conditions associated with the congenital rubella syndrome. *American Annals of the Deaf, 125*(8), 993–997.

Vernon, M., & Kilcullen, E. (1972). Diagnosis retardation and deafness. *Rehabilitation Record, 13,* 24–27.

Visotsky, H. M., Hamburg, D. A., Goss, M. E., & Lebovits, B. Z. (1961). Coping behavior under extreme stress. *Archives of General Psychiatry, 11,* 423–448.

CHAPTER 7
Behavioral Patterns, Pathologies, and Service Delivery

We feel in one world, we think and name in another. Between the two we can set up a system of references, but we cannot fill the gap.   *Proust*

Deafness produces in some individuals adjustment reactions that are relatively unique, or at least markedly more common, among those with profound hearing loss. Knowledge of these adjustment patterns is important to the psychotherapist working in deafness. From this knowledge, model services and methods of psychotherapy can be suggested which realistically and effectively assist the deaf client. Finally, the attitudes toward mental health on the part of the deaf community are covered, along with their resulting impact on the delivery of services.

SPECIFIC BEHAVIOR PATTERNS

PRIMITIVE PERSONALITY—SURDOPHRENIA

Research in this country and Scandinavia has identified a type of deaf patient who has extreme educational deprivation, almost no understanding of language, little socialization, and a generally psychologically barren life. The result is gross cognitive and social immaturity (Basilier, 1964; Grinker, 1969; Levine & Wagner, 1974; Rainer, Altshuler, Kallmann & Deming, 1963; Vernon, 1978). Most of these individauls are not psychotic, although they are frequently hospitalized for lack of any other adequate placement. Rainer et al. (1963) labeled them Primitive Personalities. Basilier (1964) independently described the same condition and used the label Surdophrenia to describe it. Such persons are different from the "feral adults" described in the next section because most, although not all, have some meager knowledge of sign language or other primitive linguistic means of communication. Primitive Personalities represent a significant percentage of deaf people needing mental health services. The situation is especially prevalent in larger inner cities. The problem is growing with the increase in inadequate mainstreaming programs in which deaf children are simply dumped into a regular public school class with 25 to 35 hearing children and told to sit in the front row and lipread (Vernon, 1980).

Not only are these deaf patients significant in terms of numbers but, more important, they pose a difficult long-term treatment-rehabilitation problem. Whereas psychotherapy for most mental patients is primarily a matter of returning the patient to previous levels of functioning, with the surdophrenic patient it is a matter of raising the individual far beyond any stage of development previously achieved. This is often an overwhelming psychological, educational, and vocational task involving the total socialization process.

The most tragic of the Primitive Personality cases are those who lived dependently with their parents until the parents die in old age or become too feeble to maintain the home. Suddenly these overprotected, defenseless deaf adults, often in their thirties or forties, face two severe traumas. One is the loss of the only people in the world with whom they have had any sort of deep human relationship. At the same time they must face coping with a job and independent living, for which they are not even minimally prepared. The result is often a psychotic break. Even without a psychosis, such persons are often placed in mental hospitals, partly because there is no alternative place for them. (See the discussion of Passive-Aggressive Personality Disorders in chapter 8 in the section on "Personality Disorders."

FERAL ADULTS

Psychology is replete with stories of so-called "wild boys" or feral children (Lane, 1976; Lane & Pillard, 1978). Allegedly "raised by wolves" or at least apart from human contact, these children appear likely to have been autistic or retarded, basically unable to learn much language or simple social coping skills. Their rearing by animals is undoubtedly a myth, although they are obviously deprived as children.

The nearest real-life approach to the classical feral child "raised in the wild by the wolves" is the person born deaf who has never attended school, had any formal education, or been exposed to sign language. Such an individual is an adult in body yet without any form of language, that is, a totally nonverbal human but not mentally retarded or asphasic.

The first author has come across 50 such individuals in his work. All were able to score about 75 to 80 on the WAIS or WAIS-R Performance Scale, but none scored higher than average. Bender-Gestalt protocols were distorted in ways suggesting brain damage or mental retardation.

These cases are interesting theoretically, because they represent a complete control over the variable of language and an overall intensive degree of deprivation. Thus they are an "experiment of nature" for studies of language development, critical stage theory, and a general nature-nurture type of question. This theoretical issue will be discussed further in chapter 13.

Along with the psychological test findings, there were interesting observations to be made with regard to the sign language learning of this group. Many of them were so accustomed to the isolation they had experienced all of their life that they rejected normal human contact. Thus they had no interest in learning language. Others, some in their early twenties, learned rudimentary sign language when briefly exposed to deaf people, but when they were then returned to their previous environments they quickly forgot what had been learned. A third group, who were identified during their teens and placed in residential schools for the deaf, mastered sign language, developed some competence in English, and acquired adequate social skills.

Because of the small number of cases and poor medical histories, it is not possible to draw definitive conclusions or to test fully the many hypotheses of the "experiment of nature" that these feral adults represent. However, in most South and

Central American countries and other underdeveloped nations there are thousands of feral deaf adults, that is, "normal" deaf human beings totally without language and severely deprived of knowledge.

CLOSET DEAF PEOPLE

Most deaf people see the value of speech, speechreading, and the use of residual hearing. They use these methods as best they can, but depend on sign language and writing in many situations. Their major social relationships are with deaf persons, but they also have hearing friends.

By contrast there are a minority of deaf people who intensely and irrationally deny the implications of their hearing loss. They attempt to "be hearing." Such individuals see using sign language as a sin or, at best, as an admission of a terrible inadequacy, that is, being deaf. They claim to have all "hearing" friends. If they acknowledge "deaf" friends at all, it is only "talking" or "oral" deaf people with whom they admit socializing. Often such deaf people have speech that is extremely difficult to understand. However, because speechreading is such an inexact and ambiguous method of communication, they try to cope in social situations by doing all the talking, thereby avoiding the stress of having to understand others through speechreading. If hearing people ask them to write or in some other way they express an inability to understand their speech, these deaf people become irate and blame some defect in the hearing person's ability or desire to understand them. If their speech is not understood and there are other deaf people around, they feel utterly humiliated. To ask such individuals to write is the ultimate put-down because it suggests they are deaf.

For obvious reasons, all but the most socially desperate of hearing people reject these kinds of extreme "oral" deaf individuals. In desperation, such persons cling to other "oral" deaf people, if they can find them. They disdain deaf people who sign, and they boast incessantly about their phantom hearing friends. The extremes to which these sad isolated people go to reject their own deafness, that is, themselves, is tragic. The following personal experience of the first author illustrates the problem.

My wife, who is deaf, and I were invited to the home of a congenitally deaf couple. He was a scientist who had earned his Ph.D. from a highly respected university and was obviously exceptionally bright. My wife, a research scientist, was excited about the opportunity to meet another deaf person in her field. When we arrived at their home, they immediately told us that they were oral and did not approve of sign language. This was especially ironic for the man because he had an eye disease which precluded effective speechreading. Thus, instead of an intellectually exciting before-dinner conversation, there were extended periods of painful silence, some subdued use of "natural" gestures, and a superficial visit to the man's laboratory. Mercifully, dinner finally was served, and along with it came some reprieve from the stressful and unsuccessful efforts at communication.

Following the meal we were ushered into the living room, where the scientist's deaf wife played the piano for her deaf husband, my deaf wife, and me. Her playing reflected years and years of practice but was esthetically lamentable. The entire effort was a sad tour de force analogous to a blind person's devoting years to learning to paint in order to appear to be sighted, that is, to deny his blindness.

This couple's entire life revolved around a denial of the implications of their deafness and an effort to be "hearing." In the process they made themselves social isolates. Had this scientist learned to sign, he could have been a professor in a college for the deaf and made a major contribution to deaf youth. Hearing people avoided this couple much as moonshiners do revenuers. Most other deaf people saw them as hostile and bizarre. A very small number of other oral deaf would occasionally visit them. At these visits, as at similar meetings of the oral deaf, a main topic of conversation is inevitably phantom hearing friends and "making it" in the hearing world. Sign language is considered as opprobrious as public masturbation. Yet inevitably, as events progress and beverages reduce inhibitions, exaggerated mouth signs and natural gestures become the dominant mode of communication. The end result is "sign language" consisting of grotesque, sometimes almost obscene, mouthing and primitive gestures that permit these people some rudimentary communication but deny them the full interaction possible from American Sign Language.

Treatment

When the stress of this denial of deafness finally brings these individuals to psychotherapy, treatment is extremely difficult. First, the presenting symptom, the ostensible reason for treatment, is never the real problem, which is denial of deafness. Second, the refusal to use sign language severely limits the communication, which in turn limits therapy.

At the heart of treatment for such individuals is a need psychotherapeutically to work through the grief and mourning over the loss of hearing (Grinker, 1969). Throughout the course of their life, these individuals have denied their loss, a denial that has resulted in a chronic repressed grief. This grief will continue to express itself as an irrational destructive denial of deafness and its implications until the reality of the loss of hearing is acknowledge. Once this occurs, and the grief and mourning over the loss are worked through, constructive ways of coping with life can begin. Sign language is learned, deaf friends are made, and more realistic relationships are formed with hearing people.

Treatment of this pathological method of coping with deafness is most effective when it is done during school or college years. When deaf persons such as these are placed in a school with a large number of other deaf people who are coping effectively with deafness, improvement generally begins. The individual with a pathological need to deny, manifested in part by refusal to sign, soon finds that, instead of having to lead a life of isolation and stressful denial of self, he or she can have friends and find self-acceptance and social acceptance as a deaf person. This process frequently occurs in residential schools and in colleges for deaf students, such as Gallaudet and the National Technical Institute for the Deaf. In these settings, closet deaf students enter as oral isolates rejecting their deafness and gradually evolve into mature individuals who accept both oral and manual means of communication and who welcome both hearing and deaf friends.

When the denial persists into adulthood, patterns of isolation become entrenched. Years have been invested in an illusion that is hard to give up. Few people are able to say to themselves, "What I have paid so high a price for in suffering all these years is nothing more than an illusion like that of the 'Emperor's Clothing.' " Thus, treatment is extremely difficult and sometimes impossible.

To go through life as a closet deaf person and survive the educational system and the world of work represents a grueling life adjustment. Most deaf people find out early in life that the anxieties and frustrations of denying the implications of deafness are so great that they face up to most aspects of it and cope more effectively; that is, they learn to sign and to have other deaf friends. Some closet deaf people who are bright, aggressive, and have parents wealthy or sufficiently persevering to see that they are tutored and sent to private schools, obtain a good education. In some instances they achieve professional success. However, frequently the terrible price they pay psychologically leaves them social isolates with solitary hobbies—eccentrics tolerated, sometimes admired for some area of achievement, but essentially social outcasts. It is unfortunate that the intellectual potential of these individuals is largely lost to the deaf community and that these individuals are denied association and companionship with others who are deaf. At an even deeper level these people are forced to live a lie involving a denial of the essence of self. In moments of insight and honesty they see the charade but are so threatened by it that defenses quickly repress awareness. Short of fairly long-term therapy, these closet deaf people live tragic, lonely lives, eventually realizing their rejection by hearing people but never completely knowing the acceptance and fullness they could have enjoyed had they opened themselves to other deaf people and to forms of manual as well as oral communication (Montgomery, 1978).

Homosexuality

Under current diagnostic criteria, homosexual behavior is not seen as a mental illness but is considered an alternative mode of sexual behavior. However, much of society and the law continue to interpret such behavior in a negative and punitive context. Thus the homosexual continues to face coping situations different from those of the heterosexual.

Homosexuality is the only atypical sexual adjustment pattern among deaf people that has been discussed in the literature in any detail. Therefore it will be discussed in this section even though it is no longer seen as psychopathological according to DSM III (Spitzer, 1980, 1987), the major diagnostic manual used in psychology and psychiatry.

Rainer et al. (1963) and Zakarewsky (1979) have provided the most complete reports on homosexuality among deaf people. The former indicate that in their outpatient clinic homosexual behavior was found fairly often. However, they do not provide any solid data indicating that this behavior is more or less frequent among deaf than among hearing outpatients.

Zakarewsky's (1979) study dealt more with the sociology of homosexuality in the deaf community. He perceives deaf homosexuals as members of two distinct minorities (handicapped and gay), thus facing a double jeopardy at the hands of the social majority. Hearing homosexuals give some support to their deaf counterparts, whereas the nongay deaf community basically rejects them. This rejection poses major problems to the deaf homosexual. Most feel a need to conceal their gayness from other deaf people. Because of the closeness of the deaf community, doing so is difficult, just as it would be for a hearing homosexual in a small town. However, there are 600 members in a national gay deaf organization, most of them located in larger cities. There are a few clubs for gay deaf people, but deaf gays lack the support systems (churches, doctors, bars, etc.) hearing homosexuals have established.

In their relationships with hearing gays, several problems arise (Zakarewsky, 1979). First, gay bars and "cruising" areas are usually dark and often loud, circumstances not conducive to communication between the deaf and hearing. Deaf gays find it somewhat difficult to establish contacts with the hearing for casual impersonal sex and almost impossible to have more lasting homosexual relationships.

Ironically, deaf gays face more parental rejection when their parents are also deaf. One reason for this rejection is the closeness of the deaf community: If a deaf couple have a homosexually active child, all their friends will know. In addition, the average deaf parent has little in-depth knowledge of homosexuality and tends to take a punitive and moralistic attitude toward it.

The following case is the actual history, in his own written language, of a bright (IQ 120) young deaf transvestite male. It gives some feeling for the life he faced as a homosexual.

My Happened History
Started 11/30/69—I Was 11 Years Old

FEBRUARY 2: I got kicked out from the school for the deaf because I was a homosexual and played with some person that counselor catched me two times so the Superintendent was afraid that I would become a bad leader of homosexual to other boys so he decided to fired me out from there and send me to my home.

MARCH 4: I entered a day elementary school for oral deaf. After the school closed for summer vacation, I looked for part-time job. But I began like to act as homosexuality so I was easy to get many men to playing sex (suck, jack off, french kisses and romance) and I got some money from them. My parents were not know that what I doing with them. Most of time I disobeyed them and make them worried and upset about me.

JULY 10: In the night I was looking around the cars parking at Body Shop and stole Oldsmobile, and started drove around town for 1 1/2 hours. Then I stopped on the street for wait signal green and suddenly police car was behind me so I was nervous and forget to stop in other street and police in car was following me and saw me that I didn't stop in signal so he arrested me and asked me "Where is your license?" I was told him liar that I left it at my home but he checked the car up. I was nervous and my heart beat so fast. He know I was liar and took me to Juvenile Hall and I was afraid to enter there because there was my first time. I went there and went to Unit 4 and stayed for overnight. Next day my parents got me and released from there and went home. I became under Probation Officer on August 2, 19—. Then I went to junior high school oral deaf class and was fine along in there but I was still acting as homosexual with other men in some places without my parents and Probation Officer know. . . .

MARCH: I stole some value things from the people's garage. I maked my face up like woman and acted homosexuality. My Probation Officer took me to Juvenile Hall again (that my third time) and stayed there for 5 days. Then I went to the court and Judge ordered me to go to the hospital.

APRIL 11: My Probation Officer took me to the County Psychiatrist Hospital and I met a nice doctor and nurse. A counselor man took me to Men's Ward and changed my clothed. I went to doctor's office and he talked to me very nice and he try to help me. My parents came and visited me every day. In the ward I was stranger to the men but I talked to them nice but a handsome man who love the homosexuality and he know me because I met him before in somewhere. So he and I went hide and had sex together without the counselors and anybody know. I was all night in there but my temper was still loving homosexuality. On April 30, I went to the Court and Judge ordered me to go other hospital in North (350 miles north).

MAY: The FBI took me from State Mental Hospital in the car and I was sad and nervous to enter there. Doctor was so mean to me and I was afraid of him. Next day I went to Examination Room for check my body up. Then I met a counselor who can use the sign language and talked with him and he was very nice to me. I stayed in Ward 3 for 1 week. Most of time we played the volleyball. A handsome man (who look like Tony Curtis) in Ward 3 was trying to playing sex with me but we did not but we just love and kiss together. Then I transferred to Ward 2 and I like there and I met a very nice guy and we talked about our life and he love to playing sex with teenage boy. He was 23 years old. I kiss and sex with him little because I was staying in Ward 2 for 2 days only. Then I transferred to Ward 5 and liked there. I got easy many friends over 18 years old. I met man who can use sign language so we became called "Cousins" together and he was not homosexuality. Counselor took me to Psychologist Therapist for Deaf every Tuesday and Thursday, with 11 deaf men. We discussed about our problem and etc. I met many homosexuality. I found several boy friends love me. I feel I was criminal homosexuality and acted so beautiful queer. I sex and kiss with some boys. I was awful crazy over it. We went to movie, clubs, school, church, party and etc. in there. I went to the Court and Judge said all men there age are over 18 years old that I was 13 years old so he wanted me to go home soon. I went home and my friend gave me a watch and some addresses and we had sex and romance together. Then I went home and released from there. I was very happy with my parents . . . .

My parents were wonder where did I go but most of time I told them liar. I disobeyed to them and was mean to them. I used makeup in my face (eyebrow, face powder, lipstick and etc.). One night I wore my mother's dress, bra, stocking, purse, shoe with high heels, jewelry and perfume when my parents were gone to visit their friends. So I wore them and walked outside and acted as cheap and beautiful girl. Suddenly a man in car stopped and asked me if I wanted to ride with him and I said yes and I know he thought I was a real lady but I was nervous. Then he drove around San Diego and stopped in the park and french kiss but he tried to try to sex with me but I won't let him because I don't want him to know that I am real a boy. So I ordered him to take me home and he did, I changed the clothes so fast and went bed.

JUNE 8: I walked outside from my home and a man in car asked me if I would like to go with him for ride so I went with him. He stopped a Liquor Store and bought a box of beers. Then he drove to mountain and hide under the dark place and got drunk and played sex together. We were having lots of fun and he took me back to my home. My mother was very angry. A telegram came to our house and said my grandma passed away so I got awful upset and cried because I can't believe that and it is real too late for me to forgive and still sorry. I know God's best way to her so I got sad and think of my beloved Gradma so often. One week later a handsome strong man was followed me by his car but I went inside home. Suddenly he came in and talked to me and he told me that he would like to sex with me for $5.00 so I accepted and had sex with him and he gave me his address with his name. So next day I went to his home and had sex again and we become love together for 1 1/2 months only but we separated and never see him again. I still go to Park for homosexuality. I stole some candy and other things from the store (secret). Then my mother and I went on our vacation from July 1 to July 30. We went to Texas first. I found a deaf homosexuality. He took me to a Downtown and met his lover boy friend (about 30 years old) and we went to Theater and then went to Airport Bowling and we had a lot of fun without being sex together. After that we went to Dallas for one week and had go to Church service most of time. On August 24 I became a christian, baptisized and joined the church for forgive my sinner in the past. Then we visited our relatives. Then we went back our home. After August 24 I went to Bible School for 4 weeks and get fine along and improved. But one day a man asked me to suck his dick (penis) for $15.00 so I did and got it from him. After I still doing homosexuality in the park again so often . . . . On september I started went to my junior high school. I started joined Bowling League. I went there every Tuesday and after that game I went to the park for sex. One time I took a deaf Mexican girl to the park and began to try to sex with her but she just showed me her breast and pussy and we got romance and little sex together. I was still doing homosexuality and was very easy got many men for sex and got money from them.

DECEMBER: My Probation Officer came to my school to questioned with me. I confessed that I was doing homosexuality with other men and sexed with a girl. So he putted me to Juvenile Hall (that my fourth time) and I got unhappy and stayed there for 2 1/4 months. I went to the Court two times and Judge ordered me to go to Children's Home about 625 miles away. In Juvenile Hall I was alright without trouble and parents. My parents visited me so often.

JANUARY 3: I released from Juvenile Hall and my Probation Officer took me to Airport and catched an airplane and flew to City and drove to Children's Home. We met ladies and I looked around there and entered my room. I met many kids and counselors and became warmly and friendly. First week I was homesick but then alright. I started worked as outside to do many things and earned $5.00 per week and went to store and movies so often. There was like home. We went for Picnic on one day at Sunday. I enjoyed there. Then I got trouble by some letters from man (homosexuality that I never see him before). So the counselor make me to stop write homosexual letters to him so I did. But I began unhappy disobeyed to counselors and fighted with him. Then I visited my brother's home for Easter vacation for 3 days only also my parents were there too so I was very happy with them. Then I went to back there. I began teaching two boys about homosexuality. They played sex with me for two times only. One night I got some whiskey from the Counselor and drank two glasses and got awful drunk and entered the counselor meeting and fall down (K.O.). They found out that I was drunk so they carried me to my bedroom in the cabin. I was eating dog food and awful acting (that the counselor told me next day).

Next day I got sick and vomited. So I don't believe that. Next week Doctor and the Counselor went to had meeting together about me so they called to my Probation Officer and told me to packed all my things to suitcase so I got stunned and they told me that I must leave there.

JUNE: My Probation Officer took me from Children's Home. So I was heart broken and missed there because there was very beautiful to me. I was wrong acting to them so why they can't keep me. I went and lived with my Brother and his family and go fine along. I wasn't understand at their advice so I became unhappy again. One day their guest came and visited us and she left her purse so she went to the kitchen. So I was curious to see her purse and opened and saw the money was over $120 so I stole $20 and put it on my pocket. On Saturday I went over a deaf boy's house and we went to downtown for shopping with my money and left $10.90. One time my brother and wife questioned me how do I got money so first I told them liar then told them truth that I stole it from their guest so they were very surprised. Then Policeman took me to Juvenile Hall for overnight and they thought I was homosexual with other boys but I was innocent but I was must be suffer and let them to give me suffer.

I released from Juvenile Hall and went to Youth Authority by car with other probation officer. I went there and was not afraid. The man ordered me to change the clothed and fingerprint with pictured of me. Then I went to Control Office and waited until noon a man ordered me to go with little kids to Cafeteria to eat lunch. Then I entered to my dormitory Drake B Mod and met a deaf boy. After a while I found out that I can't play outside of swim so I got a complained and discussed with my counselors for over 3 days. I was no patient. Next I went to see my social worker and talked with her about transferred to other unit but she said "No" so I got angry and began acted as Homosexuality. I met many friend who I know them from Park and Juvenile Hall. But one boy who is my best pal and was very glad to see him again. Next day I was angry so I was lost temper mind and hit the window and got little deep cut on right hands near thumb between wrist so the counselor saw and quickly took me to the hospital and stayed there for 1 1/2 weeks and social worker told me that I transferred to Drake A so I was very happy to make some boys to sex with me but I won't because I want to get full cured. I went to the Court and Judge was very nice talk to me and told me to go to Mental Hospital soon so I accepted as I hope I will be successful in there. One I was trying to suicide attempt but the counselor saw me scratch my wrist by glass so he took me to the hospital faster and I got a shot as dope and make me awful drunk and dizzy and went to lock up and sleep in the hospital and next day I feel sick and Doctor ordered me to go back to my unit. I learned a lesson so I won't do it again. I became unhappy in my unit because of my deafness. Then my Social Worker told me to go to State Mental Hospital today.

[NO DATE]: I released from Youth Authority and a man took me to State Mental Hospital. When I arrived there I was cried because I feel that I am mentally ill when I saw other people in there. I went to Receive Treatment and had physical examination. I met the staff and Dr._____. I stayed in Receive Men's Unit. On the night we went to the dance party and found a new girl friend and fall love in her and went steady with her. I stayed in my unit most of the time so I can't stand so I discussed with the doctors and went to Juvenile meeting and Dr._____ said wait and soon about to transfer to other unit. I started went to school and had 3 subjects (Arithmetic, History, and English). I like the school so far. After while I transferred to Unit 15 and began happy in there. I like there so much. I got partial privilege and went outside with some one who had full privilege and can go outside by myself to canteen, school, library, and etc. I dated some girls for walk to have romance and kiss as I am crazy over the girls for that. My temper was trying to sex with some men but I feel I am real cured and won't let it beat me. One day a man was trying to make me to sex with him but I won't and hit him without trouble. I began gave the card of sign language away to the people who like to talk and learn it to me. I talked to the nurses, staff and doctors some often, psychologist started work with me and I like it so much because I need someone to help me more little I feel I want to have my ears to operation to be open to hear so I asked to my staff and doctor about it but they said wait so I feel unhappy because of my begin deafness so I pray and hope I will can hear soon.

It is evident from this young man's experiences that his sexual orientation profoundly influenced his entire life adjustments. The lack of insight and the basically infantile, but moralistic perspective he and society had did not prevent his homosexual behavior, but it did cause him to see it as something wrong, a part of himself to be treated and corrected.

SUICIDE

The only formal data on suicide among deaf people was a comparative study of the number of suicides at Gallaudet University and a comparable liberal arts college for the normally hearing (Dobson, personal communication, 1976). Both colleges had two to four attempted suicides per year, mostly females taking an overdose of some potentially toxic medication. The difference was that at Gallaudet there were no successful attempts over a period of some twenty years, whereas two students at the hearing college had killed themselves. It is interesting that of those at Gallaudet who tried suicide, almost all had excellent speech skills. They were hard of hearing, adventitiously deaf, or, for some other reason, either struggling with the issue of their identify as deaf people or grieving over the loss of their hearing.

If one assumed a marked difference in the rate of depression for deaf people, this would show up in suicide rates. The limited data available are inconclusive on this point.

CHILDHOOD PATHOLOGY

Formal studies of the psychological adjustment of deaf children date back to about the time psychological tests first came into use. The research from 1930 to 1955 is summarized in Table 7.1 (p. 148). Many of measuring instruments administered in those early investigations were inappropriate because of their verbal content or the verbal nature of their directions. Some of the studies attempted to put the tests into sign language. Unless expertly done, however, this approach tends to change the meaning of the questions and hence of the responses. Considering these problems as well as other testing considerations that will be discussed in chapter 10, many of the findings of these early studies obviously have to be viewed in a somewhat dubious light.

One focus of post-1955 work on childhood psychopathology has been the assessment of the role of organic factors (Chess, Fernandez, & Korn, 1978; Hicks, 1970; Vernon, 1969). As was indicated in chapters 2 and 3, the leading causes of deafness are also major etiologies of brain damage and its resulting behavioral learning disability, hyperactivity, impulsiveness, organic psychosis, distractability, and emotional instability. The symptoms are generally most acute early in childhood, subsiding somewhat by the teenage years except in severe cases.

Three major U.S. studies have been done to assess the prevalence and to some extent the nature of psychological maladjustment among deaf children. Schlesinger and Meadow (1972) found that of their sample of 516 school-age deaf youth, 11.6 percent were severely disturbed and in need of psychiatric help. An additional 19.6 percent had lesser, but significant problems. This was five times the rate reported in a comparison group of hearing students from the same state.

Gentile and McCarthy (1973) surveyed 42,513 hearing-impaired children in the United States and found that 18.9 percent had emotional/behavioral problems. Neither Schlesinger and Meadow (1972) nor Gentile and McCarthy included children excluded from school because of psychological disturbance, but Vernon's (1969) study indicated this figure to be 9 percent for the particular school studied.

The most recent large-scale study was by Goulder and Trybus (1977). They used the School Behavior Checklist to study 150 students already identified by teachers as emotionally/behaviorally disturbed. They wanted to find the nature of the problems present in the disturbed group. Results indicate that low achievement need, aggressiveness, anxiety, and hostile isolation were the major features distinguishing the disturbed deaf child (ages 7–13) from a comparison group of satisfactorily adjusted deaf youngsters.

British research sets the prevalence of serious emotional adjustment problems at between 6 and 15 percent (Williams, 1970). For example, in the Isle of Wight study (Graham and Rutter, 1968) 15.4 percent of the deaf had psychiatric disorders, compared with 6.6 percent of the hearing.

The studies described above and others (Chess & Fernandez, 1980; Freeman, Malkin, & Hastings, 1975; Hirshoren & Rothrock, 1972; Hirshoren & Schnittjer, 1979; Levine & Wagner, 1974; Montgomery, 1978) all vary tremendously in the criteria used for psychopathology, in the type of samples studied, and in general methodology. However, there is universal agreement in this research that a higher prevalence of pathology exists among deaf children: 8 to 22 percent, compared with rates of from 2 to 10 percent for the general population of children (Meadow, 1980). One major cause of the higher prevalence among deaf children appears to be organic factors associated with the cause of deafness. The other is restrictions placed on communication by deafness, by oral education, and by societal indifference (Denmark, 1973; Meadow, 1980; Mindel & Vernon, 1971). The same basic problems seem to persist into adolescence, although data on this period of life are not extensive (Norden, 1975; Rodda, 1969; Smith, 1963).

OVERALL PERSPECTIVE OF AVAILABLE SERVICES

HISTORICAL DEVELOPMENT OF SERVICES

Until 1955 there was not a single mental hospital or clinic anywhere in the United States or the world to serve mentally ill deaf people (Rainer & Altshuler, 1971). A few schools for the deaf had been doing some basic psychological testing, but even in these schools there was no treatment for mental illness (Levine, 1981). Instead,

TABLE 7.1. Measurements of the Personality and Social Maturity of Deaf Persons (1930–1955)

Reference	Sample	Test	Results
Pintner, 1933	94 Hard-of-hearing children	Bernreuter Personality Inventory	The deaf are more introverted, neurotic, and submissive.
Lyon, 1934	87 deaf children	Thurston Personality Inventory	17% needed psychiatric help (Group F on the test). 13% were emotionally maladjusted (Group C).
Naffin, 1935	129 deaf German children	No test. He studied the children in free play.	The deaf are retarded two years socially until they reach adolescence, at which time there is no difference except in suggestibility. The deaf are more suggestible.
Timberlake, 1935		No test. Empirical observation based on years of teaching.	Suspicion, irritability, curiosity, tactlessness, shyness, deception, and naiveté are characteristics attributed to the deaf, without factual basis.
Brunschwig, 1936	Deaf children	Roger's Personality Inventory	No significant differences. Deaf children like school better; they are more afraid of other children, more withdrawn, more afraid of the dark, and feel they were happiest as babies. The overlap of answers between deaf and hearing children indicates they are not an atypical group.
Pintner, 1937	76 deaf children	Checklist of fears	The deaf checked more items. A disproportionate number checked fear of animals. This was considered a sign of immaturity.

Author/Year	Sample	Instrument	Findings
	76 deaf children	Study of wishes	The deaf children's wishes indicated their emotional maturity.
	76 deaf children	Vineland Social Maturity Scale	The deaf were 1.6 years retarded.
	Deaf college students	Bernreuter Personality Inventory; Minnesota Scale of Mechanical Ability	No significant difference. The deaf and hearing were of equal skill.
Pintner & Brunschwig, 1937	Deaf children	The Adjustment Inventory	The deaf scored considerably below the hearing. The deaf with other deaf in the family were better than deaf who had no deaf relatives.
Pintner, Fusfeld, & Brunschwig, 1937	50 college students 126 adults	Bernreuter Personality Inventory	More emotional instability and introversion and less dominance among the deaf. The deaf and hard-of-hearing were about the same. Those deafened late in life were more like the hearing.
Preston, 1937	92 deaf children ages 5–20	Vineland Social Maturity Scale	Those deaf before age 7 were 20% behind the hearing of all levels. Those deaf before age 5 showed greater variability but their means were the same as for the group deaf before age 7.
Kirk, 1938	112 deaf and hard-of-hearing children	Haggerty-Olson-Wickman Behavior Rating Scale	More problem tendencies among deaf children. Greater variation in emotional traits.
Lane 1938	48 hard-of-hearing children, grades 7, 8, and 9	Paper and pencil test	The hard of hearing were more submissive and interested.

TABLE 7.1. (*continued*)

Reference	Sample	Test	Results
Springer, 1938	377 deaf children and 415 hard-of-hearing children. An attempt was made to equate these samples for socioeconomic background.	Haggerty-Olson Wickman Behavior Rating Scale	The means were the same on Schedule A. Schedule B (behavior rating) indicated the deaf had more desirable personality traits for the deaf. The hearing children who had been selected as being of similar socioeconomic backgrounds were found to be below average.
Springer & Roslow, 1938	50 deaf children ages 12–14	Brown Personality Inventory	"Very poor adjustment."
Streng & Kirk, 1938	97 deaf children ages 6–18	Vineland Social Maturity Scale	The differences shown by the deaf were not significant.
Burchard & Myklebust, 1942a	187 deaf children	Haggerty-Olson-Wickman Behavior Scale	The deaf presented more behavior problems.
Burchard & Myklebust, 1942b	104 deaf children	Vineland Social Maturity Scale	The deaf scored an average of 18 to 20 points below the hearing.
Kline, 1945	Deaf children	A test of verbal free associations	The responses of the deaf were different from those of the hearing. The deaf failed to respond more often.
Simon, 1948		An opinion based on his life experience with deaf people	The deaf are callous, possessive, desire attention, lack foresight, lack restraint, are jealous, have tantrums, lie, are overpersistent, and are rude. He summarized these characteristics as indicating emotional immaturity.

deaf patients who were or were thought to be psychologically disturbed were dumped into regular mental hospitals, where neither the staff nor other patients could communicate with them. Such placement was and is essentially anti-therapeutic custodial isolation, more for the convenience of society than for the humane care of the deaf patient.

Finally, in the 1950's Edna Levine, Boyce Williams, and some other leaders in deafness interested psychiatrist Franz Kallmann in the condition of deafness. Dr. Kallmann's primary interest was actually not deafness, but a genetic biological theory of schizophrenia which he thought he could test by studying twins and deaf schizophrenics.

Dr. Kallman's reputation and the support of the Rehabilitation Services Administration enabled the first mental health clinic for deaf patients to open in 1955. By then, Dr. Kallmann had recruited two resident psychiatrists, John Rainer and Ken Altshuler, into his work in deafness. Hans Furth, now a professor of psychology at Catholic University, was another researcher along with Dr. Kallmann during these early years at the New York Psychiatric Institute.

In 1947, even before Kallmann entered the field of deafness, Luther Robinson, a psychiatrist at St. Elizabeth's Hospital, had started taking an interest in deaf patients. In 1963 Dr. Robinson established an in-patient program for St. Elizabeth's deaf patients, which eventually developed into the Mental Health Project for the Deaf. His efforts were totally independent of the work being done by the New York Psychiatric Institute. Today both the Mental Health Project for the Deaf at St. Elizabeth's and the work of the New York State Psychiatric Institute are world renowned.

In 1966 another psychiatrist, Roy R. Grinker, Sr., along with McCay Vernon, a psychologist in deafness, and Eugene Mindel, a child psychiatrist who had some experience at Gallaudet College, undertook a three-year study of psychosis and deafness at Michael Reese Hospital in Chicago (Grinker, 1969). They knew of the New York clinic and were building on the experience of Kallman's group.

At about this same time, in about the late 1960s, the first comprehensive treatment services for deaf children were begun at Langley Porter under Hilde Schlesinger and Kay Meadow (Schlesinger & Meadow, 1972). The former had been a dormitory counselor at the Arizona School for the Deaf and Blind, where she had begun the study of sign language. Dr. Meadow was a sociologist who brought her research and administrative skills to Langley Porter to work with deaf children.

Once these four pioneering projects began to publish their findings and present them at professional meetings, others became interested. Thirteen state hospitals in the United States established at least some basic units to serve deaf patients (Goulder, 1976). In these units they taught staff to use sign language. The work in the United States soon spread to other countries, including England, Sweden, Norway, and Denmark, all of which began to group deaf patients together and to provide them with mental health services (Montgomery, 1978; Robinson, 1978).

Despite these encouraging beginnings, today in the United States only 2 percent of the 43,000 deaf persons needing mental health services are receiving them (Robinson, 1978). Many of the programs offering services are pitifully understaffed. Most of the mental health personnel in deafness are unqualified by the professional standards held necessary to treat hearing patients (Cantor & Spragins, 1977; Curtis, 1976; Levine, 1971). Remember, only 13 of 50 states have any hospital program at all.

LACK OF CHILD TREATMENT FACILITIES

There were absolutely no in-patient services for deaf children in the United States until the late 1970s. Now two programs exist in Michigan and one in New York State. In this area is perhaps the most glaring deficiency of all. Almost every professional who works in the field of mental health with deaf people gets frequent calls from families and schools asking where a psychotic deaf child can get hospital care. Typically the answer has been, "There is no mental hospital serving deaf children." Appeals made to state and federal governments to establish such a hospital by leading scientists working in deafness have always been rejected. In the current political climate, unfortunately, no change in the pattern of rejection is foreseen.

SCHOOL PSYCHOLOGY

One study (Cantor & Spragins, 1977) indicated that there were no programs in the United States preparing school psychologists to work with deaf children. In fact, of the 178 persons who were working as school psychologists with deaf children, only 9 percent had appropriate school psychologist qualifications. In addition they had no special training to work as school psychologists with deaf children. Subsequently, Gallaudet University has started a school psychology program.

Nebulously defined "school counseling services" are more prevalent, but these are often provided by untrained staff (Curtis, 1976; Trott, 1984). Gallaudet University has established a school counseling program which includes study of such issues as the psychosocial aspects of deafness, assessment, and counseling techniques appropriate for the deaf population.

SERVICES TO PARENTS

The heart of any preventive program in deafness and mental health has to start with parents (Brown & Giangreco, 1983). What are their needs, if they are to provide appropriate psychological support for their deaf children?

First, parents need strong counseling programs to be available at the time of their child's diagnosis. These programs should involve the self-help model of Alcoholics Anonymous, that is, they should involve parents who have successfully raised deaf children in addition to, deaf adults and a therapist.

Second, parents need full awareness of the options and services available to their deaf child. Rarely is this information made known to parents early on. For example, frequently oral or Total Communication preschool programs will get a deaf child early and never tell the parents of other programs using different methods than their own. Another problem relates to hearing aids. Often parents are led to believe that these aids are a panacea to deafness when, in fact, they are relatively useless to many profoundly deaf people.

Other needs of parents are for professionals who understand deafness. For example, physicians are notoriously naive about what is appropriate for a deaf child, yet parents depend on them heavily for advice (Vernon, 1976). Teachers who are totally unable to use sign language and who have had no contact with deaf adults are given Master's degrees to teach deaf children. Parents are then dependent on them for guidance. Many rehabilitation counselors also lack sign language skills and knowledge of deafness (Tully, 1970). In addition, there is need for psychologists, social workers, and psychiatrists able to work with deaf children and adults.

OUTLINE OF MODEL PLAN

The following three services comprise the minimal requirements for a beginning state plan of mental health services for deaf and hard-of-hearing people. This plan has already been implemented in 14 states.

Identification and Centralization

Deaf patients currently in state hospitals should be identified. Then small units of 10 to 30 patients should be established for them in hospitals near large population centers. These units would serve adults and children needing inpatient services as well as those needing outpatient treatment. Such a centralization of facilities makes possible the efficient use of the limited qualified professional staff available to work with psychologically disturbed deaf people. It enables community specialists in deafness, such as educators, rehabilitation counselors, and religious workers, to coordinate their efforts at returning or maintaining appropriate deaf patients in the community. Further, state departments of mental health would then be in a position to offer school and other agencies treatment for children instead of the anti-therapeutic isolated institutionalization which now exists in most states. Then and only then will the concept of community mental health, which is the basic rationale for the state programs, be meaningful in terms of the deaf youth, their parents, and deaf adults.

Counseling

Universal counseling for parents of young deaf children should be provided in conjunction with planned early identification and education. This counseling should be patterned, in general, after other self-help groups, but with professional direction. Great care must be taken to develop in parents a realistic acceptance of what deafness is and how to cope with it in ways that help the deaf child and yield maternal/paternal satisfaction. Too many institutes for parents of deaf children have in the past raised false hopes about communication, educational achievement, and socialization that have encouraged parents to deny the handicap rather than help them cope constructively. The result has been psychological trauma and educational and social frustration.

Summer Institutes

Regular summer institutes offering information on the implications of deafness are needed to intensively educate the mental health professions (psychology, psychiatry, social work, etc.) that will serve state educational programs for deaf children.

A PREVENTION PLAN

Identification of High-Risk Children

First it is necessary to identify early those children who have psychological disorders and those who are at high risk for such problems. This can be done through appropriate psychological testing and effective training of teachers and aides in identifying potential psychopathology. Existing knowledge makes it clear that such children can be identified during the first three years in school. If they are not identified and treated, they get worse. The results of good prevention programs, however, are better school attendance, better grades, less disruptive behavior, better peer relationships, and less general pathology (Stein, Mindel, & Jaboley, 1981).

Training of Teachers and Paraprofessionals

The second part of a prevention program would be the training of teachers and paraprofessionals to work with disturbed and high-risk students in the schools (Cohen, 1980; Degrell & Ouellette, 1981). Harris, a deaf psychologist who has worked to formulate prevention programs, recommends deaf paraprofessionals in particular (Stein, Mindel, & Jaboley, 1981). These individuals, by virtue of their own deafness, would be likely to have interest, knowledge, and personal experience of great potential value in working with difficult deaf children. They would work under the supervision of a mental health professional. There is evidence from work with both hearing and deaf children that this approach is effective (Naiman, 1972; Rainer & Altshuler, 1971; Schlesinger & Meadow, 1972).

Consultants

A third aspect of a prevention program is involvement of a mental health consultant to work with and coordinate the program (Stein, Mindel, & Jaboley, 1981). Ideally such a person would have a knowledge of deafness along with mental health skills. However, it may often be necessary to use a professional who lacks knowledge of deafness. When this is the case, the following four-step orientation is mandatory.

1. The consultant should read basic selected publications orienting him or her to behavioral aspects of deafness and the use of interpreters. These readings should then be discussed with a member of the school staff experienced with deaf children.
2. The consultant should observe and interview a number of deaf children using an interpreter.
3. The children interviewed should then be discussed in a case seminar framework with the interpreter and an appropriate school official. This discussion will give the consultant a better understanding of such fundamentals as the communication, maturity, and frame of reference that characterize many children who are deaf.
4. Sign language instruction should be started.

If these steps, which represent a considerable investment, are not taken, the unique issues raised by deafness often render consultants ineffective or drive them from work with deaf children.

Once the consultant gets this basic foundation, he or she should arrange an in-service instructional program for staff, direct the school mental health services, work therapeutically with parents and children, and coordinate interaction between the school and other community mental health resources.

Often the costs of consultants can be held to a minimum by use of community mental health agencies. By law they have obligations to the community of which the school or program for deaf children is a part.

Advisory Boards

The fourth aspect of a prevention program for schools is to establish advisory boards of parents and deaf adults. These boards provide valuable extra input and support.

Pastoral Counseling

Certain religions have made conscientious efforts to serve the needs of deaf people. Others make token efforts at best. The end result is that there is a relatively small nucleus of clergymen of various faiths, some deaf themselves, who work with deaf people in religious settings. Because of the overall scarcity of services at their disposal, deaf persons tend to turn to their clergyman for everything, including psychological help. Often it is religious workers who locate cases of misdiagnosis in hospitals for the mentally ill and retarded. At other times, they are called upon as interpreters for psychotherapy.

Unfortunately, some of the religious groups that have made the greatest gains in converting deaf people to their faith are the denominations that provide the least psychological training for their pastors. Other seminaries provide excellent training in pastoral counseling. Despite the problems, any serious effort to mobilize mental health services for the deaf community should involve its religious leaders.

PROBLEMS IN PSYCHOTHERAPY

Deaf people are able to benefit from all means of psychotherapy, except for psychoanalysis that requires the patient to be on a couch with the analyst sitting behind and out of view (Brauer & Sussman, 1979). The primary problem in using various treatment approaches is not the deaf patient, but the lack of psychotherapists fluent in sign language (Bonham, Armstrong, & Bonham, 1981).

A professional who is basically competent in using signs can usually do helpful therapy with a signing deaf person who has a reasonably adequate command of English, because the signs can be used in an approximation of English syntax and key words can be spelled. This procedure slows and constricts the therapy process, but it is a feasible and reasonably effective approach.

Unfortunately, only about 25 percent of deaf people have sufficient skills in English to communicate in the half ASL/half English vernacular. The other 75 percent need treatment in American Sign Language without English syntax and without much fingerspelling. Unfortunately, if a therapist has not used ASL as a primary means of communication since childhood, it is difficult to develop the skill needed to provide treatment in ASL. This lack of skill poses several unfortunate consequences, the major one being that deaf patients needing therapy either do not get it or else receive it from someone who lacks the necessary communication skills. Sign language interpreters can be used; however, the interpreter not only must be skilled in signing but also must be extremely sensitive to human feelings and understand basic concepts of psychotherapy. Even when an interpreter has these skills, the use of a third person is a last resort. It interferes with the psychotherapeutic process by reducing rapport and depersonalizing treatment.

Ironically, hearing psychologists, psychiatrists, and social workers often have reacted to the sign language issue counterphobically. Instead of acknowledging their own understandable inadequacies in the communication skills required, they have blamed deaf patients. Often the deaf patient is described as "low verbal" or linguistically inept, when actually the individual is fluent in ASL but not English. In a true sense it is the therapist who is inept in the patient's language. Terms such as constricted personality, impoverished personality, schizophrenic, retarded, and the like have been used inaccurately to label deaf patients because of the therapist's ineptness in ASL. Real psychological difficulties have been masked and nonexistent pathologies wrongly attributed to deaf people. This is a well-documented process in regard to other languages as well. For example, it happens to Mexican-American patients seen by psychiatrists not fluent in Spanish (Rubkin, 1979).

Another counterphobic reaction of hearing therapists lacking fluency in ASL has been to say that deaf patients are incapable of "the most sophisticated verbal therapies." They are thus relegated to highly directive techniques, behavior modification, or other approaches not requiring the therapist to understand the patient's ASL. Obviously, it is unfortunate when the therapy of choice is not dictated by the patient's desires or needs, but by the therapist's inadequacy in communication. The injustice is compounded when the entire problem is blamed on the deaf patient's so-called inability to profit from verbal therapy.

Sometimes therapists will feign understanding of what a deaf patient says. Nothing is more frustrating to the deaf patient, and it soon causes the therapeutic process to break down.

There is a paradox in the communication issue because actually sign language, especially ASL, is a uniquely affective language and is thus in many respects ideal for therapy. True feelings are often revealed through the body language that is part of the signing process even when the linguistic interchange may be an evasion, an intellectualization, or other impediment to in-depth interaction. Of course, the transparency of true feelings is a two-way process. Therapy in sign language is also more revealing of the therapist's true feelings than is therapy conducted orally. This exposure can be threatening to the therapist.

One solution to the basic issue of communication with deaf patients is the training of deaf persons as psychologists, social workers, and psychiatrists. Unfortunately, there are only about 20 deaf psychologists in the United States today, although it is an increase from only 5 in 1979 (Brauer & Sussman, 1979). Only one of these is a fully qualified clinical psychologist.

Thus for deaf patients to be able to get the psychotherapy they need, not only must deaf therapists whose native language is ASL be trained, but hearing professionals must be helped to master ASL sufficiently well to serve deaf patients.

DREAMS AND HYPNOSIS

DREAMS

There have been two major studies of the dreams of deaf people (Mendelson, Siger, & Solomon, 1960; Sherman, 1970). The results are conflicting. The former group studied deaf college students and found that their dreams were more vivid, involved more color, were more easily recalled, and occurred with greater frequency than those of hearing people. Sherman's (1970) study failed to replicate the results of Mendelson et al. (1960). In fact, Sherman found no essential differences in the dreams of hearing and deaf people except that there was less sound in deaf people's dreams.

The primary reason dreams are of interest is that according to psychoanalytic theory their content mirrors in a somewhat disguised way unconscious processes and feelings. If, as Altshuler (1978) and others have theorized, deaf people have less superego function then hearing people, it would follow logically that either they would dream less often because there would be less repressed material, or the content of their dreams would be less disguised. As is the case in so many areas of research in deafness, the definitive work is yet to be done.

HYPNOSIS

Hypnosis is sometimes used as a part of psychotherapy, but until 1966 there was no report of its use with deaf people. At that time two psychiatrists (Martorano & Orestreicher, 1966) at the Rockland State Hospital Unit for the Deaf tried it on 10 deaf patients and 2 deaf ward staff. They used a machine with a black and white spiraling design on a rotating 6-inch disc for the patient to focus on visually. Communication was in sign language, with the hypnotist signing beside the rotating disc in the periphery of the deaf subject's vision. Of the 12, two developed a hypnoidal state with closed eyes and complete physical relaxation. One developed a light trance. Dehypnotization from the deep trance state proved to be a problem. It was necessary to shake the arms of the two patients, after which they responded satisfactorily.

This study indicates that hypnosis can be induced without auditory input. Thus it does offer an approach to helping deaf people. Since 1966, however, no one has reported any further use of hypnosis with deaf people.

OTHER PROBLEMS OF SERVICE DELIVERY

CATCHMENT AREA CONCEPT AND DEAF PATIENTS

A major impediment to the effective treatment of deaf patients in a state hospital/ community mental system is the catchment area concept so much in vogue today. In essence this concept says that patients should be grouped with others from their same geographic area and that hospitals and outpatient treatment centers should be as near the patient's home as possible.

The concept works directly against the deaf patient for three reasons. First, it means that he or she is likely to be isolated from other deaf patients when hospitalized. As was already indicated, this system results in essentially anti-therapeutic custodial isolation. Secondly, spreading deaf patients throughout a hospital-community mental health system precludes the training and use of specialists competent in sign language who can work with deaf patients. Obviously, every ward nurse, every ward attendant, and every ward psychiatrist in an entire state system cannot master sign language and learn to work with deaf patients. Finally, the deaf patient's community is the deaf community outside the hospital and the specialized delivery system for this community (ministers to the deaf, vocational rehabilitation specialist for the deaf, etc.).

Thus deaf patients and the deaf community should be seen as a catchment area and specialized services provided. The model plan described earlier has already been implemented in about 14 states and needs to be established throughout the United States.

DEAF COMMUNITY'S ATTITUDE TOWARD MENTAL HEALTH

The average deaf person associates mental health services with the treatment of insanity (Galloway, 1968). Even the signs used for mental health connote this association. Thus, except in cases of a complete breakdown, most deaf persons will not avail themselves of therapy or counseling unless they are specifically taught differently. They are far more likely to seek help for marriage problems, behavioral disorders, and psychological disturbances in general from a deaf person more educated than themselves, a hearing family member, or a pastor (Galloway, 1968).

There is also a tendency in the deaf community to adopt a punitive or at least a negative attitude toward those deaf persons who have been treated for a mental illness. Of course, this attitude compounds the problem of delivery of mental health services.

REFERENCES

Altshuler, K. A. (1978). Toward a psychology of deafness. *Journal of Communication Disorders, 11,* 159–169.

Basilier, T. (1964). Surdophrenia: The psychic consequences of congenital or early acquired deafness. Some theoretical and clinical considerations. *Acta Psychiatrics Scandinavia, 40* (1981). (Suppl. 180), 362–374.

Bonham, H. E., Armstrong, T. D., and Bonham, G. M. (1981). Group psychotherapy with deaf adolescents. *American Annals of the Deaf, 126,* 806–809.

Brauer, B. A., & Sussman, A. E. (1979). Experiences of deaf therapists and deaf clients. Paper given at American Psychological Association Convention.

Brown, J. D., & Giangreco, C. J. (1983). Iowa's parent–infant institute. *American Annals of the Deaf, 128,* 425–428.

Cantor, D. W., & Spragins, A. (1977). Delivery of services to the hearing impaired child in the elementary school. *American Annals of the Deaf, 122,* 330–336.

Chess, S., & Fernandez, P. (1980). Neurologic damage and behavior disorders in rubella children. *American Annals of the Deaf, 125,* 998–1001.

Chess, S., Fernandez, P., & Korn, S. (1978). Behavioral consequences of congenital rubella. *Journal of Pediatrics, 93,* 699–703.

Cohen, B. K. (1980). Emotionally disturbed hearing-impaired children: A review of the literature. *American Annals of the Deaf, 125,* 1040–1047.

Curtis, M. A. (1976). Counseling in schools for the deaf. *American Annals of the Deaf, 121,* 386–388.

Degrell, R. E., & Ouellette, S. E. (1981). The role and function of a counselor in residential schools for the deaf. *American Annals of the Deaf, 126,* 64–68.

Denmark, J. (1973). The education of deaf children. *Hearing, 70,* 3–12.

Freeman, R. D., Malkin, S. F., & Hastings, J. O. (1975). Psychosocial problems of deaf children and their families: A comparative study. *American Annals of the Deaf, 120,* 391–403.

Galloway, V. H. (1968). Mental health: What it means to a deaf person. In K. Z. Altshuler &

J. D. Rainer (Eds.), *Mental health and the deaf: Approaches and prospects.* Washington, DC: Department of Health, Education and Welfare.

Gentile, A., & McCarthy, B. (1973). *Additional handicapping conditions among hearing impaired students, United States, 1971–1972.* Washington, DC: Gallaudet College, Office of Demographic Studies.

Goulder, T. J. (1976). The effects of the presence or absence of being labeled emotionally/behaviorally disturbed on classroom behaviors of hearing impaired children, ages 7–13. Unpublished doctoral dissertation, American University, Washington, DC.

Goulder, T. J., & Trybus, R. J. (1977). *The classroom behavior of emotionally disturbed hearing impaired children.* Washington, DC: Gallaudet College, Office of Demographic Studies.

Graham, P., & Rutter, M. (1968). Organic brain dysfunction and child psychiatric disorder. *British Medical Journal, 3,* 695–700.

Grinker, R. R., Sr. (Ed.), (1969). Psychiatric Diagnosis, Therapy, and Research on the Psychotic Deaf. Final Report, Grant No. R. D. 2407 S. Social & Rehabilitation Service, Department of Health, Education and Welfare. (Available from Dr. Grinker, Michael Reese Hospital 2959 S. Ellis Ave., Chicago, IL 60612).

Hicks, E. E. (1970). Comparison of profiles of rubella and non-rubella deaf children. *American Annals of the Deaf, 115,* 86–92.

Hirshoren, A., & Schnittjer, D. J. (1979). Dimensions of problem behavior in deaf children. *Journal of Abnormal Child Psychology, 7,* 221–228.

Hirshoren, R. S., & Rothrock, I. A. (1972). Behavior problems of deaf children and adolescents: A factor analytic study. *Journal of Speech and Hearing Research, 15,* 93–104.

Lane, H. (1976). *The Wild Boy of Aveyron.* Cambridge, MA: Harvard University Press.

Lane, H., & Pillard, R. (1978). *The wild boy of Burundi.* New York: Random House.

Levine, E. S. (1971). Mental assessment of the deaf child. *The Volta Review, 73,* 80–105.

Levine, E. S. (1981). *The ecology of early deafness: Guides to fashioning environments and psychological assessments.* New York: Columbia University Press.

Levine, E. S., & Wagner, E. E. (1974). Personality patterns of deaf persons: An interpretation based on research with the hand test. *Perceptual and Motor Skills Monograph Supplement, 39,* 23–44.

Martorano, J. T., & Orestreicher, C. (1966). Hypnosis of the deaf mentally ill: A clinical study. *American Journal of Psychiatry, 123,* 605–606.

Meadow, K. P. (1980). *Deafness and child development.* Berkeley: University of California Press.

Mendelson, J. H., Siger, L., & Solomon, P. (1960). Psychiatric observations on congenital and acquired deafness: Symbolic and perceptual processes in dreams. *American Journal of Psychiatry, 116,* 883–888.

Mindel, E. & Feldman, U. (1987). The impact of deaf children on their families. In *They Grow in Silence.* E. Mindel & M. Vernon (eds.) Silver Spring, MD: National Association of Deaf.

Mindel, E. D., & Vernon, M. (1971). *They grow in silence..* Silver Spring, MD: National Association for Deaf Press.

Montgomery, G. (Ed.). (1978). *Deafness personality and mental health.* Edinborough: Scottish Workshop Publication.

Naiman, D. (1972). A model for in-service training of afterclass personnel. *American Annals of the Deaf, 117,* 438–439.

Norden, K. (1975). *Psychological studies of deaf adolescents.* Studia Psychologic et Paedagogica (Series Altera XXIX). Malmo, Sweden: Berlingska Boktryckeriet, Lund.

Rainer, J. D., & Altshuler, K. Z. (1971). A psychiatric program for the deaf: Experiences and implications. *America Journal of Psychiatry, 127,* 1527–1532.

Rainer, J. D., Altshuler, K. Z., Kallmann, F. J., & Deming, W. E. (1963). *Family and mental health problems in a deaf population.* New York: New York State Psychiatric Institute.

Robinson, L. E. (1978). *Sound minds in a soundless world.* (DHEW Publication No. ADM 77-560). Washington, DC: U.S. Government Printing Office.

Rodda, M. (1969). *Social adjustment of deaf adolescents* (Occasional Paper No. 3). London: Royal National Institute for the Deaf.

Rubkin, J. G. (1979). Ethnic density and psychiatric hospitalization: Hazards of minority status. *American Journal of Psychiatry, 136,* 1562–1566.

Schlesinger, H. S., & Meadow, K. R. (1972). *Sound and sign: Childhood deafness and mental health.* Berkeley: University of California Press.

Sherman, W. (1970). Dreams of deaf people. *Journal of Rehabilitation of the Deaf, 4,* 54–63.

Smith, G. M. L. (Ed.). (1963). *The psychiatric problems of deaf children and adolescents.* London: The National Deaf Children's Society.

Spitzer, R. L. (Ed.). (1980). *Diagnostic and statistical manual of mental disorders* (p. 195). Washington, DC: American Psychiatric Association.

Spitzer, R. L. (Ed.). (1987). *Diagnostic and statistical manual of mental disorders.* Washington, DC: American Psychiatric Association.

Stein, L. K., Mindel, E. D., & Jaboley, T. (Eds.). (1981). *Deafness and mental health.* New York: Grune & Stratton.

Trott, L. A. (1984). Providing school psychological services to hearing-impaired students in New Jersey. *American Annals of the Deaf, 129,* 319–323.

Tully, N. L. (1970). *Role concepts and functions of rehabilitation counselors with the deaf.* Doctoral dissertation, University of Arizona.

Vernon, M. (1969). *Multiply handicapped deaf children: Medical, educational and psychological considerations.* Research Monograph. Reston, VA: Council of Exceptional Children.

Vernon, M. (1976). The importance of early diagnosis. *Medical Opinion, 5,* 34–41.

Vernon, M. (1978). Deafness and mental health: Some theoretical views. *Gallaudet Today, 9,* 9–13.

Vernon, M. (1980). Perspectives on deafness and mental health. *Journal of Rehabilitation of the Deaf, 13,* 9–14.

Williams, C. E. (1970). Some psychiatric observations on a group of maladjusted deaf children. *Journal of Child Psychology and Psychiatry, 11,* 1–18.

Zakarewsky, G. T. (1979). Patterns of support among gay lesbian deaf persons. *Sexuality and Disability, 2,* 178–191.

CHAPTER 8
Deafness and Mental Illness: Categories of Nonpsychotic and Psychotic Behaviors

Nature is nowhere accustomed more openly to display her mysteries than in cases where she shows traces of her workings apart from the beaten path; nor is there any better way to advance the proper practice of medicine than to open our minds to the discovery of the normal law of nature by the careful investigation of rarer forms of disease.　　　　　*William Harvey*

One way to better understand psychological aspects of deafness is to use the "medical" model described above. By examining extremes of adjustment pathology, that is, mental illness, in the deaf population it is possible to draw inferences about normal coping behaviors used by deaf people.

First, one must realize that society usually responds inappropriately to the needs of deaf people and to the reality of deafness. Such response is the cause for a significant amount of the psychopathology seen in deaf people. Furthermore, certain normal coping responses by deaf persons are misconstrued as abnormal by the general public. The purpose of this chapter is to examine categories of nonpsychotic and psychotic behaviors in the deaf population.

CATEGORIES OF NONPSYCHOTIC MENTAL ILLNESS

In behavioral disorders of less severity than psychosis, differences between hearing and deaf people do appear. While not dramatic, they are nonetheless significant.

DISORDERS USUALLY EVIDENT IN INFANCY, CHILDHOOD, OR ADOLESCENCE

Two disorders usually first evident in youth for which there are some data comparing deaf and hearing people are mental retardation and attention deficit disorder. Two others, autism and severe organic brain syndromes, are covered later, in the section on psychosis.

Mental Retardation
While there is extensive evidence that IQ is not directly affected by hearing loss, some etiological groups of deaf children have higher prevalences of mental retardation (Vernon, 1969; also chapter 3). One group, the genetically deaf, have less retardation and higher mean IQs than the general population (Brill, 1963). The

end result is that IQs for the deaf and the hearing are, in general, similarly distributed. Deafness per se has no effect on intelligence. The major difficulty is that mental retardation is often misdiagnosed in deaf people because of their deficiency in English, the examiner's incompetence in sign language, the strange sounds made by the deaf person, inappropriate tests, and other factors (see chapter 6). It is of major importance that deaf patients not be labeled as retarded unless psychological testing has been conducted with the correct instruments by a psychologist experienced with deafness.

Attention Deficit Disorders

Because of the brain damage or endocrine disorders associated with most of the major etiologies of deafness in children (rubella, genetics, meningitis, etc.), there is an overall higher prevalence of attention deficit disorders. They are often associated with hyperactivity (Levine & Wagner, 1974; Vernon, 1969). Data on the rates of such disorders are not available in specific percentages, but the higher prevalence has been clearly established (Vernon, 1969).

SUBSTANCE USE DISORDERS

There are no patterns of substance abuse among deaf people that seem distinctly different from those found in the hearing population. For example, schools and colleges for deaf youth have problems controlling the use of alcohol, Cannabis (marijuana), cocaine, phencyclidine (PCP), heroin, amphetamines, barbituates, and similar substances, just as do regular schools and colleges.

There are deaf drug pushers who deal in large volumes and who sell to deaf and hearing users. A number of these pushers with whom the first author has had contact are bright sociopathic-type individuals with tremendous underlying hostility. One was a marginal college student who repeatedly got his brother "rehooked" after the latter had gone through drug rehabilitation. This pusher actively tried to get his mother to become a user.

In Washington there are several deaf prostitutes, one a young boy, or "chicken," who sells himself to older homosexual males. These prostitutes use drugs so heavily that there is no other way they can support their habit than through selling illicit sex. In the violent world of commercial sex and drugs, these deaf individuals are relatively defenseless. Within a period of five or at most ten years, most are dead from homicide, accidental overdose, suicide, or health problems related to substance abuse, such as liver disease.

Because of the communication problems of deafness, the deaf drug user is more vulnerable to overdoses, buying toxic drugs, and other dangers related to drugs. He does not readily pick up the street knowledge passed by word of mouth which is basic to survival in the drug culture.

There are also no data on deafness and alcoholism (Rothfeld, 1981). Existing data are conflicting. Rainer & Altshuler (1971) report that among deaf organically psychotic patients there were fewer alcoholics than in the general population of organic psychotics; among the hearing almost all organically psychotic patients were alcoholic. Hooten (1978) reports that one out of seven deaf people is alcoholic as contrasted to one out of ten in the general population. However, Hooten offers no documentation for these figures.

The first author's own clinical experience over a 25-year period suggests that drinking problems occur about equally among the deaf and hearing. However, only in a few of the large urban areas are there programs for deaf alcoholics. Whereas Hooten (1978) sees isolation, underemployment, and stress as factors leading to alcoholism among deaf subjects, Altshuler and Rainer (1970) feel that the lack of depression reduces the probability of drinking problems among deaf people.

The abuse of drugs and alcohol is especially prevalent among deaf youths who try to succeed in regular mainstreaming programs with hearing students, especially if the youth finds himself with only a very few or no other deaf students. In these settings, the deaf student often finds social acceptance only among marginal hearing students who have been rejected themselves and who are involved in drug and alcohol abuse. The following psychological evaluation describes a case of substance abuse.

Mr. X was referred for psychological evaluation to see if alcoholism had affected his cognitive functioning.

Mr. X is congenitally genetically deaf and has deaf parents and siblings. He attended a state residential school for the deaf until his junior year but was dismissed for drinking and behavior problems. Because Mr. X was an outstanding athlete and had ambitions for college, the dismissal was traumatic. Following school, Mr. X became more deeply involved in drugs and alcohol and was incarcerated several times. Between jailings there was sporadic employment at common labor. At home there was increasing friction with his parents, particularly his father, including fighting.

After much help from the Division of Vocational Rehabilitation, Mr. X was sent to the St. Paul Technical Vocational Institute (TVI), where he learned body and fender work. At TVI Mr. X functioned satisfactorily in class but had fights due to alcohol and drug use. When he returned home, he worked as a body and fender man and also had other kinds of jobs. However, drug and alcohol abuse, family friction, and his basic attitude resulted in frequent absenteeism (for example, he might show up the first three days on a job then be gone a week), and led to firings. The most recent problem had occurred in a night club when a policeman, not realizing Mr. X was deaf, warned him verbally to stop his wild behavior. When he did not comply, the policeman used force and a fight resulted. Mr. X. was sent to a state mental hospital for an evaluation.

Mr. X was brought to the current evaluation by his rehabilitation counselor. His appearance has changed considerably over the last three years. He is now puffy, overweight, and less responsive to questions. However, he retains a basic capacity to relate to others, although with some defensiveness. Anxiety level is high, as evidenced by chronic nail biting, smoking, and muscular tension. Mr. X is fluent in manual communication but does not use speech nor lipread. Reading and overall educational level is estimated to be fifth to sixth grade. At the time of testing he was on psychotropic medication.

Administration of the WAIS Performance Scale yielded an IQ of 107 with excessive subtest scatter. His Ravens Matrices percentile was also in the average range. However, the quality of his responses and certain high subtest scores (e.g., Block Design Scaled Score of 14) indicated Bright Normal intelligence (IQ 110–119). His work habits reflect a lack of determination, impulsiveness, and low frustration tolerance.

The Minnesota Paper Form Board Test and his WAIS subtest pattern indicated spatial perception (used in drafting, body and fender work, art, etc.) as being in the upper 10 percent compared with factory workers his age. Drawings also indicated good artistic potential.

Interviewing, case history, and projective testing (Draw-A-Person and Bender-Gestalt) gave clear indisputable evidence of an addictive personality. Defensiveness is of such intensity that there is little or no insight and an almost total psychological denial or projection of his problems. Compounding the pathology is his family situation: An older brother repeatedly encourages alcohol and drug use (and supplies these substances), and his father continual reminds Mr. X of his current and past failings. Thus the family triggers his substance abuse, activates his acute feelings of failure, and in general exascerbates his pathology.

Bender-Gestalt and WAIS protocols gave no clear evidence of brain damage affecting visual motor function. However, mental status-type questioning in sign language revealed a slight diminishing of some higher cognitive functioning such as short-term memory, flexibility of thought pattern, and overall alertness. It is not possible to determine the extent to which this represents early stages of Karsachov's syndrome or effects of medication which he had taken shortly before testing.

In sum, Mr. X is an addictive personality. At the current stage of his alcoholism and drug use he is unable to admit the degree of his problem and is now rejecting his need for antibuse. Until he acknowledges his addictiveness and seeks help (antibuse and therapy), the prognosis is totally negative for employment and basic rehabilitation.

ANXIETY DISORDERS

These disorders include phobias, obsessive-compulsiveness, anxiety states, and posttraumatic stress disorders. All are found among deaf people, and clinical impressions suggest that they exist there in about the same proportion among the hearing. Posttraumatic stress disorders may be a little more common, as a consequence of either late onset deafness or the loss of a parent. Disorders due to the latter usually occur in unmarried deaf adults who have had a lifelong dependency on their parents. When the parents die, the deaf persons are often left totally alone, frightened, depressed, and helpless. Frequently such individuals, although not psychotic, are committed to state hospitals in lieu of appropriate available alternatives.

SOMATOFORM DISORDERS

Somatoform disorders consist of physical symptoms, such as backache or stomach pains, for which there is no apparent organic basis. They are caused by psychological factors but are not under voluntary control, as in the case of malingerers. Basically, these disorders represent a somewhat immature defense mechanism. In the first author's clinical experience, he has found that these disorders are as common among the deaf as among the hearing, but there exist no research data to substantiate this fact. It was Grinker's view (1969) that because deafness closes out much sensory input, there is a greater internal focus on body functions, resulting in increased somatoform disorders.

The somatoform disorders of functional deafness and hearing loss deserve attention. In England (Denmark & Eldridge, 1969) it was found that 3 out of 170 cases of deaf patients in British mental hospitals were functionally deaf. One was a case of Munchausen's syndrome, a condition typified by people who habitually present themselves to hospitals with different psychogenic diseases.

The most common form of functional deafness involves those with a childhood history of middle ear infections resulting in variable and essentially temporary loss of hearing. In some cases the secondary gains from these losses (more attention, staying home from school, preferential seating, etc.) may lead the individual to "become hard of hearing," that is, experience a conversion hearing disorder. Generally these are not rigidly fixed states and can be dealt with by appropriate audiological testing and brief counseling. Getz (1955), Vernon (1969), and Malmo, Davis, & Barza (1952) report cases of functional deafness that are part of overall severe adjustment problems such as autism.

Cases in which there is a complete severe conversion disorder are reported by Knapp (1948, 1953), and the first author has seen them in his own work. Such patients are difficult to treat. The following case reports illustrate the problem.

Jeffrey C. was 13 years old and ill when suddenly he complained that he could not hear. After all efforts at treatment had failed, Jeffrey was transferred to a residential school for the deaf. From there he went, at a young age, to a college for the deaf. There pathological drinking and gambling on his part led to dismissal. However, after transferring to a college for hearing students, Jeffrey was able eventually to complete graduate school and become employed as a laboratory scientist in a hospital. Through a pathologist friend and drug user, Jeffrey was able to get narcotics. Being an addictive personality, he was soon abusing opiates. Finally he overdosed. Found at the point of death, he was taken to a hospital, where he recovered. Psychotherapy was ordered. The therapist used a sodium pentothal interview, and under this medication, with Jeffrey's defenses down, it was discovered that he had normal hearing. When confronted bluntly with this fact (a terrible therapeutic error), the confrontation compounded other problems and led to his suicide.

Lyman H. had "lost" his hearing at age 15. Now 17 and totally rejecting his own deafness, Lyman was an obvious misfit in a school for the deaf. In addition, he strongly identified with the Nazis, although he had a Jewish girlfriend. Obviously bright, he easily passed the entrance exams for college. During the summer before starting college he was hypnotized, and in the hypnotic state he was able to understand speech with no difficulty. The hypnotist ended the session, never told Lyman what happened, and refused to see him again. Once out of the "trance," Lyman reverted to his functional deafness. He went on to a college for the deaf, graduated, and was employed by a large corporation, still "deaf." Over the years he became increasingly paranoid, left his job, and started to badger lawyers to sue a multitude of people as well as the corporation, all of whom he perceived were "against him."

In both of these cases the individual had a severe underlying disturbance which manifested, in part, as a conversion disorder. Each professed a total deafness, which made routine audiological detection of the functional nature of the disorder unlikely, although impedence measures or brain stem techniques would have revealed normal hearing.

A key factor in treatment is that a defense as drastic as a conversion disorder deafness should never be taken away from a patient until psychotherapy has prepared the individual for the loss of this defense. A failure to recognize this fact in the case of Jeffrey led to his suicide.

DISSOCIATION DISORDERS

This category includes amnesias, fugue states, multiple personality, and depersonalization. There is no information in the literature on deafness that gives specific prevalence rates for these disorders. In 30 years of clinical work with deaf patients, the first author has seen amnesias, fugues, and multiple personalities only as dimensions of psychotic disorders. In such cases the appropriate primary diagnosis is the psychosis, not the dissociative disorder.

Depersonalization independent of a psychotic illness is seen in deaf people. It involves ego alien feelings, that is, the individuals feel self-estrangement. They may think that their extremities have changed in size or that these extremities are functioning mechanically, as if in a dream. Such feelings in deaf patients are most common in adolescence.

PSYCHOSEXUAL DISORDERS

There are not a lot of data on sexual adjustment among deaf people. Just like the hearing, most marry and have children, although there is a somewhat higher rate of single persons among the deaf (Schein & Delk, 1974). There is also considerably less sexual knowledge, especially among deaf youth (Altshuler, 1978; Fitzgerald & Fitzgerald, 1978; Grinker, 1969; Shaul, 1981). This lack of information sometimes leads to naive behavior and self-destructive experimentation.

Gender Identity Disorders

Persons with this disorder have an incongruence between anatomic sex and gender identity. For example, they may deny their gender or they may want to be surgically changed from a male to a female or vice-versa.

Transexualism

Transexualism does occur among deaf persons. With rare disorders such as this, there are little or no reliable prevalence data for the hearing and none for the deaf. However, the following case illustrates the disorder in a deaf patient.

> Carlton R. is a deaf adolescent with deaf parents and siblings. He was dismissed from a residential school for deaf youth for repeatedly dressing in women's clothing. Later Carlton was caught shoplifting female items from a store and he is currently under court jurisdiction for this. He frequently goes to New York City to interact with transexual friends there, and from them he learned about sex change surgery. He is now trying to make arrangements for this to be done

when he becomes of age. Repeated efforts at psychotherapy have failed to alter his transexual pattern, but the family refuses to accept him as a girl. They forbid his cross-dressing and use of cosmetics. The result is continual friction in the home. Recently he has obtained a Civil Service job and moved out of the home. Without the active conflict situation with his parents and the school, Carlton is able to dress and act appropriately while working and he can restrict his transexual behavior to settings where it creates fewer adjustment problems.

Paraphilias

Transvestism is similar in some ways to transexualism, but the transvestite does not have a wish to have anatomically the genitals of the opposite sex, nor is the person homosexual. The major feature is an intense need to cross-dress. Sexual excitement is felt as part of this process. Transvestism is seen in deaf persons. One patient with whom the first author has had contact came from a family in which the father practiced bondage with his wife. The deaf son, who also had Usher's syndrome, practiced clandestine transvestism starting early in adolescence.

Other paraphilias such as fetishism, pedophilia, exhibitionism, voyeurism, masochism, and sadism occur fairly often in the general population. In the first author's clinical experience these paraphilias seem to be present at about the same rate among deaf people. No research data exist on the prevalence rates. The same is true of the number of cases of psychosexual dysfunctions and other psychosexual disorders.

Lately the treatment methods of Masters and Johnson have been brought to the field of deafness, primarily by Fitzgerald and Fitzgerald (1978). There is also an increase in sex education in residential schools for deaf children, which may help resolve some of the adjustment problems that exist.

FACTITIOUS DISORDERS

Factitious disorders are characterized by physical or psychological symptoms that are "made up" by the patient and are under voluntary control. For example, the individual may study the symptoms of appendicitis and then present himself or herself to a surgeon with this disorder. Sometimes such patients are convincing enough to fool medical authorities, gain admission to hospitals, and be operated upon. The factitious disorder is different from malingering because there is no goal, that is, the individual does not invent a backache to get an insurance award.

The first author has never identified a factitious deaf patient nor read of one in psychological literature. However, such deaf patients probably exist, although the medical sophistication required for this disorder to be convincing is relatively rare in the deaf population.

GENERAL DISORDERS OF IMPULSE CONTROL

For years professionals have cited research and clinical evidence indicating impulsivity to be far more common among deaf than hearing people (Altshuler, 1978; Freeman, Malkin, & Hastings, 1975; Hess, 1960; Levine, 1956; Myklebust, 1960; Rainer, Altshuler, Kallmann, & Deming, 1963; Robinson, 1978). In fact, the term was used so often it almost seemed an intrinsic trait of deaf people. More definitive studies (Chess & Fernandez, 1980 a & b; Harris, 1976; Levine & Wagner, 1974; Vernon, 1969) have indicated that it is not deafness per se, but factors associated with deafness that create the problem in certain types of deaf persons. For example, impulsive behavior is a major symptom in multiple-handicapped prenatal rubella-deafened children (Chess & Fernandez, 1980 a & b) and a lesser but still significant problem among prenatal rubella-deafened children as a group (Chess & Fernandez, 1980 a & b; Vernon, 1969). In these individuals there is often an organic basis for the problem. Others (Harris, 1976; Levine & Wagner, 1974) have shown that when factors such as linguistic competence (primarily due to early exposure to sign language), high levels of academic achievement, or deaf parents are present, there is no more impulsiveness among the deaf than among the hearing population.

In sum, the research indicates that deafness does not directly cause impulsiveness. Instead, this trait seems more common than average only among certain subgroups of deaf people. In these groups, impulsiveness is due primarily to organic factors, especially those associated with rubella, and to a lack of language competence.

Clinically there are some other obvious reasons why a deaf person might tend to be impulsive. Whereas a hearing person driven by an impulse usually has many opportunities to discuss it with others and to work it through verbally without acting it out, the deaf person so afflicted does not. The latter often has no chance to "let off steam" verbally or get another viewpoint. Instead, the feelings tend to build up inside with no opportunity for catharsis or feedback through discussion. The result can be increasingly idiosyncratic thinking or an explosion or other impulsive acting-out reaction. The cause is not deafness per se, but the communication problem fostered by the failure of parents and other key individuals to learn sign language. As was indicated earlier, it is frequently acts of aggressive impulsiveness growing out of this kind of situation that precipitate confinement in a mental hospital for deaf patients.

Other impulse control problems such as pathological gambling, kleptomania, and pyromania, are seen among deaf patients but there are no data on prevalence rates. Clinical experience and research (Altshuler, Deming, Vollenweider, Rainer, & Tendler, 1976; Grinker, 1969; Robinson, 1978) indicate that explosive disorders may occur with more than average frequency.

ADJUSTMENT DISORDERS

This category refers to a maladaptive reaction to some major life stress. Deaf people are at least as susceptible to such disorders as others because of the added stresses created by deafness and because of the limitations deafness places on coping options.

In the diagnosis of adjustment disorders, the current emphasis is on the response: for example, adjustment disorder with depressed mood, or adjustment disorder with disturbance of conduct. This type of diagnosis is in contrast to the pre-DSM III period, when the stresses were the focus: for example, adjustment disorder to adolescence.

PSYCHOLOGICAL FACTORS AFFECTING PHYSICAL CONDITION

Certain physical conditions, such as epilepsy, some type of ulcers, rheumatoid arthritis, asthma, obesity, and others can be brought about or exacerbated by psychological factors. Clinical experience indicates that such precipitating stress factors definitely occur among deaf people. However, in these patients it is much more difficult to diagnose the underlying psychological factors because few physicians can communicate sufficiently well in sign language to be able to establish the dynamics involved. Thus there is an absence of research or other literature on the extent to which psychological factors affect physical conditions in deaf people.

PERSONALITY DISORDERS

When an individual's personality traits (habitual ways of perceiving, relating, and thinking) are maladaptive and inflexible in ways that significantly impair social or occupational functioning or cause subjective distress, the pathology is termed personality disorder (Spitzer, 1980). This is an important diagnostic category and will be examined in some detail.

Cluster I

Included in this group are Paranoid, Schizoid, and Schizotypal Disorders. Persons in these categories appear off or eccentric.

The Paranoid Personality Disorder deserves special attention because of the frequent references to "the paranoid deaf" in professional and lay literature. Even DSM III is guilty of this error (Spitzer, 1980), despite a lack of objective evidence in the literature showing that deaf people are paranoid.

Frequently deaf people are taken advantage of by hearing people. These experiences usually start with siblings, then peers, and later include job and business associates. Consequently, they have a reality-based suspiciousness of hearing people. Low educational levels (most read at about a fourth-grade level) and other disadvantages of deafness increase the deaf person's vulnerability to exploitation. Thus, to some degree, an attitude of suspiciousness is adaptive in those who are deaf. However, when the suspiciousness is pervasive, and the deaf person refuses to abandon it even when presented with convincing contradictory evidence, a Paranoid Personality Disorder is present. Clinical experience and research (Zimbardo & Anderson, 1981) indicate that the disorder is more common in the hard-of-hearing or in those who become hard-of-hearing or deaf later in life than among the congenitally deaf.

There *is* evidence that at a less than psychotic level more suspiciousness exists among deaf people (Knapp, 1948, 1953; Vernon, 1980). However, much of this suspicion is reality based, because hearing people do consistently take advantage of deaf people, talk about them in front of others, and, in general, exploit their own advantage of hearing. This practice starts in childhood with teasing, with using hearing to gain an unfair advantage in games like hide and seek, and it continues through life. For example, when the supervisor of food services approaches a group of kitchen workers and tells them someone must clean the grease trap, inevitably what is communicated to the deaf employee is that it is *his* assignment. Similarly, when the deaf person goes to buy a used car, he is often taken advantage of because he cannot hear the broken muffler roar or the defective piston slap against the cylinder wall. Obviously after years of these kinds of experiences deaf people become very leery of their hearing peers. The problem is compounded by the huge amounts of general information they miss and by the isolating aspects of deafness. The end result is that deaf people learn not to trust those who hear. Their scars are so deeply ingrained that even in close relationships between deaf and hearing people, trust by the deaf is slow to develop.

In understanding why deaf people would be more likely to have considerable suspiciousness, Grunebaum and Perlman's (1973) theory of paranoid thinking is helpful. In their view such thinking grows out of naiveté, that is, out of a misperception of the behavior of others. They also theorize that paranoids lack social skills. This deficiency in part grows out of habitually dealing with problems in solitude by brooding, puzzling, and ruminating. Individuals with such behavior patterns tend to turn to increasingly idiosyncratic frames of reference inconsistent with reality. All of us have had the experience of becoming angry with a person. As our anger mounts, we "build a case" against the offending individual, making him out to be, in our hostile fantasy, an ogre on whom we wreak horrendous hostility. All of this is done in righteous indignation. However, once we talk out the experience that caused the anger, we are brought back to reality. The deaf person is usually denied the opportunity for this verbal reality testing.

In Grunebaum and Perlman's theory, most paranoid thinkers suffer from huge gaps in their life experiences. These gaps lead to projection, confabulation, and other manners of defensive coping which then distort the interpretation of subsequent events. Granted the validity of this theory, it is certainly understandable why deaf people would develop suspiciousness. They have the requisite gaps in their life experiences, breakdowns in communication, and isolation, all of which contribute to paranoid thinking according to Grunebaum and Perlman's theory.

In the more widespread theory of paranoid thinking developed by Freud, the implications for deafness are different. Freud argues that the paranoid process has its basis in repressed homosexuality which is projected or denied in ways that lead to excessive suspiciousness and feelings of reference (everybody is looking at me). Associated with these dynamics is a perception of paranoia as a regression to a narcissistic level (Zeckel, 1942). Some research supports Freud's views (Wolowitz, 1971). While there is no strong evidence demonstrating more homosexuality or regression among deaf than among the hearing, there are data showing a greater degree of immaturity among those who are deaf.

Recent research on hearing losses of late onset indicates that these types of loss are related, at least to some degree, to paranoid ideation (Zimbardo & Anderson, 1981). This is especially true in the initial stages, when the loss is present but the individual is as yet unaware of it. In trying to interpret a world where people are saying things they cannot understand and are rejecting them socially, they understandably undergo an increase in anxiety and suspiciousness.

Schizoid personalities are characterized by chronic aloofness, coldness, and indifference to the feelings of others (e.g., praise or criticism) which are not due to psychosis. The Schizotypal disorder involves magical type thinking (magical thinking, telepathy, clairvoyance, etc.), ideas of reference, social isolation, vague and overelaborate speech, suspiciousness, coldness, undue social anxiety, and hypersensitivity.

Schizoid and Schizotypal Personality Disorders appear somewhat more frequently among rubella-deafened children (Vernon, 1969), and those of low birthweight (Vernon, 1969). Incidentally, low birthweight hearing children are also at risk for schizophrenia. Other than a slightly higher prevalence in these two etiological groups, no difference in prevalence has been reported for these disorders among the deaf than among the hearing.

Cluster II

Histrionic, Narcissistic, Antisocial, and Borderline Disorders comprise this cluster. Histrionic personalities are overly dramatic and reactive individuals who tend to be shallow, egocentric, vain, demanding, and dependent. Many are prone to manipulative suicidal threats. Clinically, this disorder appears to be quantitatively and qualitatively the same in deaf and hearing people, but research data are lacking.

Narcissism consists of a grandiose sense of self-importance or uniqueness, fantasies of unlimited success, a need for constant attention and praise, overreaction to either criticism or indifference from others, and interpersonal relationships involving little reciprocity and excessive expectations. The Narcissistic Disorder may be encountered more often in the deaf than in the hearing. However, narcissism in deaf patients generally results from their immaturity and naiveté rather than from the more typical psychodynamics. Antisocial Personality Disorders may differ slightly in deaf people because resentment over their deafness and society's response to it often plays a causative role. This is also one of the few disorders seen with some frequency in deaf children of deaf parents.

A common family pattern involves parents who exercise either too little discipline or discipline that is inconsistent and sometimes physically abusive. Even more important, these parents support their child in all altercations the child has with outside agencies of authority. For example, if the school punishes the child, the parents fault the school, support the child, and undermine the entire disciplinary effort. Similarly, should the police apprehend the child, the parents inevitably side with the child, demean the police, and help the child "beat the rap." Often the child's deafness is used to gain leniency. The end result is a child who has no respect for authority, is highly manipulative, feels immune from punishment, and most important, has little feeling of guilt or remorse.

The occurrence of such dynamics with hearing parents often indicates that they are acting out their guilt over having a deaf child. By defending their child, they feel that they are doing their duty. With deaf parents the dynamics are more often an acting out, through the child, of deep-seated resentment about their own deafness and their treatment at the hands of agencies, schools in particular, and hearing authority figures.

Psychiatrist Roy Grinker, Sr., who did extensive work on both the Borderline Personality Disorder (Grinker, Werble, & Drye 1977) and deaf mentally ill patients (Grinker, 1969), does not report seeing this illness among deaf patients. While there are numerous cases of deaf people with impulsiveness, rage responses, and other basic traits of the Borderline Disorder, the first author and his associates did not see any individuals during the three years of research at Michael Reese Hospital who met the full criteria for this disorder (Grinker, 1969). Nor is its presence noted in other research on deafness. Of course, its absence may be due to the newness of the diagnostic category and the diagnostic difficulty it poses rather than to its nonoccurrence in deaf people.

Cluster III

Avoidant Personality Disorder involves hypersensitivity to potential rejection, humiliation, or shame; an unwillingness to enter interpersonal relationships unless given certainty of acceptance; and low self-esteem. The social dynamics created by deafness result in a rather high prevalence of this disorder among deaf people. It is one of the causes of the isolation seen in many who are deaf.

Just as the psychodynamics of deafness contribute to Avoidant Personality Disorder, they also result in a higher than average rate of Dependent Personality Disorder (Grinker, 1969; Rainer, Altshuler, Kallmann, & Deming, 1963; Robinson, 1978). Many admissions to mental hospitals are deaf individuals who remained at home with their parents well into adulthood. Some worked in a family business in a token way. Many had never been employed. In this protected environment, such individuals are able to get by, but in a highly dependent or hostile dependent way. When their parents die or become too old to manage, the deaf person's total dependency comes to the attention of authorities and hospitalization is often recommended (Grinker, 1969). Many of these individuals are "closet people," hidden away from society and essentially unknown to anybody but the immediate family until parental death brings them to public attention.

Although the deaf population does have many compulsion traits, they do not have an especially high rate of Compulsive Personality Disorders. For example, the preoccupation with trivial details, rules, schedules, and the like that seems to dominate organizational functions of deaf people is a compulsive trait. Yet the full spectrum of such traits required for a person to be classified as a Compulsive Personality Disorder is no more common among deaf than among hearing people (Grinker, 1969; and Robinson, 1978).

The picture with Passive-Aggressive Personality Disorder is especially interesting. Because a deaf person often must respond to authority figures with whom he cannot communicate, frictions build up, there are misunderstandings, and resistances develop. Sometimes these are acted out in direct impulsive ways, such as tantrums, quitting a job without notice, striking a supervisor, or otherwise lashing out. However, in other instances the result is a Passive-Aggressive Personality Disorder. This is seen more in adults than children. Often it is found in those who as children were more direct and impulsive in their oppositionalism. Having found that direct acting out created more problems than it solved, they withdraw into passive compliance, beneath which there is subtle resistance, sometimes involving theft, alcoholism, minimal effort on the job, abuse of sick leave, and similar behaviors. These same behaviors are obviously seen in Passive-Aggressive hearing persons.

Now we turn to more severe personality disorders: those involving psychosis.

PSYCHOSES

Psychoses are mental disorders indicating a gross impairment in reality testing, in ability to think, to perceive the world, and to behave appropriately. Persons with such disorders often require hospitalization, at least for certain periods during their lifetime.

When we look at the research on psychotic disturbance among deaf people, the results are somewhat contradictory. In the sections, that follow, these findings will be carefully examined relative to the major psychotic disorders.

SCHIZOPHRENIA

Schizophrenic illness is generally characterized by hallucinations, delusions, disorganization of personality, and a breakdown in reality contact and cognitive function. It is the most common of all psychoses, accounting for about half of the patients in mental hospitals.

Most of the more thorough studies, especially those using North American diagnostic practices, find that the proportion of deaf hospital admissions for schizophrenia are about the same as for the hearing (Altshuler, 1978; Grinker, 1969; Rainer, Altshuler, Kallman, & Deming, 1963; Robinson, 1978; Vernon, 1978, 1980). However, both the North American studies and those of Central Europe and Scandinavia indicate that there are proportionately more deaf schizophrenics in mental hospitals (Basilier, 1964; Matzker, 1960; Remvig, 1969, 1972). The reason for this apparent discrepancy is that deaf patients tend to get little or no treatment and are frequently misdiagnosed as not only schizophrenic but also mentally retarded or paranoid. Thus they tend to be placed in the worst hospital wards. In addition, because no one can communicate with them, they often remain inpatients much longer even though their rate of admission corresponds to that of the hearing.

Some Central European and Scandinavian studies (Basilier, 1964; Denmark & Eldridge, 1969; Matzker, 1960; Remvig, 1969, 1972) indicate more schizophrenia among deaf people or a higher overall rate of hospital admissions. The reason for this may be the somewhat different standards used in Europe to diagnose schizophrenia.

The overall picture of schizophrenia derived from the above research and the consensus of the scientists who did it is that schizophrenia is essentially the same illness in deaf and hearing people. It occurs at about the same rate in both populations but, because of errors in diagnosis and lack of treatment, the deaf hospital patients tend to be more chronic than their hearing counterparts.

Current research from the field of general psychiatry strongly indicates that schizophrenia is, to a significant degree, a genetic biochemical disorder (Berger, 1978). These findings support the results of the New York Psychiatric Institute (Rainer & Altshuler, 1971), which indicated that the rate of schizophrenic siblings of deaf schizophrenics was about the same as that for siblings of hearing schizophrenics. Were environment the major causative agent of schizophrenia, the stresses of deafness would result in more deaf twins being schizophrenic where one of the pair could hear. Consequently, in addition to revealing something about schizophrenia in the deaf population, these data give strong support to the view that a major determinant of schizophrenia is not environmental but organic.

PARANOID DISORDERS

Paranoid disorders involve persistent delusions of being persecuted, feelings of grandiosity and reference, intense resentment, anger, delusional jealousy, and social isolation. Behaviors such as writing hate letters, complaining of imagined injustices, and frequent threatening of lawsuits are common. Paranoid disorders of a psychotic degree are relatively rare, but many psychoses do involve paranoid dimensions (Retterstöl, 1966). For example, about half of schizophrenics have feelings of grandiosity, reference, and elaborate paranoid thought patterns. They are diagnosed as having a paranoid form of schizophrenia, not paranoid disorders.

One of the oldest myths in psychological and psychiatric literature is that deaf people are paranoid, that is, overly suspicious. This has been found to be untrue in the sense that research shows no greater proportion of paranoia or paranoid schizophrenia among deaf than among hearing psychotics (Basilier, 1964; Grinker, 1969; Remvig, 1969, 1972; Robinson, 1978). Despite data to the contrary, the myth is so strong that the classic diagnostic manual, DSM III, indicates that deaf people are prime risks for paranoid disorders (Spitzer, 1980).

AFFECTIVE DISORDERS

Affective disorders are essentially disorders of emotion and feeling involving conditions such as depression, extreme euphoria, hyperactivity (mania), low self-esteem, and withdrawal.

There is some controversy in the research regarding the rate of depression among deaf people. It is the position of the New York Psychiatric group (Altshuler, 1971) that the guilt, reproach, and other forms of self-depreciation and self-hate which psychoanalysis feels are basic to depression are rare in deaf people. Their view is that the development of a strong superego (the "child" irrational conscience) occurs primarily through hearing parental and societal values and demands early in life. Most deaf children are not exposed to these societal pronouncements and parental admonitions. Thus there is less superego and little resulting depression. It is reported (Altshuler, 1971; Knapp, 1948, 1953) that even among involutional patients where depression is most common, the deaf involutional is more likely to be paranoid, anxious, agitated, or psychosomatic than depressed. However, the researchers did recognize what they termed "superficial" depression, especially over the fact of being deaf (Altshuler, 1971; Knapp, 1948, 1953).

Other researchers (Grinker, 1969; Remvig, 1969, 1972; Robinson, 1978) do not report depression as being any different qualitatively or quantitatively in the deaf population. The manic phase of manic depressive psychosis is seen in all hospital programs serving deaf patients.

ORGANIC PSYCHOSES AND PERVASIVE DEVELOPMENTAL DISORDERS

Organic brain disorders and pervasive developmental disorders as they relate to deafness and psychosis are explained in chapters 2 and 3. However, in brief, the major causes of deafness in children are also leading causes of brain damage: for example, meningitis, low birthweight, genetic syndromes, complications of Rh factor, prenatal rubella, and sexually transmitted diseases. Thus there are proportionately more chronic brain syndromes resulting in pervasive mental disorders and psychoses among the deaf than among the hearing. Autism is an example.

Autism

Autism is a psychosis involving pervasive lack of response to other people, gross deficits in language development, either no speech or pathological speech, and bizarreness. This most severe of all psychoses is clearly more common among persons deafened by prenatal rubella. The prevalence for the rubella group is 7.4 percent versus about 0.7 percent for the general population (Chess, 1977; Chess & Fernandez, 1980 a & b). In these children, autism is clearly an organic psychosis and not the result of poor parenting (Chess, 1977). However, in the Chess study, of 17 cases diagnosed at ages 2 to 5 years, 6 had recovered by the age of 8 or 9. Others not previously autistic became so. These findings by Chess (1977) yield two important conclusions. First, they establish the major cause of autism among deaf children to be rubella. Considering that an estimate of 12.5 percent of deaf students currently in school programs had prenatal rubella as their etiology of deafness and that their rate of autism is over 7 percent, the problem is obviously one of significant magnitude. One point of caution is needed in interpreting the data. Most of the autistic deaf children in the Chess study were also blind, mentally retarded, or otherwise severely multiply handicapped. Thus they would not have been in most regular school programs for deaf children, but in programs for the retarded or mentally ill or in separate programs for deaf-blind youth.

The second interpretation of Chess' longitudinal study offers a generalization that goes far beyond deafness. It clearly proves that autism can be caused organically. Theories about functional causes attributed to "refrigerator parents" and other parenting flaws, while not totally ruled out, are certainly tentative at best in view of Chess's findings. This point is a major consideration for those working with parents, who can be devastated by guilt over autism and financially crippled by the inappropriate parental psychotherapy growing out of such theories. Such a case is vividly represented by psychiatrist John Kysar (1968), who despite his professional status, was, as a parent of an autistic child, the victim of this kind of diagnostic and treatment error and exploitation.

Autism is not known to exist disproportionately among deaf people whose etiology is other than prenatal rubella. The first author has seen two deaf autistic youths where there was evidence that the etiology of the hearing loss was genetic. In one of the families both parents were deaf and there were three deaf children. However, in neither case could the added factor of prenatal rubella be ruled out. Yet these two cases raise the possibility of genetic syndrome involving hearing loss and autism.

Organic Factors

As was indicated earlier, many of the leading causes of deafness are also major etiologies of brain damage (Vernon, 1980). Some of this damage, such as encephalitis resulting from meningitis, can lead directly to chronic brain syndromes causing psychosis in and of itself. In almost any large state mental hospital there will be one or two deaf patients of this type. They are also found in hospitals for the retarded. Remvig's (1969, 1972) and Vernon's (1969) work have documented clearly the significance of organic psychoses that are associated with the causes of deafness.

These organic factors also play a more subtle role in mental disturbance among deaf people. Brain damage in itself is associated with a variety of other behaviors, such as increased impulsivity, short attention span, learning disability, rigidity, unstable emotionality, and hyperactivity. Such behaviors when compounded by deafness make life far more stressful and create added behavioral disturbances. Consequently, brain damage plays a major role in a variety of mental problems and common abnormal behaviors present in deaf people, and not only as a cause of chronic brain syndrome psychoses.

GENERAL FACTORS RELATED TO PSYCHOTIC ILLNESS IN DEAF PATIENTS

HALLUCINATIONS

Hallucinations are present in several mental disorders but are most common in schizophrenia. Evidence indicates that about half of deaf schizophrenics hallucinate (Rainer, Abdullah, & Altshuler, 1970). This is the same percentage as with hearing schizophrenics. They "hear" people talking about them, they "hear" the Devil telling them to do bad things, and so on. The hallucinations of deaf schizophrenics also involve sign language: Some deaf patients report that God signs to them.

Ross (1978) reports musical hallucinations in deaf people which tend to be permanent and which enable them to foretell the advent of wet weather in much the same way that people with arthritis can predict dampness. Thus the musical phenomenon seems to have a physiological base and may be related to tinnitus. Altshuler (1971) also proposes an organic cause for hallucinations but he adds that they can be induced by dreams too.

MISDIAGNOSIS

It is clear from chapter 6 that psychological misdiagnosis is a common problem with deaf patients. Among deaf psychotics, the difficulties are compounded a hundred-fold. For example, Denmark and Eldridge (1969) found that one-third of hospitalized deaf patients were misdiagnosed. Others have reported similar findings (Altshuler, 1971). Solely on the myth of "the deaf paranoid," many deaf patients are given this diagnosis with no factual basis.

The other most frequent diagnostic error is the assumption that the deaf psychotic patient is also mentally retarded, because of the problems with written English and with reading. For example, in the study of the New York State Mental Hospital system, for about one out of five deaf patients, there was added to the major diagnosis the label "with mental retardation"—for example, paranoid with mental retardation, or schizophrenic with mental retardation (Rainer, Altshuler, Kallmann, & Deming, 1963). Actually, only one of nine of these patients was mentally retarded when retested with appropriate instruments. The diagnosis of psychotic with mental retardation usually results in placement in a "chronic ward," where the subject receives relatively little treatment and the prognosis is assumed to be poor. Thus the application of such an incorrect label to a deaf person minimizes any hope for appropriate care.

Errors in diagnosis often come about because the written language and the general behavior of certain deaf patients are misinterpreted as psychotic. The writing of many perfectly sane deaf individuals is characterized by such syntactical confusions and incorrect uses of vocabulary that it may approximate the jumbled language of schizophrenics or those with other thought disorders. Similarly, the vocal sounds and gestural behavior of some people who are deaf often seem psychotically bizarre to naive diagnosticians.

Finally, deaf patients are often the victims of the projections of the psychologist, social worker, or psychiatrists making the diagnosis. Because communication is limited, it is often difficult to obtain the thorough data needed for accurate diagnosis. Thus the deaf person becomes a "neutral stimulus" analogous to a Rorschach Inkblot. The diagnostician tends to project his or her own repressed pathology onto such a patient rather than making an objective diagnosis. It has been said that if you read 20 psychological evaluations of deaf persons, all done by the same diagnostician, you may know little about the patients but will have a full understanding of the diagnostician's pathology.

ADMITTING SYMPTOMS

One point brought out in all of the research on psychosis and deafness is that impulsive aggressive acts and medical procedures are the major presenting symptoms or precipitating incidents leading to hospitalization (Altshuler, 1978;

Basilier, 1964; Grinker, 1969; Matzker, 1960; Rainer, Altshuler, Kallmann & Deming, 1963; Remvig, 1969, 1972; Robinson, 1978; Vernon, 1978, 1980). Deaf patients often lack the opportunity to talk through their stresses and gain insight and coping skills. Thus feelings build up to intensive levels which lead to explosive, impulsive acts and hospitalization. For example, Fred S. was a young deaf man who could not communicate with his parents because they did not know sign language. For years he had had a hostile-dependent relationship with them. Finally, one day finding himself at home alone, he vented his cumulative anger by destroying every antique in the house. The collection was worth hundreds of thousands of dollars and represented a lifetime of professional collecting and most of the family savings. Had he been able to vent his feelings in sign language, this tragedy could probably have been avoided.

The other factor frequently precipitating psychotic breaks is some critical medical problem, often one requiring surgery. Most deaf people have a history of negative experiences with doctors and hospitals. As children, they are often taken into surgery or undergo other painful and frightening medical procedures with no preparation, foreknowledge, or explanation. Doctors often fail to explain even to their adult deaf patients what they are going to do or why. Of course, the major reason for the problem is that most doctors and most families of deaf children cannot communicate adequately in sign language. The following case from the work at Michael Reese Hospital illustrates the problem (Grinker, 1969).

> A young deaf man was told by some gross "home" signs and pointing to get into the car, with no other explanation than that the family was going out to get some ice cream. Instead, they stopped at a hospital, where he was ushered into a room, still with no explanation other than that he would sleep there overnight. The family then left. The next morning the young man was taken into surgery to correct a double hernia, still with no explanation, with nobody around with whom he could communicate, and with no understanding of what had been done to him. When he awoke from anesthesia and discovered that major surgery had been performed in his genital area, his behavior became bizarre. Ten days later, when home, he became blatantly psychotic. This time his parents reacted to the need for hospitalization by gesturing that they were going to take him to town for a job. Instead, he was brought to a psychiatric hospital, put on an elevator, and then placed in a unit for severely disturbed patients.

AGE OF ONSET OF HEARING LOSS

There is agreement that in general when the deafness occurs later in life, the sense of loss is much more intense (Knapp, 1948, 1953; Pochapin, 1965; Vernon, 1980). For example, a middle-aged individual, already married and established in a career, who is struck by sudden deafness experiences an intense trauma over the loss of his hearing. By contrast, a child born deaf who has never know hearing rarely experiences this sort of acute grief. (See chapter 12 for a discussion of adjustment to a late onset hearing loss.)

When deafness occurs during the preschool, or even as late as the college years, if the deafened youth is transferred to a school program for deaf students, he learns sign language and establishes an identity as a deaf person. Under these circumstances the overall adjustment to deafness is usually satisfactory. Career and marriage are planned with the fact of deafness in mind. There is an initial intense shock and period of grief, but a new social and educational life emerges. Problems arise if these individuals reject their deafness, sign language, and other deaf people. Such rejection is a form of denial which ultimately leads to isolation and maladjustment.

By contrast, deafness acquired during postschool years frequently results in a total loss of one's existing career and a concomitant need to prepare for a new profession or job. Frequently, spouses find that living with a deaf person is a stressful and well-nigh unendurable experience. Such marriages often end in divorce. The overall consequence for the deaf individual is depression and isolation. Some reactions might be compulsiveness, anxiety, and hypochondrical states.

A different type of patient, but one of particular interest, is the individual who avoids stapedectomy (middle ear surgery to correct hearing loss). Such individuals share with many psychogenically deaf people a certain secondary gain from their hearing loss and a rigid fear of change (Stone, 1969). Surgeons selecting candidates for stapedectomy need to consider these and other psychological factors, because for some people, restoration of hearing results in depression (Draf, Draf, & Kley, 1972).

Although the picture yielded by research on deafness and psychosis is far from definitive, the basic conclusion is that most psychotic disorders are distributed in the deaf population in essentially the same proportion as among the hearing. The qualitative nature of the processes also seems identical. The exception is the category of organic psychoses and major developmental disorders, which are more common among deaf people.

The major implication of these findings for the field of mental health is the suggestion that the leading psychotic disorders may have an organic cause. If environment played the major role, so psychologically traumatic a condition as deafness would result in a different picture of psychosis in this population. Such is not the case.

REFERENCES

Altshuler, K. Z. (1971). Studies of the deaf: Relevance to psychiatric theory. *American Journal of Psychiatry, 127,* 1521–1526.

Altshuler, K. Z. (1978). Toward a psychology of deafness. *Journal of Communication Disorders, 11,* 159–169.

Altshuler, K. Z., Deming, W. E., Vollenweider, J., Rainer, J. D., & Tendler, R. (1976). Impulsivity and profound early deafness: A cross cultural inquiry. *American Anals of the Deaf, 121,* 331–345.

Altshuler, K. Z., & Rainer, J. D. (1970). Observations on psychiatric services for the deaf. *Mental Hygiene, 54,* 534–539.

Basilier, R. (1964). Surdophrenia: The psychic consequences of congenital or early acquired deafness. Some theoretical and clinical considerations. *Acta Psychiatrics Scandinavia, 40*(Suppl. 180), 362–374.

Berger, P. A. (1978). Medical treatment of mental illness. *Science, 200,* 974–981.

Brill, R. G. (1963). Deafness and the genetic factor. *American Anals of the Deaf, 108,* 359–372.

Chess, S. (1977). Follow-up report on autism in congenital rubella. *Journal of Autism and Childhood Schizophrenia, 7,* 69–81.

Chess, S., & Fernandez, P. (1980a). Impulsivity in rubella deaf children: A longitudinal study. *American Annals of the Deaf, 125,* 505–509.

Chess, S., & Fernandez, P. (1980b). Neurologic damage and behavior disorder in rubella deaf children. *American Annals of the Deaf, 125*(8), 998–1001.

Denmark, J. C., & Eldridge, R. W. (1969). Psychiatric services for the deaf. *Lancet, 14,* 259–262.

Draf, W., Draf, U., & Kley, W. (1972). Der operierte Schwerhorige. *Zeitschrift fur Laryngologic Rhinologie-Otologie und ihre Greuzgebiete, 51,* 351–354.

Fitzgerald, D., & Fitzgerald, M. (1978). Sexual implications of deafness. *Sexuality and Disability, 1,* 57–69.

Freeman, R. D., Malkin, S. F., & Hastings, J. O. (1975). Psychosocial problems of deaf children and their families: A comparative study. *American Annals of the Deaf, 120,* 391–405.

Getz, S. B. (1955). AL psychological aid in the diagnosis of deafness of emotional origin. *Annals of Otolaryngology, 61,* 217–219.

Grinker, R. R., Sr. (Ed.). (1969). Psychiatric diagnosis, therapy, and research on the psychotic deaf. Final report, Grant No. R.D. 2407 S. Social & Rehabilitation Service, Department of Health, Education and Welfare. (Available from Dr. Grinker, Michael Reese Hospital, 2959 S. Ellis Ave., Chicago, IL 60612).

Grinker, R. R., Sr., Werble, B., & Drye, R. (1977). *The borderline syndrome.* New York: Basic Books.

Grunebaum, H., & Perlman, M. S. (1973). Paranoia and naiveté. *Archives of General Psychiatry, 28,* 30–32.

Harris, R. I. (1976). The relationship of impulse control to parent hearing status: Manual communication and academic achievement in deaf children. Unpublished Doctoral Dissertation, New York University.

Hess, D. W. (1960). The evaluation of personality and adjustment in deaf and hearing children using a non-verbal modification of the Make-A-Picture Story (MAPS) Test. Unpublished doctoral dissertation, University of Rochester.

Hooten, K. J. (1978). Double handicap: The deaf alcoholic. *Vibrations, 6*(11), 9–10.

Knapp, P. H. (1948). Emotional aspects of hearing loss. *Psychosomatic Medicine, 10,* 203–222.

Knapp, P. H.(1953) The ear listening and hearing. *Journal of American Psychoanalytical Association, 1,* 672–689.

Kysar, J. E. (1968). The two camps in child psychiatry: A report from a psychiatrist-father of an autistic retarded child. *American Journal of Psychiatry, 125,* 141–147.

Levine, E. S. (1956). *Youth in a soundless world.* New York: New York University Press.

Levine, E. S., & Wagner, E. E. (1974). Personality patterns of deaf persons: An interpretation based on research with the Hand Test. *Perceptual and Motor Skills Monograph,* (Suppl. 4-V39).

Malmo, R., Davis, J. and Barza, S. (1952). Total hysterical deafness: An experimental case study. *Journal of Personality, 21,* 188–204.

Matzker, V. J. (1960). Schizophrenia and deafness. *Zeitschrift fur Laryngologic Rhinologie-Otologie, 39.*

Myklebust, H. (1960). *The psychology of deafness.* New York: Grune & Stratton.

Pochapin, S. W. (1965). Some emotional aspects of deafness. *Larynogascope, 75,* 57–64.

Rainer, J. D., Abdullah, S., & Altshuler, K. Z. (1970). Phenomenology of hallucinations in the deaf. In *Origins and mechanisms of hallucinations* (pp. 449–465). New York: Plenum Press.

Rainer, J. D., Altshuler, K. Z. (1971). A psychiatric program for the deaf: Experience and implications. *American Journal of Psychiatry, 127,* 1527–1532.

Rainer, J. D., Altshuler, K. Z., Kallmann, F. J., & Deming, W. E. (1963). *Family and mental health problems in a deaf population.* New York: New York State Psychiatric Institute.

Remvig, J. (1969). Deaf-mutism and psychiatry. *Acta Scandinavica, Supplementum 210,* Munksgaard, Copenhagen.

Remvig, J. (1972). Psychic deviations of the prelingual deaf. *Scandinavian Audiology, 1,* 35–42.

Retterstöl, N. (1966). *Paranoid and paranoic psychoses.* Springfield, IL: Charles Thomas.

Robinson, L. D. (1978) *Sound minds in a soundless world* (DHEW Publication No. ADM 77–560). Washington, DC: U.S. Government Printing Office.

Ross, E. D. (1978). Musical hallucinations in deafness revisited. *Journal of American Medical Association, 240,* 1716.

Rothfeld, P. (1981). Alcoholism treatment for the deaf: Specialized services for special people. *Journal of Rehabilitation of the Deaf, 14,* 14–17.

Schein, J. D., & Delk, M. T. (1974). *The deaf population of the United States.* Silver Spring, MD: National Association of the Deaf.

Shaul, S. (1981). Deafness and human sexuality: A developmental review. *American Annals of the Deaf, 126,* 432–439.

Spitzer, R. L. (Ed.). (1980). *Diagnostic and statistical manual of mental disorders* (3rd ed.). Washington, DC: American Psychiatric Association.

Stone, C. B. (1969). Deaf psychiatric patients who avoid stapedectomy. *Psychosomatics, 10,* 314–317.

Vernon, M. (1969). *Multiply handicapped deaf children: Medical educational and psychological considerations* (Research Monograph). Reston, VA: Council of Exceptional Children.

Vernon, M. (1978). Deafness and mental health: Some theoretical views, *Gallaudet Today, 9,* 9–13.

Vernon, M. (1980). Perspectives on deafness and mental health. *Journal of Rehabilitation of the Deaf, 13,* 9–14.

Wolowitz, H. M. (1971). The validity of the psychoanalytic theory of paranoid dynamics. *Psychiatry, 34,* 358–377.

Zeckel, A. (1942). Research possibilities with the deaf. *American Annals of the Deaf, 87,* 173–191.

Zimbardo, P. G., & Anderson, S. M. (1981). Induced hearing deficit generates experimental paranoia. *Science, 212,* 1529–1531.

CHAPTER 9
Attitudes and Deafness: The Authoritarian Personality and Other Prejudicial Attitudes

Anti-Semitism has nothing to do with Jews.
Leo Lowenthal, "The Authoritarian Personality"

The most significant aspect of any human being, his *self-concept,* is formed primarily by the attitudes people have toward him (Vash, 1981). Thus the deaf person's attitude about his deafness and about himself is in large measure determined by the feelings the handicap arouses in hearing persons, especially parents and teachers. This chapter examines the authoritarian personality and other prejudicial attitudes which adversely affect deaf people.

THE AUTHORITARIAN PERSONALITY

Attitudes toward deaf people and prejudicial attitudes in general are determined largely by the emotions, needs, and fears of human beings, not by their reason. Lowenthal's statement above makes the same basic point: attitudes arise more from the personality structure of the individual making the judgment than from characteristics of the ethnic, political, or disability group toward which they are directed. Read, for example, the following case history.

A. H. was raised in a rigidly strict family, where he was subjected to corporal punishment. In A. H.'s home, father's word was law. Any questioning or discussion of this authority was forcefully squashed. A. H.'s parents were socially conscious, status-seeking, middle-class people.

Religion loomed as a club over A. H.'s head. For example, he was frequently threatened that if he did not love and respect his parents, God would be angry and he might go to hell. Consequently, he became highly anxious and fearful about the possibility of going to hell because of some particular thought or act he may have directed against his parents. Later in life A. H. thought about becoming a priest, but then he changed ideologies, maintaining that Christianity was for weaklings.

A. H.'s father made certain that his son would grow up to be a "man" by teaching him boxing, hunting, and other so-called manly pursuits. During these boxing sessions A. H. was often pummeled unmercifully and would fearfully plead with his father to stop. His father berated him about how horrible it was to be such a sissy weakling; he indicated that real men do not cry and forced

A. H. to continue fighting. In an effort to please his father and prove himself a man, A. H. would fight back his tears and continue to box. For this he was highly praised. Later he taught boxing to younger neighborhood children. When they cried, A. H. would lecture them even as his father had lectured him.

The lectures of A. H.'s father also dealt extensively with the problem of unemployed people. They were all seen as lazy, shiftless bums living off the state. References to them were filled with hostility and descriptions in subhuman terms.

Sex was taboo in A. H.'s home. However, A. H. knew that it was important to play the stereotyped male role. He learned to call nonmasculine boys sissies or fags. He was told that it was commendable to tease them and beat them up.

Despite a veneer of conformity, A. H. felt tremendous inner frustration and rage. This hostility grew out of his rigidly strict parental discipline. However, it was frantically repressed because, had it ever come out, it would have resulted in more parental physical punishment, increased admonishments to "honor thy father and mother," and more threats of eternal damnation. Consequently, A. H. appeared to be a very respectful child and always spoke most appreciatively of what his parents had done for him. Never was he able to verbalize his anger or discuss his parents in terms of their human weaknesses and strengths.

A. H.'s one desire was to paint. However, his father demeaned this activity as a pastime for women and fags. Mr. H. tried to force his son to take a respectable government job. After the death of his father, as a counterreaction to paternal pressures, A. H. decided to pursue art and a somewhat Bohemian lifestyle. He applied to an institute for advanced instruction in painting, but he failed the entrance examination, losing out to some of the very same "lower-class" children whom his family had said he would avoid because of their inherent inferiority and different ethnic backgrounds.

Key aspects of A. H.'s history are frighteningly similar to most peoples'. A. H.'s case is actually a brief biography of Hitler. It illustrates in a cursory way some of the dynamics that lead to the authoritarian personality. Unfortunately, authoritarians are common in all societies. The authoritarian traits which reside to varying degrees in all of us bring special tragedy upon deaf people and other minority groups and represent a basic ingredient in the inhumanity that people impose upon their fellow human beings. So crucial is this concept to understanding public, professional, and parental attitudes toward deafness, that A. H.'s case history is going to be followed by a more didactic examination of the development of authoritarian personalities.

AUTHORITARIANISM

CHARACTERISTICS

Most authoritarians come from strict, status-seeking parents. The emphasis is on "Do as I say." The use of reason and flexibility are minimal. There is also a preoccupation with maintaining an impressive front or veneer. Inner values are not as highly regarded as is keeping up with others. Showy cars, the right clubs, and a good neighborhood are paramount.

Religion tends to be used as a tool of hostility. Acts of brutality or insensitivity to others are explained away with clichés such as "it's God's will" or "an eye for an eye." The religious beliefs of many authoritarians are ultra-fundamentalistic. Children are terrified and controlled by threats of "hellfire and brimstone."

This conceptual framework creates a tremendous need to deny personal weakness within authoritarian families. Normal aspects of sexuality, hostility, doubt, ambivalence, and similar feelings are misconstrued as weakness. The need to deny and repress these universal aspects of humanity places the authoritarian in the position of fearing insight and self-examination because these introspective processes may result in an awareness of what is repressed. Rather than look inward for a solution to their problems, authoritarian personalities prefer to make use of such psychological defense mechanisms as denial, rigidity, and projection.

Authoritarians are anti-introspective. For example, they are hostile to psychotherapy and psychology because of their deep-seated fear of what lurks within their own inner psychic processes (Sales, 1972). Self-awareness threatens to expose the blunted sensitivity and narrow range of awareness upon which their precarious psychological adjustment is based. They are "ego alien" in the sense that they cannot be self-critical; this trait is characterized by the expression, "It was not I who did it, but the devil in men." Introspection may be avoided by recourse to the common rationalization, "Just keep busy and you can get it off your mind." This avoidance of insight also causes authoritarians to somaticize anxiety rather than deal with it in more mature ways; for example, they tend to get psychosomatically ill under stress. Somatization, like projection and denial, is a primitive defense mechanism.

Weakness is intolerable to the authoritarian. Thus he bullies weaker persons, both to reaffirm his perception of himself as strong and to punish in others the weaknesses he sees as evil and threatening to his own ego. The primary emphasis on these basic coping mechanisms fixes personality development into a pattern having pathological manifestations in many areas of behavior.

The authoritarian tends to equate being different with being weak. Blacks, homosexuals, Jews, foreigners, Catholics, disabled persons, and other minorities are seen as threats for this reason. To allay the anxieties they symbolize, he calls them "niggers," "queers," "kikes," "gooks," or "freaks." Such labeling helps depersonalize these minorities, making the rationalization of atrocities wrought upon them in the name of "purity," "love of country" or "God's will" acceptable to the authoritarian's moral code. Moral righteousness, however bizarrely rationalized, is inevitably used by authoritarians to explain their behavior. For example, the Nazis, the Ku Klux Klan, and the Manson Family all claim pure altruistic motives and in many instances "spiritual" support.

To further cope with his own fear of weakness, the authoritarian identifies with strong "in-groups" while condemning or punishing "out-groups" (Sales, 1972). Thus the Nazi storm troopers epitomized the German authoritarian's ethnocentric desire for power and his need to destroy the Jew, who symbolized the "weakness" which threatened him from within. Unfortunately, the power and status symbolized by uniforms and by the structure of the police and the military magnetize authoritarians into these fields. Given the power of such organizations, authoritarians become the type of self-righteous sadists characterized by Herman Göring, Adolf Eichmann, and others.

By exaggerating the importance of power, dominance, and force in human relationships, the authoritarian conceals his own weaknesses. Because disabled persons and minority groups are usually thought of as different, inferior, or pitiable, they are seen as deserving the lower status usually assigned them. They are perceived similarly to unknown situations or ambiguous stimuli and thereby activate the authoritarian's projections of his own difficulties. He attributes to them the problems that are in his own psyche. Through such psychological mechanisms, the authoritarian is made anxious by handicapped people and racial minorities, and he reacts with rationalized hostility to such anxiety. For example, the authoritarian will project his own sexual fears and lack of motivation onto a minority group and label them moral degenerates and worthless loafers. He can then justify punishing them, denying them social services, forcing segregation, and so on.

The authoritarian tends to overglorify his parents instead of seeing them as real people with normal strengths and weaknesses. This view grows out of the combination of fear and repressed hostility that authoritarians felt toward their parents when they were children. The notion predominates that "if I must love, obey, and worship my parents without questioning, they must be 'godlike.' " This overglorification of parents generalizes to the institutions for which they stand—motherhood, country, flag, hard work. Thus the authoritarian tends to be a superpatriot, a strong nationalist, and a driving worker. He represses his own hostility and is unable adequately to acknowledge even normal aggression. Instead, such feelings are initially repressed and then self-righteously projected and rationalized as punishment of Jews, welfare cheaters, hippies, and blacks.

Similar dynamics operate in the area of sexuality. Normal sensuality is denied or repressed because it is seen as a self-indulgent weakness. This sort of defensiveness results, in turn, in a compartmentalization and projection of the authoritarians' own sexual feelings. They manifest themselves in a narrowing of rules for sexual conduct in neurotic reactions such as the "Madonna–Prostitute" complex. For example, a male with this complex is impotent with his wife because she symbolizes the horror of his repressed sexual feelings toward his mother and other "decent" women whom he feels should not be thought of in sexual terms; however, he can seduce a prostitute because she represents the debased role he attributes to sexuality and to women in whom these impulses are present.

In the authoritarian, courtship must feed power needs, not desires for tenderness and love. It becomes a matter of how many women he can seduce, the number of impressive names he can drop, and the quantity of "right" friends whom he can claim. A female counterpart might voice such clichés as, "I'd like to marry a doctor" or "My ex-husband came from a good family, but he did not have the drive I would like." Close human relationships between the sexes are given only perfunctory attention. Sexual attitudes of this sort combined with the hatred of a minority lead to notions that it is acceptable for a white man to use a black woman but it is a crime worthy of lynching for a black male to have intercourse with a white female.

In the more general area of friendships and human relationships, there is the tendency to put these interactions in the service of status-seeking rather than closeness and love. The authoritarian judges a friend by, "What can he do for me?" not by standards suggesting a balanced, healthy relationship.

Ambivalence bothers the authoritarian because it represents doubt and thus weakness. He assumes a "black and white" attitude: anything his country, group, or family does is one hundred percent right but what is done by foreigners, outgroups, or nonconformists is automatically regarded with suspicion and doubt. This need for certainty and the intolerance of ambivalence are reasons why even people of high intelligence often resort to simplistic, dogmatic explanations in emotion-laden realms of human interactions. Authoritarians' capacity for objectivity is blinded because concepts having strong emotional overtones are not allowed to enter conscious awareness lest they create anxiety.

As administrators or persons in positions of power, authoritarians prefer totalitarian systems which brook no criticism over more democratic approaches. By avoiding criticism, they escape the feeling of weakness it engenders and the anxiety weakness arouses. Hitler's Germany is a classic example. There, dissent or objectivity about the Nazi government was punished by torture and death. At a less extreme level, authoritarians surround themselves with an administrative structure that shields them from criticism. "Yes-men" predominate and a military-like discipline is maintained that reinforces an absolute loyalty to the leader. Authoritarian administrators like doers, not thinkers, because the latter tend to look inward and be critical whereas doers ask few questions and move obediently.

In our own country, leadership that emphasizes hatred of the press (which can dissent), hostility to minority group needs, overemphasis on law and order, and the creation of special "police" groups such as the Ku Klux Klan illustrates the same underlying authoritarian dynamics.

The more marginal a person is, the more authoritarian he is likely to be. For example, the newly promoted corporal or the bureaucrat on the lower fringes of the administrative power chain usually brandishes his authority more than the four-star general or Cabinet Secretary. In the deaf community, the hard-of-hearing person who seeks to cling to "the hearing world" is often the most "anti-deaf," just as the light-skinned black trying to "cross over" as a white person is frequently the most "anti-black."

Superstition and cynicism also characterize authoritarians. For example, Hitler and Göring consulted astrologers. Superstition is a primitive defense mechanism used to shift responsibility from within the individual to outside influences. Cynicism and contempt for other human beings is a projection of the authoritarian's own undesirable impulses and, in this respect, they are highly self-deceptive (Scarr, 1970).

AUTHORITARIANISM, A COGNITIVE STYLE

Authoritarianism is a cognitive-affective process, not a political position. For every ultraconservative Dr. Stranglelove, Adolph Hitler, or Bull Connor, there is an authoritarian counterpart in a racist Black Panther, a hippie who demeans all who choose to be straight, or a revolutionary "Stalin" stereotype who, as soon as he gains power, institutes all the totalitarian techniques against which he ostensibly revolted. It is the dominant use of projection, denial, and repression which determine the style known as authoritarianism, not the ideology to which the style happens to be attached.

AUTHORITARIANISM AND DEAFNESS

Extensive space has been devoted to the concept of authoritarianism because the dynamic it represents is pervasive in our culture and most countemporary societies. In fact, significant elements of authoritarianism are basic to the way almost all of us cope with life. Thus, authoritarians are common. They are also the type of person who makes life extremely difficult for deaf children and adults.

We have seen that authoritarians commonly come from families in which submission to parents was demanded. The adult authoritarian generalizes this exaggerated "need to submit" to life in general. A statement such as "Every person should have a deep faith in some supernatural force higher than himself to which he gives total allegiance and whose decision he obeys without question" reflects this need to submit at an abstract level. The comments of some of the defendants in the Nuremberg and Watergate trials, which consisted in essence of "I did it because those in authority told me to," illustrates the same dynamic. The exaggerated need to submit is a trait associated with those who are likely to be "anti-deaf."

First, authoritarians tend to be antagonistic to groups other than their own. They equate being different with being bad because that is the message their rearing has communicated to them. Since deaf people are different, authoritarians are threatened by them. Furthermore, they equate being handicapped with being weak, a characteristic they cannot tolerate. Weakness in others symbolizes weakness in themselves and thus causes them anxiety. Because deaf people make them uneasy, they prefer not to have them around. For example, the authoritarian may give $5.00 to a benefit for deaf children, but he will not hire a deaf person and thereby have to face the inner anxieties a deaf colleague would arouse in him.

Imagine what happens when authoritarian personalities become the parent or teacher of a deaf child. The first thing they might try to do is eliminate the deaf child's difference, that is, try to make him just like a hearing person. Obviously, doing this necessitates eliminating sign language. In addition to its being the most visible of the deaf person's differences, a "secret" language taxes the authoritarian's insecurities and projectional tendencies, sometimes causing a paranoid-type reaction. Another reason for authoritarians' resistance to sign language is that it makes visible a lot of primary process (affective) material that is repressed in authoritarians.

A second characteristic of authoritarian personalities affecting their reaction to deaf people is the high level of repressed anger and hostility which grows out of a strict upbringing that prevented the normal expression of these aggressive and oppositional feelings. Authoritarians tend to direct this repressed aggression against minorities, who are "different" and therefore "bad." Once so stigmatized, minority groups can be depersonalized. For example, the Nazis were able to do horrible things to Jews because they rationalized that Jews were different, thus not really human. Once depersonalization took place, ghastly atrocities were committed under the guise of self-righteousness. Guilt feelings were minimal because the depersonalized group was seen as not having the same feelings and needs as other human beings.

Some of the brutality that occurs toward deaf children stems from this kind of logic. For example, some educators think it is all right to deny deaf children a usable means of communication, that is, language, even though signs are necessary if the children are to be able to communicate with their family or peers. This denial of the human right to communicate has implicit in it a depersonalization of both the deaf child and his parents. The essential tragedy is that the authoritarian is not consciously aware of his motives and often means well.

Depersonalization is also illustrated in some schools for deaf children where administrators and staff have a luxurious meal served on tables with tablecloths while inferior menu and decor are provided for the children. In some cases, high-level administrators living on school grounds use school funds to purchase exotic imported foods and wines. When they are asked about the difference between their own dining and that of the children, a not uncommon answer is, "They (the children) don't know the difference anyway." This is the essence of depersonalization. Fortunately, it is a rare or isolated occurrence.

Another trait of authoritarians which has direct relevance to deafness is that they see racial and religious minorities as deserving an underprivileged status, and these minorities then tend to become the object of a set of negative attitudes. Part of this attitude grows out of the authoritarian's aforementioned need to divide the world into the strong and the weak, good and bad, right and wrong, and so on. In these dichotomies, handicapped groups are associated with the bad.

A corollary characteristic of authoritarians is that they tend to repress their undesirable feelings and project them to others, especially groups that are different. For example, an extremely lecherous and authoritarian used car salesman, whose business was across the street from a school for the deaf, was certain that all deaf women were oversexed. He was attributing his own sexual preoccupations to deaf schoolgirls. Projection of this sort is easier when the somebody else is a "foreigner," a "kike" or a "deaf-mute."

The point to be made from this overview is that many of the attitudes toward and reactions to deaf children and adults are due to the personality structures of those involved. They are seldom the result of a reasoned conviction or a simple lack of information. The public's attitude is seldom to be changed merely by providing it with logically persuasive arguments or more information. We are faced with the far more profound challenge of creating a society in which structure and social institutions alter the values and psychodynamics that create authoritarians.

ATTITUDES TOWARD DEAFNESS AND DISABILITY

The concepts concerning the authoritarian personality underlie much of the research on attitudes toward deafness and other handicaps. The classic work of Adorno, Frenkel-Brunswik, Levinson, and Stanford (1950) in the 1940s provided a basic hypothesis that has been tested, refined, and developed by years of subsequent investigation. Other theories involving somato-psychological approaches, body image/self-concept ideas, and subcultural hypotheses also deserve consideration for an understanding of attitudes toward deafness (Schroedel & Jacobsen, 1978).

VISIBILITY OF DISABILITY

In general, the more invisible a disability, the less people understand its effects (Jones, Farina, Hastorf, Markus, Miller, & Scott, 1984). Because deafness is the most invisible of all major handicaps, it is the least understood by the general public. For example, "Do you read Braille?" is one of the more common questions asked of deaf persons. When a deaf individual manifests difficulty in speech, it is often a source of amazement to others. When he has trouble hearing what is said, the reaction is frequently one of annoyance rather than understanding. For example, college professors are often suspicious of hard-of-hearing students with intelligible speech who use interpreters in class. By contrast, since cerebral palsy is highly visible, its effects are more readily grasped. Thus the cerebral palsied person is not expected to thread a needle, whereas deaf people are often expected to understand conversational speech they cannot hear. A failure to do so is seen as willfulness ("He hears what he wants to"); yet people do not charge the blind man who asks for help in crossing a busy intersection with "seeing only what he wants to"!

Obvious disadvantages grow out of this invisibility of deafness. Among these are inappropriate educational and rehabilitation programs. For example, many deaf children have been misdiagnosed and placed in institutions or classrooms for the mentally retarded (see chapter 6).

The advantage afforded by the invisibility is that deaf people are not the object of the pity that devastates the blind, cerebral palsied, and others. Since nothing is more demeaning than pity, this is a significant, though far from complete, compensation. Instead of pity, deafness tends to arouse humor, illustrated by the classic theatrical jokes associated with the earhorn, hearing aids, and the humorously irrelevant but humuliating responses of the deaf person who does not understand what is said.

DEAFNESS SEEN AS MINOR LOSS

The public's perception of deafness as a minor loss is characterized by clichés such as "Deaf people just miss out on music, that's all" or "If you are totally deaf, all you have to do is learn to lipread" or "They could understand if they wanted to." This last remark suggests that deafness is a willful act. All who have been around hearing-impaired people have on occasion been guilty of this kind of thinking. By the same token, most who are deaf have on occasion used their hearing loss to feign ignorance for purposes of personal convenience.

There is an almost universal annoyance at having to raise one's voice or repeat oneself. Here again the deaf person is the object of anger or disparaging jokes rather than understanding. To avoid arousing such feelings, the deaf person often smiles and nods to suggest understanding rather than asking the hearing person to repeat. This practice leads to misunderstanding and other problems. The basic dilemma has no clear resolution and is at the heart of the problem of interaction between deaf and hearing people.

The public's confusion between the deaf and the hard-of-hearing also contributes to a perception of deafness as a minor loss. For example, deaf people are repeatedly told by well-intentioned hearing friends of some "deaf" individual they know who lipreads perfectly and who has very clear speech. The implication to the deaf person is, "Why aren't you like this?" Inevitably, the "deaf" person who speaks and lipreads so well turns out to be hard-of-hearing, not deaf. The current use of "hearing-impaired" as a blanket term to describe both deaf and hard-of-hearing adds to the problem, but seems to please those who wish to deny the implications of deafness.

STIGMA OF BODY DISTORTION

There is wide inclination to believe that the more the body is distorted, the more unhealthy the personality. The novelist Victor Hugo used this myth to create the image of depravity in *The Hunchback of Notre Dame.* Because deafness is invisible, that problem does not arise here, but the myth does have relevance for two reasons. First, deafness is sometimes associated with disfiguring conditions such as cerebral palsy or skin disorders. Second, the deaf person, because he is different and because he does not speak, tends to be like a "Rorschach Blot" in that he is a somewhat ambiguous stimulus into which many may project their own problems, including depravity.

Hostility from Insecure and Unstable

In general, people who are insecure or unstable tend to be hostile toward the handicapped and made anxious by them, because of the authoritarian dynamics discussed earlier. An irony of this is that, because the stresses of deafness tend to adversely affect personality development, there exist within the deaf community itself some authoritarians whose attitudes toward deafness are destructive. These attitudes that exist from within as well as from without have major implications.

Insecure and unstable people who also have some special problem often have negative attitudes toward a specific related handicap. For example, those with a communication difficulty such as stuttering may be especially negative toward deaf individuals. Paranoid-type persons have been shown by research to have highly negative atttitudes toward deaf people (Grinker, 1969). They feel that people who use sign language are talking about them, that is, they project their own negative thoughts onto the deaf.

Nature of Contacts as a Factor

A major determinant of a person's attitude toward deafness is the quality of his contacts with deaf people, not the quantity. Unfortunately, the deaf person the public is most likely to see is the peddler (beggar). He communicates an extremely negative image of deaf individuals, yet it is the image that tends to be pervasive.

It is interesting that teachers and other professionals who work with deaf people often develop negative attitudes because of the nature of their contacts with the deaf. For example, a teacher who spends 20 years in the classroom dwelling on speech, speechreading, and composition is dealing with deaf students in the areas of their greatest weakness. Such teachers tend to have the attitude that deaf youth cannot learn well and do not know much (Schroedel & Jacobsen, 1978).

Contacts that result in the most positive attitudes are usually close personal, social, or colleague interactions. For example, adult hearing students who work on class projects with peer adult deaf fellow students may develop relationships based on mutual interests rather than on "hearing helping the deaf." On the other hand, medical settings, rehabilitation programs, and sibling relationships tend to generate negative attitudes. Brief casual contacts generally yield no attitudinal change.

Research indicates that when there is extensive interaction between hearing and deaf children, several things tend to happen (Donaldson, 1980). First, the hearing youth begin to see the deaf as less independent and weak. Second, hearing children's perception of deaf individuals becomes more homogeneous. As a corollary, it has been shown that younger children who start out with the most aversive attitudes have them favorably modified (Rapier, Adelson, Corey, & Croke, 1972).

Congenital Versus Adventitious Handicaps

Most people think that being born with a handicap predisposes that person to a more warped personality than if he acquired the disability later in life. Although there are some differences between those born deaf and those whose onset of hearing loss is later, there is no evidence that the former have more personality problems. In fact, some would make just the opposite point (Tringo, 1970). However, the tendency of those with late onset deafness to have more normal speech reinforces the idea that congenital deafness results in more personality difference.

FEAR OF CONTACT

A fear and avoidance attitude toward deafness can have a twofold cause. First, the deafness is perceived as punishment for some evil deed, and so the handicapped person is thought to be bad. Some religions foster such thinking and go so far as to claim that the failure of the deaf person to respond to efforts at "healing" is due to a deficiency in faith. Second, as was indicated earlier, deaf people are often the object of the psychological projection of one's own unacceptable desires. In this context, they can be seen as evil or dangerous people to be avoided.

The breakdown in communication that occurs when hearing people cannot understand "deaf speech" and deaf people cannot speechread is extremely stressful. (See chapter 5). It creates, on the part of many, the feeling of being "stuck with a deaf person" in a social situation, a concern often shared equally by the deaf individual. The major responsibility for reducing this stress lies with the deaf person because it is he who will continually face it. Thus he benefits most by learning how to cope.

There are a number of related problems. For example, an error commonly made by deaf people who are especially proud of their speech is to continue to use only speech when it is obvious that they are not being understood. The hearing person, who struggles to understand but cannot, is humiliated and frustrated. Likewise, the deaf person is embarrassed and angered that his speech is not intelligible. Often the problem is compounded by background noises. The problem can be coped with if the deaf person remains flexible and resorts to pad and pencil when it is obvious he is not being understood. Unfortunately, educators often communicate to deaf children the erroneous idea that to use writing instead of speech is bad and makes them less competent.

A related concern about social interaction with deaf people are noises some deaf people make, such as eating noises, sounds associated with having dentures, slamming doors, grinding teeth, and compulsive vocalizations. Some are unaware they are making these sounds, some do not know the extent to which they demean their image and irritate hearing people. It is crucial that deaf persons be made aware of these seemingly trivial annoyances. Like poor personal hygiene, such disturbances can devastate social or work relationships.

AGE AND ATTITUDES TOWARD DEAFNESS

Adolescents are generally the most negative toward deaf people because they tend to be the most insecure themselves. Their insecurity leads to authoritarian-type dynamics, which are manifested in a preoccupation with conformity, belonging to the "in group," and a great fear of being different. Ironically, integrating or mainstreaming deaf students into schools with the hearing is most widely implemented at the high school level. Other than during adolescence, age does not seem to be related to attitude toward deafness (English, 1971a&b).

EDUCATIONAL LEVEL

The generalization that the higher the educational level, the less the authoritarianism is supported by research findings (Yuker, Block, & Young, 1970). However, a critical look at these data, especially the attitude tests upon which they are based, suggests that the more educated person is simply better able to see through attitude measures and give "acceptable" answers. There is also evidence to suggest that whereas the less educated individual may join the more transparently authoritarian groups such as the Ku Klux Klan, the same underlying authoritarianism manifests itself among the educated in subtler forms such as the paternalism of the "white liberal" Urban League Leader.

OTHER PERSONAL FACTORS THAT AFFECT ATTITUDE

There is a high correlation between personality type (such as authoritarians) and attitudes toward handicapped people. The person who stereotypes the deaf ("the deaf are happy people") and who places a high value on strength, authority, and status is likely to have a negative attitude toward deaf children and adults. Those who are basically hostile are more likely to be anti-deaf. Those with positive self-concepts accept deafness more readily (English, 1971a&b).

Women generally accept deafness and other disabilities better than men. Mothers in general are more realistic and more active in coping than fathers, who often run from the problem in the sense of avoiding involvement.

Airline stewardesses, models, weightlifters, and others in fields that tend to place great emphasis on physical attractiveness generally reject deaf people more often than do others. Imperfection is to them more threatening (English, 1971a&b).

DIMENSIONS OF ATTITUDES

There are several dimensions of the negative attitudes held toward the disabled. One is a feeling of physical revulsion. For example, some persons meeting an amputee respond with comments such as "seeing one makes me sick in the stomach" (Siller, Ferguson, Vann, & Holland, 1967). Because deafness is invisible, the revulsion dimension is not important, except for multiply handicapped deaf persons such as those with cerebral palsy or genetic syndromes involving dermatological conditions.

Siller and Chipman (1967) found that, of all handicapped people, the deaf and blind were reacted to most favorably. Strongest aversion responses were to skin disorders and body deformations. Muscular dystrophy and cerebral palsy were the least socially acceptable of the conditions rated.

Interaction Strain

A second dimension of attitudes toward the disabled is interaction strain (Siller, Ferguson, Vann & Holland, 1967). People feel a social awkwardness when the cerebral palsied person has trouble holding his coffee cup or the blind individual cannot locate a chair. Deafness poses a major problem in this regard because speechreading and the speech of deaf persons often causes a communication breakdown that is tremendously stressful to both the hearing and deaf party.

Rejection of Intimacy

A third dimension of attitudes, "rejection of intimacy," is a willingness to interact with handicapped people in certain situations but not those involving intimate behavior such as dating or marriage. For example, people who are confined to a wheelchair for life as a result of an accident are often rejected by their girlfriend or boyfriend. Persons with disabilities are often dehumanized by others, who consider them not eligible for courtship because of their physical limitations (Vash, 1981).

Attitudes vary as a function of environmental circumstances. This phenomenon is illustrated in professional football, where players may have close positive interracial ties on the field yet have totally different attitudes about social interactions after practice. Frequently deaf persons are regarded as fine co-workers but the attitude toward socializing after hours is negative. Usually, but not always, it is the communication problem, rather than prejudice, that is responsible for this attitude.

HIERARCHY OF PREFERENCE

Usually, the most negative attitudes are held toward groups who are felt to be morally responsible for their problems, such as the alcoholic or the mentally ill. The physically disabled are, in general, the more preferred group because they are not seen as having caused their own difficulty. However, there are exceptions. The disfigured lose preference because of physical revulsion. (Tringo, 1970). The attitude toward deafness is generally one of indifference or blandness. It involves even less negativism than that shown to most physically disabled groups (Cowen, Rockway, Bobrove, and Stevenson, 1967).

STEREOTYPING

It is undesirable to stereotype, regardless of the nature of the stereotype. Often, in the case of disability groups, there is a tendency to take the lowest common denominator and hang this categorization on every one in the group: for example, "All the deaf are paranoid" or "All mongoloids grow up to be obese." Even stereotypes such as "Blind people possess special gifts" are negative because they take from the handicapped person his or her individuality.

ATTITUDES OF EMPLOYERS

Employers tend to choose handicapped workers primarily in terms of their estimated productivity rather than on the basis of their physical appearance (English, 1971a & b). For this reason, amputees and paraplegics are often preferred over deaf applicants, who are in turn hired before persons with brain-related disorders such as cerebral palsy, epilepsy, or mental retardation. Of course, all of the other attitudinal dimensions also apply to employers. In the end, their decision about hiring is a result of the interaction of these dimensions, coupled with their perception of the productive capacity of the deaf applicant.

Negative attitudes toward deafness often surface in the employment situation. One reason is that personnel work attracts many authoritarian personalities because, in having control over who will or will not be given work, they have the kind of unchallenged power that meets some of their pathological needs. When a deaf person is confronted by an authoritarian personnel officer, negative attitude can usually be anticipated. Any appeal on the basis of the worker's qualifications is wasted because the decision is going to be made in terms of the personnel officer's personality structure. Inevitably, the officer is not consciously aware of the dynamics underlying his opposition to the deaf applicant and goes into extensive rationalization about insurance laws, safety, and the like.

CONDITIONS CAUSING AUTHORITARIAN RESPONSES

Certain situations trigger authoritarian responses. Knowing these is helpful for one trying to understand and anticipate attitudes the deaf person may face. Such knowledge can also help the deaf person cope with the social environment.

In general, conditions involving threat evoke authoritarian responses. For example, when people are afraid, they turn to strong leaders who can defend them and they develop an intolerance toward outgroups. During times of threat, weakness and ambiguity are despised. For example, in the turmoil of the Reconstruction Period, where the loss of an entire way of life threatened white Southerners, there was a turning to the Ku Klux Klan and to brutality. Similarly, Hitler and the Nazis came to power at a time when the German government was tottering and inflation was threatening the economic survival of almost every German. In times of economic depression in our country, we see a rise in cynicism, fundamentalist religions, cults, interest in astrology, and witchcraft. Such behavior is characteristic of the superstition and the reliance on leaders who project power on the part of people who feel threatened and helpless (Sales, 1972).

Minorities, including deaf people, are victimized by situations that threaten the majority. For example, during World War II, when jobs were plentiful, deaf employees were welcomed into industry and unions. In fact, Akron, Ohio, attracted deaf war workers from all over the United States. However, when the postwar recession set in, people became afraid for their jobs. Factories and unions then decided that deafness precluded workers from doing the same jobs they had been successfully performing until then.

Thus, deaf people, like every minority, have to live with the reality that people who are threatened by economic or psychological circumstances generally respond by becoming more authoritarian. They will turn to the powerful and autocratic for leadership. Simultaneously, those who are weak or different will be treated as scapegoats. The deaf suffer terribly as a result. Historically, the process has been illustrated many times over by the Jewish minority, who have faced persecution in one country after another when conditions threatened the majority (Greenberg, 1963).

The deaf community can try to combat such behavior through public education. It can also cope with the reality of what happens to minorities by trying to become an integral part of the power structure and joining the important organizations in the social structure.

ATTITUDES OF PROFESSIONALS

Deaf people (and other handicapped groups) often comment that a significant proportion of the professionals who are paid to teach and rehabilitate them have negative, paternalistic, and authoritarian attitudes, that is, that they are essentially anti-deaf (Mitchell, 1971; Schreiber, 1973; Vernon & Makowsky, 1969). Research has shown there is some basis for this viewpoint (Scarr, 1970). For example, students and practitioners in special education and rehabilitation are more authoritarian than the general public (Scarr, 1970; Yuker, Block, & Young, 1970). They tend to be somewhat immature, insecure, hostile, prejudiced persons who have a need to feel psychologically superior (Scarr, 1970). Some of these individuals seek to gain feelings of superiority by working with deaf people. Since it is normal for human beings to get satisfaction from feeling superior, the trait becomes pathological only when it is extreme or when it is acted out in hurtful ways.

Most professionals enter work in deafness with a wide range of motives varying from a genuine desire to help others to the mundane need for a job and salary. The competent professional with a sincere commitment makes life-altering contributions to hundreds of deaf individuals and their families. By contrast, the parasite who feeds on deaf persons for financial and psychological gratification leaves a path of irreversible human exploitation. What follows is a rather hard look at professional attitudes and some of the conditions that influence them.

INTERACTION OF PROFESSIONALS AND DEAF PEOPLE

It is tragically ironic that professionals, as a group, rarely have more than a superficial contact with deaf people outside of working hours. Yet these same professionals have major roles in determining what happens to deaf people. In other words, those who have the professional power to exercises primary control over the sociological and psychological fate of adult deaf persons frequently have little or no real experience with the deaf adult population. For example, there are many teachers who make life-determining educational decisions about deaf children who have no idea of what life is like for deaf adults. The failure of the education of deaf youth is a direct result of this omission on the part of professionals. The failure to interact with deaf people reflects strongly the obvious attitude of many professionals toward deaf people.

This inexperience with the lifestyle of the adult deaf that is characteristic of many professionals in deafness is, in a sense, analogous to ghetto schools where classes are taught by middle-class suburban whites who likely have only a theoretical knowledge of what it means to be black and poor in the city. Similarly, Indian reservations typically have non-Indians in positions of authority. Only recently have blacks assumed significant roles in programs affecting them. A look at the attitudes and the sociological and psychological state of the Indian, the black, and the deaf vividly reveals the price paid when a minority group is not involved in its own rehabilitation or when professionals fail to establish close personal and social contacts with the groups they are "serving."

The reluctance of hearing professionals to prepare deaf students for professional roles or to allow deaf adults to play important roles in serving other deaf persons clearly indicates their attitudes (Vernon, 1972). The contrasting success of minorities such as Mormons, Jews, and American Orientals is in large part due to attitudes which have led to people from these groups being in professional positions enabling them to control.

Ironically, the very professional groups that exclude deaf persons from representing the deaf, do not choose outsiders to represent *them*. For example, the

American Speech and Hearing Association (ASHA) does not have chiropractors representing them in Washington, nor is ASHA's governing board comprised of specialists from other fields. Similarly, Israel is not run by Aryans, Brigham Young University does not have a Baptist President, no recent Pope has been Jewish and the IRA does not have an English commander. Yet deaf people have had almost no decision-making roles in the professional, governmental, religious, and other institutional groups that decide their fate. Public and professional attitudes about deafness are a primary reason for this. An example of this situation was seen in the recent election of the president of Gallaudet University. A hearing person who had no experience in deafness or knowledge of sign language was initially elected over three deaf applicants.

Exclusion of deaf people from decision-making roles is a more direct statement of professionals' attitudes toward them than is the sum total of euphemistic slogans generated by these professionals during "Hire the Handicapped Week" or at annual conventions. Because this problem is so major, it is important to illustrate with examples.

In education, the statement from oralists has for years been for the full integration of the deaf into the hearing community. However, these same professionals often refuse to integrate their own teaching and administrative staffs by accepting deaf members, or they do so only in very token numbers. Rarely do these advocates of integration see deaf people socially, belong to organizations of deaf people, or learn sign language in order to communicate with the deaf who cannot speak. The little integration that does occur is inevitably with the deaf person gifted in speechreading and speech. Such ostracism is not limited to oralists. Some advocates of total communication are equally guilty. In fact, deaf children often think that all deaf people die young, because they never see any deaf adults employed in the schools they attend.

In rehabilitation, the professionals' attitudes toward deaf people has been slightly better than in education. Rehabilitation has been more open to accepting and training deaf counselors and involving them as leaders in professional organizations. Much of this acceptance stems from the influence of Boyce Williams, a deaf man himself, who had an important federal position relative to the funding of training programs and other rehabilitation endeavors. He was able to use his influence to open opportunities for deaf professionals and students. However, there remain many high-level rehabilitation administrators whose attitudes toward deaf people are so insensitive and ill-conceived that they fail to realize that deaf clients need counselors skilled in sign language (Tully, 1970). The fact that many professionals who administer rehabilitation programs fail to realize that the counseling process cannot function without counselors who "sign" is stark evidence of their lack of positive attitudes or knowledge about deafness.

Physicians

For every doctor, audiologist, or speech pathologist who responds in a negative way toward deaf people, there are many physicians who offer compassionate treatment and deep understanding. Unfortunately, in medicine, we see the effect of authoritarianism on deafness rather vividly (Vernon, Griffin, & Yoken, 1981). The prestigious and lucrative aspect of being a physician has an almost universal appeal to authoritarian personalities, and so many authoritarians become doctors. Occupying positions of tremendous power over patients and their families, they exhibit condescending attitudes and denigrating behavior toward patients. In fact, this problem with doctors is one of the primary complaints of parents of deaf children and of deaf people.

Part of the difficulty is that irreversible deafness symbolizes to the physician, especially the otolaryngologist, his inability to treat and cure a disease, that is, his failure in a professional activity to which he has devoted most of his adult life. Such failure is threatening and tends to trigger in the physician denial, hostility, and other defense mechanisms, which are devastating to the parents and deaf persons toward whom they are directed. Speech pathologists and audiologists may have similar dynamics. Just as some ophthalmologists cringe at the impression created by a waiting room full of people with white canes, so some professionals in deafness cringe at the thought of serving patients with irreversible hearing losses.

Professionals with Deafness in Their Family

A significant number of professionals in deafness have parents, siblings, or close relatives who are deaf. Such persons have many advantages over others in that they generally know sign language fluently and have intimate experiences with what it means to be deaf. For this reason, some of the greatest contributions to deaf people have been made by those having deaf relatives.

Unfortunately, some of these hearing persons, especially the children of deaf parents, have strong negative feelings toward those who are deaf, because of the limitations and responsibilities imposed upon them by having had deaf parents. Most of these hearing children grow up to enter fields entirely separate from deafness. Others have repressed their negative feelings and coped with them by reaction formation. They enter work in deafness, where they spend a lifetime acting out their pathological feelings upon deaf people. The court interpreter Comstock, in Joanne Greenberg's novel, *"In This Sign,"* (1970) best characterizes such a person.

The problem of the attitudes of professionals toward deafness is not restricted to some educators, audiologists, speech therapists, rehabilitation administrators, and physicians. It is also shared by psychologists and even by some deaf professionals (Schroedel & Jacobsen, 1978).

EFFECTS OF PUBLIC ATTITUDES ON DEAF PEOPLE'S SELF-CONCEPT

There have been numerous studies showing that, in general, the self-concept of deaf people is more negative than that of the general population (Myklebust, Neyhus, & Mulholland, 1962; Roy, 1962; Randall, 1969). This negative self-image is both a direct and a subtle outgrowth of public attitudes.

For example, deaf children of hearing parents show a significantly worse self-image than those who have deaf parents (Fleming, 1967). This is so because hearing mothers and fathers generally reflect the feelings of the general public toward deafness. The stigma embodied by the parental attitudes is communicated to the child and, in turn, affect his self-perception. By contrast, deaf parents' attitudes tend to be based more on their own life-experience as deaf people and thus their attitudes are more positive. These positive feelings are communicated to the deaf child and create in him a better self-image. There are other variables involved in the case of deaf parents but certainly the attitudinal one is major. Relative to this issue is the question of whether or not skills such as speechreading and speech are related to self-concept. Educators place great emphasis on these skills, yet results of research on their role in self-image are conflicting (Sussman, 1973).

The educational process has also played an indirect role in regard to the deaf person's self-image. For years the strong emphasis in schools for the deaf has been on speech development and oral communication. The deaf student, however, is foreordained to failure in such a discipline just as the blind or partially sighted would be in their efforts at painting. The attitudes of educators which have brought about such a curriculum have resulted in a consistent pattern of failure and frustration for deaf children. (See chapter 11). Few activities are more belittling to self-esteem than spending three to five hours a day from infancy through adolescence trying to develop skills, the mastery of which is precluded by deafness.

Deaf adults are sensitive to the tremendous impact the attitudes of hearing people have. They feel themselves the object of ridicule and of other forms of disparaging behavior, including pity, that make them feel inferior (Heider & Heider, 1941). A tiny minority understand that these difficulties are related more to public attitudes than to the reality of deafness (Barker, 1948). Unfortunately, the over-whelming majority of deaf people come to feel that many of the negative judgments of society about them are correct.

In sum, the self-concepts of deaf people tend to be poorly developed and negative. They frequently involve strong feelings of inferiority and a low level of self-worth (Sussman, 1973). The marked defensiveness noted in many deaf people is, in part, a reaction to these feelings. Some of the paranoia reported to be common among deaf people may be best explained as a reality-based reaction to the collective beliefs of hearing people about deafness (Sussman, 1973).

REFERENCES

Adorno, T. W., Frenkel-Brunswik, E., Levinson, D. J., & Sanford, R. N. (1950). *The authoritarian personality.* New York: Harper.

Barker, R. G. (1948). The social psychology of physical disability. *Journal of Social Issues, 4,* 28–38.

Coopersmith, S. (1967). *The antecedents of self-esteem.* San Francisco: W. H. Freeman.

Cowen, E. L., Rockway, A. M., Bobrove, P. H., & Stevenson, J. (1967). Development and evaluation of attitudes to deafness scale. *Journal of Personality and Social Psychology, 6,* 183–191.

Donaldson, J. (1980). Changing attitudes toward handicapped persons: A review and analysis of research. *Exceptional Children, 45,* 504–514.

English, R. W. (1971a). Combatting stigma towards physically disabled persons. *Rehabilitation Research and Practice Review, 2,* 19–27b.

English, R. W. (1971b). Correlates of stigma towards physically disabled persons. *Rehabilitation Research and Practice Review, 2,* 1–17a.

Fleming, J. M. (1967). Body image and learning of deaf and hearing boys. Unpublished doctoral dissertation, University of Florida, Gainsville.

Greenberg, J. (1963). *The king's person.* New York: Holt, Rinehart and Winston.

Greenberg, J. (1970). *In this sign.* New York: Holt, Rinehart and Winston.

Grinker, R., Sr. (Ed.). (1969). Psychiatric diagnosis, therapy, and research on the psychotic deaf. *Final report,* Grant No. RD 2407 S, Social and Rehabilitation Service, Department of Health, Education, and Welfare.

Heider, F., & Heider, G. M. (1941). Studies in the psychology of the deaf. *Psychological Monographs* (No. 2, 53). Evanston, IL: American Psychological Association.

Jones, E., Farina, A., Hastorf, A., Markus, H., Miller, D., Scott, R. (1984). *Social stigma: The psychology of marked relationships.* New York: W. H. Freeman.

Mitchell, S. H. (1971). The haunting influence of Alexander Graham Bell. *American Annals of the Deaf, 116,* 349–456.

Myklebust, H. R., Neyhus, A., & Mulholland, A. (1962). Guidance and counseling of the deaf. *American Annals of the Deaf, 197,* 383–408.

Nagel, R. F. (1962). Audiology and the education of the deaf. *Journal of Speech and Hearing Disorder, 27,* 188–190.

Randall, L. H. (1969), A comparison of the self-concept and personality characteristics of deaf high school students with norms for the hearing and norms for delinquents. Unpublished master's thesis, University of Tennessee, Knoxville.

Rapier, J., Adelson, R., Corey, R., & Croke, K. (1972). Changes in children's attitudes toward the physically handicapped. *Exceptional Children, 39,* 219–223.

Roy, H. L. (1962). Vocational counseling aspects of deafness. *American Annals of the Deaf, 197,* 562–565.

Sales, S. M. (1972). Authoritarianism. *Psychology Today, 7,* 94–98, 140–142.

Scarr, S. (1970). How to reduce authoritarianism among teachers: The human development approach. *Journal of Educational Research, 68,* 367–372.

Schreiber, F. C. (1973). The meaning of deafness. *The California News, 89,* 4–6.

Schroedel, J. G., & Jacobsen, R. J. (1978). *Employer attitudes toward hiring persons with disability: A Labor Research Model.* Albertson, NY: Human Resource Center.

Siller, J., & Chipman, A. (1967). Attitudes of the non-disabled toward the physically handicapped. *Final Report,* Grant No. RE 707. Vocational Rehabilitation Administration: Department of Health, Education and Welfare.

Siller, J., Ferguson, L., Vann, D. H., & Holland, B. (1967). *Structure of attitudes toward the disabled* (p. 104). New York: New York University School of Education.

Sussman, A. E. (1973). An investigation into the relationship between self-concepts of deaf adults and their perceived attitudes toward deafness. Unpublished doctoral dissertation, New York University, New York.

Tringo, J. L. (1970). The hierarchy of preference toward disability groups. *Journal of Special Education, 4,* 295–306.

Tully, N. L. (1970). Role concepts and functions of rehabilitation counselors with the deaf. Doctoral dissertation, University of Arizona, Tucson.

Vash, C. (1981). *The psychology of disability.* New York: Springer Publishing.

Vernon, M. (1972). Mind over mouth: A rationale for total communication. *Volta Review, 74,* 529–540.

Vernon, M., Griffin, D. H., & Yoken, C. (1981). Hearing loss. *The Journal of Family Practice, 12*(6), 1053–1064.

Vernon, M., & Makowsky, B. (1969). Deafness and minority group dynamics. *Deaf American, 21*(11), 3–6.

Yuker, H. E., Block, J. R., & Young, J. H. (1970). *The measurement of attitudes toward disabled persons.* Albertson, NY: Human Resources Center.

SECTION III SUMMARY

Chapter 6 examined the emotional reactions of the family and professional when a child is discovered to be deaf. It showed diagnosis is often delayed or mistakenly labeled as mental retardation. The coping mechanisms parents typically adopt to deal with deafness in the family were listed and explained. Grief and depression were shown to be healthy, normal, responses. Finally, the counseling needs of the family were outlined and examples of model programs were presented.

Chapter 7 described specific behavioral patterns found in the adult population. It was emphasized that verbal tests should not be used to determine the psychological adjustment of children. Finally, an overall perspective was given for available services that treat psychologically disturbed deaf individuals.

Categories of nonpsychotic and psychotic mental illnesses in the deaf population are covered in chapter 8. The chapter showed that most psychotic disorders are distributed in the deaf population in the same proportion as among the hearing but there are significant differences between hearing and deaf people among behavior disorders of less severity than psychosis.

Chapter 9 focused on the negative attitudes hearing people have towards deafness. Deaf people's attitude toward themselves is largely determined by the feelings the handicap arouses in hearing persons, especially in parents and teachers. Authoritarianism was discussed, a cognitive-affective process found in many personality types who work with deaf people. Finally, it was explained why it is important for professionals to have positive attitudes toward deaf people and how their attitude affects self-concept, education, and rehabilitation.

REVIEW QUESTIONS

1. What are the effects on the child and the family when the diagnosis of deafness is delayed?
2. How does the professional's feelings toward deafness affect the child's treatment and rehabilitation?
3. Why are many of the studies on childhood psychopathology in deaf children inaccurate and unreliable?
4. What kind of services do parents need to help them cope with their child's deafness?
5. Impulsivity and deafness are often cited as being closely related. Explain how this is a complex issue. Why might a deaf person tend to be impulsive?
6. How does the distribution of psychotic and nonpsychotic forms of mental illness in the deaf population compare with that in the hearing population?
7. How is an authoritarian personality style detrimental to the development of deaf persons?
8. Why is it important for professionals to have healthy attitudes toward deaf people and their deafness?

SECTION IV

Evaluation and Teaching

OVERVIEW

Chapter 10 is closely linked to chapters 2 and 3 on etiologies and chapter 6 on diagnosis. Numerous published tests that can be used with deaf persons are listed and evaluated. To prevent the danger of misdiagnosing deafness as mental retardation, there is a warning against the use of verbal tests for the deaf and hearing-impaired populations. Finally, the components of a complete psychological evaluation are given.

Chapter 11 focuses on helping deaf children to learn. It stresses that since academic achievement levels of deaf students do not measure up to their intellectual potential, changes in the school curriculum are warranted. A bilingual/bicultural approach is described whereby the child learns to function effectively in the deaf and hearing communities. Chapter 1 on the deaf community and chapter 4 on sign language are linked to this chapter.

Chapter 12 examines the major variables that determine the psychological adjustment of hard-of-hearing persons. While the hard-of-hearing population is large, occurring in about 7 out of 1,000 school children, their needs have been neglected. At the core of this lack of attention is the misunderstanding among families, professionals, and the lay public as to the significance of partial hearing. For this reason, the audiological assessment and implications for this population are extensively discussed in the chapter. Their predominant coping mechanisms are discussed, and recommendations for rehabilitation are given.

CHAPTER 10
Psychological Evaluation

Do not persist, then, to retain at heart
One sole idea, that the thing is right
Which your mouth utters, and nought else beside.   *Sophocles*

The broad scope and tragic nature of misdiagnosing deaf people needs thorough discussion. Consider first the following case study.

> Susan F. was almost 2½ years old and not talking. Other symptoms such as delayed motor development (crawling, walking, raising hand, etc.) were causing her parents, a physician and his wife, concern. Referral was made to a psychologist, who administered the Stanford-Binet Intelligence Test and obtained an IQ of 29, indicating severe mental retardation.
>
> The family was in shock. The psychologist and several physician friends advised them to hospitalize Susan in a facility for the mentally retarded, which they did immediately. Susan remained there for seven years. Finally, a new psychiatrist on her unit began to question whether Susan was mentally retarded. She was nine years old and still not speaking, her coordination indicated mild cerebral palsy, and she had a significant hearing loss. She also seemed to reason better than the other hospital patients her age.
>
> The psychiatrist called the nearby state residential school for the deaf and requested that their psychologist evaluate Susan. The resulting IQ obtained from an appropriate test for hearing-impaired children (not the Stanford-Binet), was 113. In other words, Susan had college level intelligence.

A gross misdiagnosis often results in irreversible psychological and educational damage, as is the case of Susan. She was immediately transferred to the state school for the deaf. The adjustments of the initial three years there were traumatic for Susan and the school. Her behavior was unmanageable in a classroom setting. On several occasions Susan was almost dismissed and referred to a psychiatric hospital. However, eventually her behavior improved and Susan went on to graduate from the state school. She then completed a two-year community college program and received a college degree from an art institute. Now Susan is married and has begun her professional career. Nothing can ever compensate Susan for the seven years of her early childhood spent institutionalized with severely mentally retarded patients. The bitterness she feels, the devastation of family ties, and the irreversible psycho-educational damage done will remain with Susan all her life. And whereas she was able to compensate remarkably for her losses, many cannot.

What happened to Susan is not an isolated situation. The misdiagnosis of deaf children and adults as mentally retarded or psychotic is an all too common occurrence. There is not a state hospital system nor large city school program that does not have a number of deaf individuals as grossly misdiagnosed as Susan F.

THE LANGUAGE-COMMUNICATION ISSUE

Language communication is at the heart of the misdiagnoses that occur with deaf and hard-of-hearing people. It must be understood in full, as described in chapters 4, 5, and 11, but will be cursorily summarized here. In essence, most prelingually deaf people (and many who are hard-of-hearing) lack a mastery of the syntax and vocabulary of English because they have not heard it or been given sufficient exposure to it. Their situation is somewhat analogous to the average American college student who has studied French for a semester or two. If such a student were given a verbal psychological test in French, the responses would not reflect IQ, psychological adjustment, interests, aptitudes, and the like. Instead, they would mirror the student's failure to understand French because of limited contact with it. Giving a Mexican-American preschool child of Spanish-speaking parents English language tests is another situation analogous to that faced by most deaf children who are given English language psychological tests.

Most prelingually deaf people are fluent in ASL. When communicated with in this language, they are fully capable of responding to complex, abstract tests such as the Rorschach, TAT, Hand test, and others (Levine & Wagner, 1974). The problem is that few of the mental health professionals who evaluate deaf people know how to communicate through ASL (Sullivan & Vernon, 1979). In a survey of 172 psychologists working with hearing-impaired children in 48 states, little was found in the professional backgrounds of a majority of the respondents that would qualify them to perform psychological services with deaf youth (Levine, 1974). Specifically, 83 percent had no special preparation for their work. Some had "learned on-the-job." Some 90 percent were unable to communicate in sign language. Obviously, most school psychologists are unqualified to work with deaf children. The same lack of qualification exists with psychiatrists and social workers. It is an even more severe problem with regard to mental health professionals who work with deaf adults.

LEGAL FACTORS

CHILDREN

Psychological tests and testing procedures in the evaluation of hearing-impaired children, as well as the services provided by psychologists, come under the purview of P.L. 94–142, the Education for All Handicapped Children Act of 1975. A clause of P.L. 94–142 defines nondiscriminatory testing and requires that materials and procedures utilized for the evaluation and placement of handicapped children be selected and administered in a manner that is neither culturally nor racially discriminating (Section 612). The law further states that these materials and procedures must be administered in the child's native language or mode of communication. Native language was later defined in the specific case of a hearing-impaired child to be the *normal mode of communication used by the child,* namely, sign language or oral communication (Federal Register, 1977). Additionally, evaluation tests must be selected and administered in a manner that ensures that children with impaired sensory, manual, or speaking skills not be penalized for their linguistic difference (Federal Register, 1977).

There are several implications of this legislation for psychological testing procedures for hearing-impaired children. Those who have been taught only by an oral/auditory methodology and who do not know sign language should be tested in a communication mode that emphasizes speech, speechreading, natural gestures, and mime. Those who have been taught by a total communication methodology should be tested in a communication mode that entails the simultaneous use of speech, signs, and/or finger-spelling. If the child has been taught by the Rochester Method, then only fingerspelling combined with speech should be employed. Finally, tests and other criteria measures that require language facility between tester and testee should not be used if the examiner is not skilled in total communication. In cases where children do not know sign language, oral communication may be attempted. However, if, after numerous questions are asked, it is found that the child's skills in oral communication are not adequate, then continued testing is invalid.

In-service training programs mandated by P.L. 94–142 are designed to remedy the difficulties encountered by school psychologists who lack specific expertise in servicing the hearing impaired. Realistically, this is a herculean task. Attending in-service workshops and depending on cookbook articles are not adequate. Too often, the school psychologists find themselves relying on speech/language pathologists, audiologists, and teachers of the hearing impaired to administer and interpret tests and to render psychological services to hearing-impaired youth.

ADULTS

Legal protection for deaf adults in mental health settings and decisions regarding legal competency stem primarily from the Vocational Rehabilitation Act of 1973, which guarantees equal access to all. Without interpreting services, mental health workers able to communicate in sign language, and other supportive services, deaf people are being denied basic access to public institutions and services (Vernon & Coley, 1978). This lack of access is against the law. Unfortunately, these laws have not been adequately enforced and too few test cases have been raised.

The legal issues involved in commitment proceedings, confinement in mental hospitals, legal competence, and so on of deaf children and adults are not totally clear, but recent court decisions and the Vocational Rehabilitation Act of 1973, especially section 504, do ensure that sign language interpreters will be provided when needed in order to ensure full communication (Vernon & Coley, 1978).

GENERAL CONSIDERATIONS IN PSYCHOLOGICAL EVALUATION

Certain fundamental considerations are crucial to the psychological evaluation of deaf and hard-of-hearing youth and adults. Failure to be aware of them can result in the kind of gross psychodiagnostic errors and tragic consequences described in the case of Susan. Misdiagnosis is not as unusual as one might imagine. The following general principles are basic to psychodiagnostics with deaf persons.

VERBAL TESTS

Psychological tests or interviewing procedures that depend upon the use of verbal language to measure intelligence, personality, or other attributes almost inevitably measure the hearing-impaired person's language difficulties rather than his intelligence, psychodynamics, interests, or aptitudes (Vernon, 1976; Zieziula, 1982). A valid measure of intelligence may be obtained from a nonverbal performance type of instrument (Sullivan & Vernon, 1979). However, not all performance tests are appropriate, because some require verbal directions.

Administration Modifications

Modifications that have been recommended for the administration of the Wechsler Performance Scales include pantomime (Graham & Shapiro, 1963) and visual aids (Reed, 1970). These alternate techniques, however, result in significantly lower scaled scores on the WISC-R than when the tests are administered in the medium of total communication. These lower scores apply to deaf people whose communication mode is sign language.

Speechreading/Lipreading

The benefits of speechreading and hearing aids are often misunderstood. As was indicated in chapter 5, speechreading is a learned skill that entails attempts to derive meaning from partial and nonexistent clues obtained by watching the rapidly moving lips, tongue, facial expressions, and other articulators (Cox & Lloyd, 1976). It is an extremely difficult task. Only 33 percent of English speech sounds are visible (Hardy, 1970). The best lipreaders get only 25 percent of what is said even in ideal one-to-one situations with good lighting and clear speakers. Most deaf children get about 5 percent of what is said to them through speechreading (Vernon, 1972). Thus speechreading obviously has markedly limited effectiveness as a mode for receptive language in psychological testing as well as other activities. The media have contributed to gross misconceptions concerning lipreading ability by depicting deaf people in movies and on television as being able to understand perfectly every word spoken to them.

Oral Communication

The speech of most persons deafened before age 3 or 4 is usually understandable only to those who have become accustomed to it. Even then only part of what is said is intelligible. By contrast, the speech of those who are hard-of-hearing is generally intelligible, even though it contains many articulation errors.

Hearing aids are not magical devices that enable a hearing-impaired individual to hear as normal people do. Aids do not restore regular hearing for the ear in the same way that spectacles give normal vision to the eyes. Their usefulness depends on the often idiosyncratic interaction of type and degree of loss, age at onset, previous auditory training, and ability to perceive meaningful acoustic signals from an impaired inner ear mechanism. Ross (1976) provides an excellent review of amplification systems.

Psychologists who depend upon speech during psychological assessments of deaf youth and adults must recognize the limitations and adverse effects on the validity of test results. The deaf individual will frequently not understand what is expected, and conversely, the examiner will frequently not understand the deaf person's speech. However, according to law, spoken communication should be employed if the deaf youth has been exposed only to this methodology (Federal Register, 1977).

Because oral communication places such great stress on most deaf people, this mode of communication tends to prevent rapport and create much anxiety on the part of both parties involved. However, when oral communication is to be used, the following techniques are helpful.

Make sure the deaf person is watching your face. A failure to make certain of full visual attention is the most common mistake made by those not trained in working with the hearing impaired. Also, if the person being tested has a hearing aid or auditory training unit, it should be worn. In the case of children, the classroom teacher might ensure that it is working properly. Many hearing-impaired children turn their aids or units off, so it must be checked before testing begins.

A pleasant face is easiest to lipread. It does not help to make exaggerated lip movements. It does help to speak as clearly and distinctly as possible. Mustaches, beards, gum, cigarettes, or other objects in the mouth, as well as hand movements covering the mouth, make speechreading difficult. Make sure there are no obstructions blocking the view of your lips. Optimal distance between tester and testee is 2 to 3 feet. A light source, such as a window or lamp, that is *behind* the speaker shadows the speaker's face, makes lipreading ineffective, and places great stress on the deaf person.

With younger children and uneducated adults it is imperative to speak in short, simple sentences. It will usually be necessary to repeat instructions, especially if the testee does not respond as directed. If you do not understand what the deaf person is saying, be honest and say so. Do not nod your head affirmatively when you have no idea what is said.

Because hearing aids amplify all sounds in the environment, care should be taken not to make excessive noise when scrambling blocks or handling other test materials. Also testing should be done in settings free of background noises. Perhaps the most helpful thing the examiner can do is use natural gestures and mime in giving directions. Extra sample items can help too. For example, in giving the WAIS Picture Completion and Picture Arrangement subtests, it is helpful to use items from the WISC Picture Completion and Picture Arrangement to illustrate what is expected. There is also available specially made sample items for the Wechsler Tests (Ray, 1979, cited in Zieziula, 1982).

SIGN LANGUAGE INTERPRETERS

The use of interpreters who express the psychologist's directions in fingerspelling and sign language is a questionable procedure. Such an interpreter must be fluent not only in manual communication but also in psychology and testing (Sullivan & Vernon, 1979). Obviously, an individual trained at such a high level of expertise would be doing the examining himself and not interpreting it for another. Therefore, results are not likely to meet high standards of validity. This is especially true when complex projective testing is required. However, until enough psychologists learn sign language, it will be necessary to use interpreters. Their use is certainly preferable to the complete breakdown which occurs when the psychologist cannot sign and the deaf person cannot communicate in any other mode.

TIME FACTORS

Complete and valid psychodiagnostics with hearing-impaired persons often require more time than is needed with hearing children (Vernon, 1976). Several introductory trials and examples of the task may be needed before actual testing begins in order to help ensure an understanding of what is to be done. As was indicated earlier, sample items from alternate forms of tests may be used for this purpose.

Tests emphasizing timed responses are often not as valid as other types (Zieziula, 1982). Hearing-impaired children, in particular, often react to being timed by trying to finish as quickly as possible even if their work is incorrect. In general, their attentive set toward being timed differs from that of hearing children (Vernon, 1976). These difficulties must be taken into account in planning and scheduling. Several testing sessions may be required to ensure valid results.

TOTAL COMMUNICATION

The superiority of total communication as an administration mode for psychological testing with deaf children is demonstrated by research (Sullivan & Vernon, 1979). Its use is also specified in the Federal Guidelines (1977) of P.L. 94–142 for children in school who use total communication or who know sign language.

It is not unreasonable to expect psychologists serving hearing-impaired people to learn total communication. It is a necessary condition for adequate evaluation in terms of assessment and programming. Classes in sign language are available in most communities at schools, churches, and numerous colleges. Teachers of the hearing-impaired often conduct classes in total communication for interested professionals within their schools.

The psychologist is in a unique position to be an advocate in fostering total communication skills among professionals in schools and other facilities. Too often, for example, mainstreamed hearing-impaired children or rehabilitation clients are sent, for disciplinary reasons, to administrators who are unable to communicate with them.

TESTING YOUNG HEARING-IMPAIRED CHILDREN

Test scores on preschool and primary school hearing-impaired children tend to be extremely unreliable (Sullivan & Vernon, 1979). For this reason, low scores should be viewed as questionable in the absence of other supporting data, such as comparable performance on a measure of adaptive behavior and additional performance-type intelligence tests. The diagnosis of mental retardation should be rendered with extreme caution and in accordance with American Association of Mental Deficiency (AAMD) criteria. These include scores that fall in a range greater than two standard deviations below the mean on a standardized nonverbal intelligence test, combined with equally poor functioning on a measure of adaptive behavior. The psychological evaluation of very young children presents special challenges in choice of appropriate tests, administration/behavior difficulties, and predictive validity of scores obtained. (See Table 10.1.) These children should be reevaluated periodically to ensure appropriate placement.

MISCELLANEOUS FACTORS

Factors for Low-Functioning

There are a variety of factors and circumstances that can lead hearing-impaired people to function below capacity on tests. These include poor attending behaviors, impulsive response patterns, inappropriate assessment instruments, inexperienced examiners, a lack of understanding of the task expected because of poor communication between the examiner and the deaf testee, and others. Therefore there is always the danger that a low IQ score may be invalid. It is particularly important to note that tests given to hearing-impaired persons by inexperienced psychologists are far more likely to be in error than those administered by a psychologist familiar with deaf people (Sullivan & Vernon, 1979).

Group Testing

Group testing should generally be avoided with hearing-impaired people (Levine, 1981; Sullivan & Vernon, 1979; Zieziula, 1982). There are many reasons for this. One is the difficulty in getting and keeping deaf people's, especially children's, attention for involved test directions. The second major reason is that group testing frequently requires high reading levels for an understanding of the directions, levels above those of many deaf people.

MULTIPLE MEASURES AND MULTIDISCIPLINARY APPROACH

Multiple measures and comparisons are the most effective assessment approaches with deaf and hard-of-hearing people. In the case of intelligence testing, for example, it is usually necessary to give two tests, because with many tests such as the Wechsler Scales, the performance items are only half the test; therefore, to sample an adequate amount of behavior and approach the validity of a full intelligence test, it is recommended that at least two performance scales be administered.

The assessment needs of hearing-impaired individuals are best met with a multidisciplinary team. This approach in the evaluation of exceptional children is also mandated by P.L. 94–142 (Federal Register, 1977). Matkin, Hook, and Hixson (1979) have proposed ideal primary and secondary or consultant teams. The primary evaluation team would consist of the otologist, the audiologist, the psychologist, and aural rehabilitation specialist, the speech/language pathologist, and the learning disabilities specialist. The teacher of the hearing-impaired might also be involved in the assessment process through diagnostic teaching implemented within the classroom. Secondary or consultant team members whose input might be requested include pediatrician, ophthalmologist, neurologist, physical and occupational therapists, geneticist, and audiologist specializing in electrophysiological measurements. Unfortunately, law or no law, the fact is that the ideal of the multidisciplinary team is rarely met.

ADDITIONAL HANDICAPPING CONDITIONS AND TESTING ISSUES

As we discussed in chapter 3, the leading etiologies of deafness frequently leave the victim with disabilities in addition to the hearing loss. Conditions such as prenatal rubella, meningitis, genetic complications of Rh factor, and prematurity, which account for over 90 percent of all deafness of early onset, are also known to be associated with brain damage, learning disabilities, aphasia, mental illness, and other disorders (Vernon, 1969). In the case of the deaf person, the very presence of a sensorineural hearing loss is already evidence of major neurological damage, a condition that increases the probability of other pathology within the nervous system. In fact, one-third of deaf children are reported to have additional handicaps deemed "educationally significant" (Karchmer, 1985). Thus it is especially important to identify learning strengths and weaknesses, and these needs must be taken into consideration in the selection and use of psychological tests and the supplementary information obtained on the deaf child or adult.

The most difficult of all psychological testing involves the deaf-blind person. For a thorough discussion of this topic the reader is referred to Vernon, Blair, and Lutz (1979) and Vernon and Green (1980) for information on the evaluation of deaf-blind children and adults, respectively.

INTELLIGENCE TESTING

Assuming a full understanding of the general considerations just discussed, there are a number of intelligence tests that are useful with deaf children and adults (Tables 10.1 and 10.2, pp 212–214). Age ranges, publishers, and an evaluation of each test are given in order to help the psychologist, the purchaser of psychological services, or the consumer of such services determine the appropriateness of various tests for deaf children and adults.

INAPPROPRIATE TESTS

Two tests that are not recommended in Table 10.1 need special discussion. The Stanford-Binet Intelligence Scale (Terman & Merrill, 1973) is totally inappropriate for use with hearing-impaired children because of its heavy emphasis on language ability. Unfortunately, the probability of its use is quite high, especially because of the mandate of P.L. 94–142 to identify handicapped children at the preschool level. Any child who scores low on the Binet should be given an audiological examination routinely, because the low verbal functioning often reflects partial hearing. Mild to moderate hearing losses frequently go unidentified for years, and in the interim the hearing-impaired are either educationally misplaced or do not receive appropriate support services.

The Goodenough-Harris Drawing Test (Harris, 1963) is of dubious value with deaf youth. Normative data are inadequately described, hearing-impaired subjects were not included in the sample, only one aspect of intelligence (detail recognition) is measured, and standardization and scoring criteria regarding dress are dated (Salvia & Ysseldyke, 1978). These limitations offset the advantage of ease of administration with hearing-impaired children.

ADAPTIVE BEHAVIOR SCALES

The diagnosis of mental retardation is appropriately based on dual criteria involving cognitive deficits and adaptive behavioral deficiencies. Failure to use both criteria have led to the erroneous placement of children in classes for the mentally retarded. The President's Committee on Mental Retardation and Education for the Handicapped coined the term "six-hour retarded child" to describe children who were retarded only in school and functioned adaptively in society.

Professionals serving hearing-impaired children may be interested in assessing the adaptive behavioral parameters of independent functioning, personal responsibility, and social responsibility. Probably the major value of behavior scales for most psychologists is its use with deaf children who, for some reason, are untestable. With these scales it is possible to use an informant (parent, teacher, etc.) to obtain evaluation data. The major problem associated with using such scales is communication. Only the Brunschwig has been normed on the hearing-impaired.

Psychologists in residential schools for the deaf may wish to employ adaptive behavior scales in in-service workshops for counselors and dormitory personnel. Some counselors have unrealistic expectations in terms of age-appropriate behaviors, particularly for elementary school children. The scales presented in Table 10.3 (p. 215) may be used as criterior-referenced assessment measures, that is, checklists reporting whether the child does or does not exhibit the described behavior. They may be used in a variety of settings (residential, day, and public school placements) and with the entire gamut of the hearing-impaired population (hard-of-hearing, deaf, and multiply handicapped).

To repeat, a statement of adaptive behavioral deficiencies should accompany diagnoses of mental retardation. Results from these scales may also foster some behavioral objectives for a given child's Individual Education Program (IEP).

PERSONALITY ASSESSMENT

Personality evaluation of deaf persons is a far more complex task than is IQ testing. For this reason, test findings should be carefully interpreted in light of case history data, personal experiences with the client, and behavioral observations of the client by people knowledgeable about deafness. In fact, it is often wise for professionals with sophistication and long experience in the field of deafness to view with skepticism results reported by examiners unfamiliar with deafness when these findings sharply contradict their own impressions of a deaf child.

Because of the inherent communication problems, most personality tests are inappropriate for use with deaf people (Levine & Wagner, 1974; Sullivan & Vernon, 1979). Not only do most of these tests depend on extensive verbal interchange or reading skill, but they also presuppose a rapport and confidence on the part of the subject that is difficult to achieve when the examinee may not fully understand what is being said or written. Paper and pencil personality measures are perhaps suitable for hearing-impaired youth with well-developed expressive and receptive language ability; however, such individuals are the exception, and even here the problems of test administration and interpretation make the results highly fallible (Levine & Wagner, 1974; Sullivan & Vernon, 1979). If projective measures such as Rorschach or Thematic Apperception Test are used, fluency in sign language by the examiner is mandatory.

Rosen (1967) demonstrated that hearing-impaired persons whose academic achievement scores are comparable to the level required by the Minnesota Multiphasic Personality Inventory (MMPI) to take the test are still unable to understand many of the test questions. This difficulty is due in part to the idiomatic nature of most MMPI items. Idioms are the aspect of English most difficult for deaf

TABLE 10.1. Intelligence Tests for Deaf and Hard-of-Hearing Children[a]

Tests	Age	Publisher
The Arthur Adaptation of the Leiter International Performance Scale (1952)	4–12 years (also suitable for older mentally retarded deaf subjects where a qualitative picture of functioning is desired)	Chicago: Stoelting Co.

Evaluation: Interest appeal is high. Thus it can be used to test disturbed or hyperactive deaf children who would otherwise be untestable. The Leiter is expensive. Validation studies on deaf children are adequate (Vernon & Brown, 1964). Only a few of the subtests are timed, which is a major advantage. The test is one of the best available for deaf children within the age range of 4 to 9. Items above this level involve a narrow range of intellectual functioning and penalize impulsiveness excessively.

Bayley Scales of Infant Development (Bayley, 1969)	2–30 months	New York: Psychological Corporation

Evaluation: The Mental Scale, Motor Scale, and Infant Behavior Record are well-standardized developmental measures for hearing children and meet satisfactory reliability standards. Although not valid for predicting later functioning or achievement, the three scales provide valuable estimates of current developmental status that may be used with hearing-impaired infants. Approximately 36 of the 163 items on the Mental Scale require auditory or language skills. Correction for these items should be made in final scoring according to the procedure employed on the Merrill Palmer Scale of Mental Tests (Stutsman, 1931). However, the items may be attempted in order to yield data on language skills. Many hearing-impaired children will fail most auditory/language related items. All items are arranged developmentally. If the deaf child passes a performance item at a higher level than a language item, the language item(s) should be credited that precedes the successfully completed performance item.

Developmental Activities Screening Inventory (DASI) (Du Bose & Langley, 1977)	6 months–5 years	New York: New York Times Teaching Resources Company

Evaluation: A valuable performance *screening* measure of cognitive development. It taps a variety of skills, including fine-motor coordination, cause–effect, and means–end relationships, number concepts, size discrimination, and association and seriation abilities. Limitations include an inadequate description of normative data and procedures in the manual. The composite developmental quotient is also a psychometrically weak quantification of test performance. Concurrent validity appears to be adequate. Reliability is not reported. Items are untimed, easily administered, and do not penalize children with auditory impairments or language disorders. The test appears to be appropriate for use with multiply handicapped hearing-impaired children, including those with visual losses. Instructional suggestions for the concepts assessed are included.

[a] A number of older tests, many of which are no longer available, difficult to get, or almost anachronistic, were not included in this Table. For ratings on the WISC Performance Scale, Ontario School Ability Examination, Nebraska Test of Learning Aptitude, Chicago Non-Verbal Examination, Grace Arthur Performance Scale, Goodenough Draw-A-Man Test, and Randalls Island Performance Tests, see Vernon & Brown (1964).

TABLE 10.1. (*continued*)

Tests	Age	Publisher
Hiskey-Nebraska Test of Learning Aptitude (Hiskey, 1966)	3–17 years	Lincoln, NE: Union College Press

Evaluation: The Hiskey is one of the best tests available for use with hearing-impaired children. Norms for both the hearing impaired and the hearing are provided. Comparisons, when appropriate, can be made. Deaf norms should be used, regardless of the child's degree of hearing loss, when directions are pantomimed. Hearing norms should be used when the verbal directions or total communication is employed. At age levels 3 and 4 years the Hiskey should be supplemented with another measure. Pantomime directions are easy to master. Although normative data are poorly described, reliability and concurrent validity are adequate.

Tests	Age	Publisher
Merrill-Palmer Scale of Mental Tests (Stutsman, 1931)	2–5 years	Chicago: Stoelting Co.

Evaluation: Requires a skilled examiner with a thorough knowledge of the psychology of hearing impairment. Although the norms are dated, the item variety offers interest appeal for hearing-impaired children. Adjustments in scoring can be made for items that are refused, omitted, or failed because of language difficulties. The time factor in some items is a weakness in its use with hearing-impaired children. The Merrill-Palmer is best seen as a screening test for developmental functioning and as a supplemental performance measure for another IQ test. It is one of the few tests with an adequate number of 2- and 3-year-olds in the standardization sample. Subtest instructions are best given in pantomime or total communication.

Tests	Age	Publisher
Ravens Progressive Matrices (Raven, 1948)	5 years through adulthood	Los Angeles: Western Psychological Corporation

Evaluation: There are various forms of Ravens Progressive Matrices, some designed for children as young as 5 and others for adults of exceptionally high intelligence. They are best used as a second IQ test giving supplementary evidence for a more comprehensive measure of intelligence. They have the advantage of being easy to administer and score. Care must be taken to ensure that the child is not responding in a hasty, almost random way; this can happen especially with young or difficult-to-test cases. Such responding totally invalidates results as an indicator of IQ.

Tests	Age	Publisher
Smith-Johnson Nonverbal Performance Scale (Smith & Johnson, 1977)	2–4 years	Los Angeles: Western Psychological Corporation

Evaluation: This is an absolutely outstanding test for young hearing-impaired children. Norms for hearing and deaf children are provided by gender. The hearing-impaired normative sample included 36 percent with profound hearing losses and 64 percent with mild and moderate losses. Thus the majority of hearing-impaired subjects were hard-of-hearing rather than severely and profoundly deafened. Subject directions are presented in pantomime and many repetitions may be given. Total communication is suggested, although it is not necessary, in the administration of this test to children who use this communication mode. Fourteen categories of subtests are presented and the child's average in comparison to peers of the same sex and chronological age. As may be expected in preschool measures, test-retest reliabilities are low. Both reliability and validity data with hearing-impaired children are inadequately described in the manual.

TABLE 10.1. (*continued*)

Tests	Age	Publisher
Wachs Analysis of Cognitive Structures (Wachs & Vaughn, 1976)	3–6 years	Los Angeles: Western Psychological Corporation

Evaluation: Based upon Piagetian theories of cognitive development, it is primarily nonverbal in format. It appears to have promise for use with the hearing impaired, although they were not included in the normative sample. This test might be used to supplement another measure on this table.

Wechsler Preschool and Primary Scale of Intelligence Performance subtests (Wechsler, 1967)	3 years, 11 months to 6 years, 8 months	New York: Psychological Corporation

Evaluation: This scale is not recommended for use with hearing-impaired children. Most subtest directions are difficult to explain to deaf children.

Wechsler Performance Scale for Children-Revised (Wechsler, 1974)	6–16 years	New York: Psychological Corporation

Evaluation: An excellent test for use with school-age hearing-impaired children. Norms exist on deaf children (Anderson & Sisco, 1977). Total communication should be used in administration rather than pantomime and visual aids if the child and the psychologist know total communication. All six subtests should be administered.

TABLE 10.2. Evaluation of Some of the Intelligence Tests Most Commonly Used with Deaf and Hard-of-Hearing Adults

Tests	Age	Publisher
Wechsler Performance Scale for Adults—Revised (1981)	16–70 years	New York: Psychological Corporation

Evaluation: The Wechsler Performance Scale is at present the best test for deaf adults. It yields a relatively valid IQ score and offers opportunities for qualitative interpretation of factors such as brain injury or emotional disturbance (Wechsler, 1955, pp. 80–81). It has good interest appeal, is relatively easy to administer, and is reasonable in cost.

Progressive Matrices (Raven, 1948)	9 years to adulthood	Los Angeles: Western Psychological Corporation

Evaluation: Raven's Progressive Matrices is good as a second test to substantiate another, more comprehensive intelligence test. The advantage of the Matrices is that it is extremely easy to administer and score, takes relatively little of the examiner's time, and is very inexpensive. It yields invalid test scores for impulsive deaf subjects, who tend to respond randomly rather than with accuracy and care. For this reason, the examiner should observe the client creafully to ensure that he or she is making a genuine effort. (See Table 10.1 for additional information).

The Revised Beta (Levine 1960, pp. 203, 206, 269)	Adults	New York: Psychological Corporation

Evaluation: The Revised Beta is a nonlanguage test involving mazes, spatial relations, matching, and similar performance type items. It provides an adequate measure of the intelligence of adults who are deaf. However, it has some dated items.

TABLE 10.3. Adaptive and Behavioral Scales

Tests	Age	Publisher
AAMD Adaptive Behavior Scale (Nihira, Foster, Shellhaus, & Leland, 1974)	Norms range 3–69 years	Washington, DC: American Association of Mental Deficiency

Evaluation: The AAMD is standardized on mentally retarded, nonretarded public school children, and children in special classes for the handicapped. Part I measures items such as independent functioning, physical development, economic activity, domestic activity, self-direction, responsibility, socialization, etc. Part II has measures of maladaptive behavior related to personality, i.e., antisocial behavior, withdrawal, self-abusive behavior, inappropriate interpersonal mannerisms, etc. The entire scale has excellent applicability for all ages and categories of deaf and hard-of-hearing children. Scoring is somewhat tedious and should be completed by an experienced examiner from a knowledgable informant or on the basis of direct observation. The scale yields relevant data for behavioral and instructional objectives as well as therapy goals.

Alpern-Boll Developmental Profile (Alpern & Boll, 1972)	Birth to 12 years	Indianapolis: Psychological Development Publications

Evaluation: This scale is standardized on normal subjects. Assessed content areas include physical development, self-help, social development, pre-academic, academic, and communication skills. It is applicable for the hearing-impaired population and for the multiply handicapped. Academic and communication sections may be omitted. Used as a criterion referenced scale, it yields valuable data for behavioral and instructional objectives.

Balthazar Scale of Adaptive Behavior (Balthazar, 1971)	All ages of mental retardation	Champaign, IL: Research Press

Evaluation: This scale is most applicable for multiply handicapped hearing-impaired children. It can be used to gather baseline data prior to initiation of behavior training/ management techniques, for an assessment of appropriate target behaviors, as an aid in task analysis for identifying components of a given behavior, and in the evaluation of intervention effectiveness.

Brunschwig Personality Inventory for Deaf Children (Brunschwig, 1936)	School age	See Brunschwig reference (1936)

Evaluation: This is the only scale specifically normed on deaf subjects. It has been widely used and has value. The problem is that the norms and items are based on 1936 standards.

Cain-Levine Social Competency Scale (Cain, Levine, & Elzey, 1963)	5–14 years	Palo Alto, CA: Consulting Psychologists Press

Evaluation: This scale was standardized on the mentally retarded. It is appropriate for use with multiply handicapped hearing-impaired children. It assesses self-help, initiative, social skills, and communication skills, intended to lead to self-sufficiency and social contributory behavior. The interview method from parent or teacher is employed.

Haggerty-Olson-Wickman Behavior Rating Schedules (Kirk, 1938; Myklebust, 1962).	School ages	See Myklebust (1962) reference

TABLE 10.3. (continued)

Tests	Age	Publisher

Evaluation: Next to the School Behavior Checklist, this is the most widely used behavioral rating scale with deaf children. Relative to what is available, it is satisfactory, but based on old normative data and test items.

School Behavior Check List (Miller, 1974)	Children grades 1–6	Louisville, KY: University of Louisville Press

Evaluation: This is the best available instrument for use with deaf school-age children. It has been used in national studies (Goulder & Trybus, 1977) by knowledgable psychologists, who choose it out of all available scales.

Vineland Social Maturity Scale (Doll, 1953)	1–25 years	Princeton, NJ: Educational Testing Service

Evaluation: This scale is usable in the assessment of the social maturity of hearing-impaired youngsters. However, it needs revision. Norms and some items are dated. Language-related questions make it difficult to adapt to deaf youth. A lot of time is required to master the Vineland, and a sophisticated examiner is needed.

Behavior Rating Scales	Age	Publisher
Child Behavior Profile (Achenbach, 1978)	6–16 years	Bethesda, MD: Laboratory of Developmental Psychology
Devereux Child Behavior Rating Scale (Spivak & Spotts, 1966)	6–12 years	Devon, PA: Devereux Foundation Press
Devereux Elementary School Behavior Rating Scale (Spivak and Swift, 1966)	6–12 years	Devon, PA: Devereux Foundation Press
Devereux Adolescent Behavior Rating Scale (Spivak, Spotts, & Haines, 1967)	12–18 years	Devon, PA: Devereux Foundation Press
Walker Problem Behavior Identification Checklist (Walker, 1976)	8–12 years	Los Angeles: Western Psychological Services

Evaluation: All of these rating scales have demonstrated value in work with hearing children but have not been used with the deaf enough to have known empirical validity. However, they do have face validity relative to deaf children.

Behavior Problem Checklist (Quay & Peterson, 1967)	6–18 years	Champaign: University of Illinois Press

Evaluation: In an extensive evaluation of behavioral rating scales, Goulder (1976), an experienced psychologist in deafness, chose this scale as by far the best of those available. His own work and that of others (Goulder, 1976) fully supports this evaluation. There are normative data on its use with deaf children (Goulder & Trybus, 1977).

people (Conley, 1976; Giorcelli, 1982; Payne, 1982). Rosen (1967) gave the MMPI to entering deaf students at Gallaudet University, and all profiles suggested extreme psychopathology. Since the subjects were the intellectual elite of the deaf population and were not exhibiting adjustment difficulties, it is obvious that the MMPI is not appropriate for use with the deaf. Specific items such as "My hearing is apparently as good as that of most people" and "While on trains and buses, I often talk with strangers" further indicate how grossly inappropriate the MMPI is for most deaf people.

There is some question as to whether the norms for the personality structure of hearing people are appropriate for deaf and hard-of-hearing subjects (Sullivan & Vernon, 1979). Conceivably, deafness alters the perceived environment sufficiently to bring about an essentially different organization of personality, so that normality would differ from what it is for a person with normal hearing. Although this issue is presently unresolved, it is frequently raised by scholars in the field of deafness and should be considered in any discussion of the personality of those with severe hearing loss.

In connection with personality evaluation, it is important to note that the syntactical confusion and apparent disassociation frequently reflected in the writing of deaf persons rarely indicate a deranged thought process. It is usually only the result of English language difficulties. Psychologists unaware of this have been known to equate the atypical written language of many deaf persons with that of the schizophrenic. Unfortunate misdiagnoses have been made based in large part upon this confusion.

USEFUL TESTS

Despite the problems involved and the dangers inherent in assessing psychological adjustment in deaf people, there are tests that can be useful (Table 10.4). However, extreme caution is advised. Because of the dangers of misdiagnosis discussed above, interpretations should not be speculative. They should be conservative and limited to what is irrefutably clear in the protocol. Where test findings conflict with case history, with the views of people experienced with deaf children, or with clinical judgment, such conflicts should be clearly stated and the tenuous nature of the findings frankly communicated.

RATING SCALES

Because of the many problems inherent in the use of conventional personality tests, behavioral rating scales are often the best measures (see Table 10.3). They enable a psychologist not experienced with deaf children to get extensive additional input from those who have in-depth contact with the child. The Behavioral Problem Checklist is especially highly recommended (Quay & Peterson, 1983).

REPORTING RESULTS

A practical dilemma faced by psychologists is how to report findings in a manner that is in the best interest of both the subject and the referring agency. For example, destructive labeling frequently occurs in the reporting of psychosexual adjustment. Psychologists who are struggling with their own problems in this area or who are anxious to impress others with their understanding of psychodynamics are likely to report conditions such as latent homosexuality, guilt over masturbation, or sexual fantasies. These are common traits in adolescents and are also present in many adults. Little value is gained by describing deaf people in these terms except in the rare case where a specific referral for therapy is in order. More important, when

TABLE 10.4. Personality Tests

Tests	Age	Publisher
Draw-A-Person (Machover, 1949), House-Tree-Person (Buck, 1949), and Bender-Gestalt (Bender, 1938)	Childhood through adulthood	New York: Psychological Corporation

Evaluation: Because drawing tests largely circumvent the communication problems inherent in testing deaf persons, they are widely used. The three above are helpful as gross screening devices capable of identifying extremes of mental illness. They are not definitive instruments for the precise diagnosis of most pathology. In fact, their reliability and validity are tenuous at best (Sullivan & Vernon, 1979).

Education Apperception Test (Thompson & Jones, 1973)	School age 6–12 years	Los Angeles: Western Psychological Services

Evaluation: Although no publications exist on the use of this scale with deaf children, it seems to have potential.

Make-A-Picture-Story Test (MAPS) (Schneidman, 1951)	School age 6–12 years	New York: Teachers College Press

Evaluation: This test has been used with deaf children and proven to be of value (Hess, 1960). It does require sign language skills on the part of the examiner and child or excellent oral communication skills by both parties.

Rorschach Ink Blot Test (Rorschach, 1942)	Can be given to deaf subjects if they are able to communicate fluently manually or communicate with exceptional skill orally	New York: Psychological Corporation

Evaluation: In order for the Rorchach to be used, it is absolutely necessary that the psychologist and the deaf subject taking it be fluent in manual communication. Even under these circumstances it is debatable whether it has great value unless the subject is of above-average intelligence. It would be possible, with a very bright deaf subject who had a remarkable proficiency in English, to give a Rorschach through writing, but this would be a dubious procedure.

Thematic Apperception Test (TAT) or Children's Apperception Test (CAT) (Bellak & Bellak, 1974, 1975)	Can be used with subjects of school age through adulthood who can communicate well manually or communicate skillfully in written language	New York: Psychological Corporation

Evaluation: These are tests of great potential, if both the psychologist and the deaf subject taking them can communicate with fluency in manual communication. Otherwise they are of very limited value unless the subject has an exceptional command of language. The tests could be given through an interpreter by an exceptionally perceptive psychologist, although they are far more effective if the psychologist can communicate in sign language.

these kinds of descriptions are sent to employers, educators, or others who are repressed or are otherwise struggling with similar problems, the deaf person is often perceived as a sort of sexual monster and thus arouse all sorts of hostile rejecting behavior.

The same basic problem of dubious labeling occurs in other personality and adjustment areas. Paranoia is perhaps the most widely misapplied diagnosis. Almost invariably, both normal and mentally ill deaf people are so labeled. Such labeling is generally incorrect (Rainer, Altshuler, Kallman, & Deming, 1963).

ACADEMIC ACHIEVEMENT

Some measure of academic achievement is an essential component of many psychological evaluations. In interpreting results, it is important to recognize that the achievement levels of the hearing impaired, particularly in reading, are significantly below those attained by hearing peers (Moores, 1987). Achievement tends to be lowest in areas that rely on knowledge of English, such as reading, social studies, and science, and somewhat higher in spelling and arithmetic computation (Moores, 1987). The mastery and processing of standard English presents particular problems to deaf people, and most acheivement tests presuppose these abilities.

Specific group and individual achievement tests are presented in Table 10.5 (p. 220). Of those listed, the version of the Stanford Achievement Test by the Office of Demographic Studies is by far the best.

NEUROPSYCHOLOGICAL ASSESSMENT

As has been discussed, many causes of hearing impairment also cause learning difficulties that are independent of hearing loss. For this reason, most thorough psychological evaluations of a hearing-impaired person should include some neuropsychological measures. This assessment can also be useful in the description of cognitive strengths and weaknesses, even when there may be no reason to suspect damage to or dysfunction of the nervous system.

The basic objective of any neuropsychological assessment is to identify cognitive strategies rather than content, that is, *how* the individual comes to know what he or she knows or does rather than *what* is known (Lezak, 1976). Accordingly, a variety of cognitive variables are assessed. These include aspects of language function: visuo-spatial and visuo-perceptual functioning; various aspects of visual and auditory memory including recognition, retrieval, and recall in immediate, short-term and long-term memory stores; verbal learning and mediation strategies; and the mental status variables of attention, alertness, affect, and cooperation. Thus cognitive strategies, response tempos, and behavioral correlates are measured.

There are several assessment parameters in a neuropsychological evaluation (Lezak, 1976). These include differential patterns of performance within and between measures, differences in laterality of performance, assessment of the qualitative aspects of performance, comparison with normative test standards, and longitudinal comparisons whenever possible.

Testing must always involve recognition of the severe limitations of psycho-

TABLE 10.5. Educational Achievement Tests

Group	Level	Publisher
Metropolitan Achievement Test (Durost, Bixler, Wrightstone, Prescott, & Belaw, 1971)	Kindergarten—9th grade Age 6—16 years	New York: Harcourt Brace Jovanovich

Evaluation: The MAT is a group-administered achievement test normed on hearing and hearing-impaired children. Reading, language, spelling, math, science, and social studies subtests are included. However, this test has been criticized for an inadequate normative sample and no reported validity data in the manual for hearing children (Salvia & Ysseldyke, 1978). These same criticisms apply for the hearing-impaired when performance is compared with hearing norms. The MAT is a norm-referenced and multiple-skill achievement test.

Group	Level	Publisher
Gates-MacGinitie Reading Tests (Primary A, B, and C Batteries) (Gates & MacGinitie, 1972)	All ages and categories of hearing-impaired children (6 years +)	New York: Teachers College Press

Evaluation: These tests are suitable for all ages and categories of hearing-impaired children because of their format. Vocabulary is tested by requiring the child to circle a word, from a series of four, that corresponds to a given picture. The comprehension subtests have a similar format. The child is required to mark a picture that best depicts a stimulus sentence. Resulting grade-equivalent scores may be used to compare a hearing-impaired child with hearing children in grades 1, 2, and 3. This test may be used with young hearing-impaired children (6—12) and with the multiply handicapped (all ages). It is easy to administer and practice items are provided. If the child is multiply handicapped, the teacher may need to make more practice trials to make sure the child understands the task. It is best administered individually to these children because many have difficulty doing the items sequentially and mark answers on the test booklet at random. Individual administration minimizes these difficulties. However, it can be administered in small groups. This is a norm-referenced and single-skill achievement test.

Group	Level	Publisher
Stanford Achievement Test, Special Edition for Hearing-Impaired Students (Madden, Gardner, Rudman, Karlsen, & Merwin, 1972)	8 years and above	Washington, DC: Office of Demographic Studies, Gallaudet College

Evaluation: This is currently the best test available for measuring the academic achievement of hearing-impaired children and adults. Normative, validity, and reliability data are exemplary for those of school age. Age-based percentile norms are provided for comparisons with all hearing-impaired students on a given battery. Grade-equivalent scores are available for comparisons with hearing students. The SAT is both a norm- and criterion-referenced multiple-skill achievement test. It may be administered either individually or in small groups.

Group	Level	Publisher
Brill Educational Achievement Test for Secondary Age Deaf Students (Brill, 1977)	Secondary level 13—20 years	Northridge, CA: Joyce Media

Evaluation: This is a fair test for use with secondary level hearing-impaired youngsters. It has been criticized regarding item development, reliability, correlative validity, lack of individual age norms, and typographical and grammatical errors on protocols (Grant, 1978). It may be used as a screening test with adolescents but should be supplemented with other measures.

TABLE 10.5. *(continued)*

Group	Level	Publisher
Peabody Individual Achievement Test (Dunn & Markwardt, 1970)	Kindergarten—12th grade (6–16)	Circle Pines, MN: American Guidance Service

Evaluation: The PIAT is an individually administered, norm-referenced, and mutliple-skill achievement test. Both grade norms are provided for hearing children. This easily administered test should be given in total communication if the child communicates primarily through this mode. The PIAT is a useful screening device to compare the achievement of the hearing impaired with that of hearing peers.

Group	Level	Publisher
Wide Range Achievement Test (Jastak & Jastak, 1978)	5 years to adult	Wilmington, DE: Guidance Associates

Evaluation: This is a quick screening device that may be used to garner an estimate of grade-level sight word recognition, spelling, and arithmetic computation skills. The reading and spelling subtests should be used only if the examiner is fluent in total communication skills. The WRAT should be supplemented with another achievement measure.

Group	Level	Publisher
Standard Reading Inventory (McCraken, 1966)	6 years to adult (tests to 7th-grade reading level)	Klemath Falls, OR: Klemath Printing Co.

Evaluation: Total communication is the administration procedure of choice because measures may be garnered for oral performance (expressive sign language), silent performance, and vocabulary. Word recognition errors are easily discernible in the expressive sign language of the child. Comprehension is also easily checked. Valid estimates of the child's independent, instructional, and frustration reading levels may be derived as well as implications for programming, appropriate textbooks and reading series to implement.

Group	Level	Publisher
Key Math Diagnostic Arithmetic Test (Connolly, Nachtman, & Pritchett, 1971)	6 years to adult	Circle Pines, MN: American Guidance Service

Evaluation: This is an excellent individually administered test that is ideally given in total communication. It is appropriate for all ages and categories of hearing-impaired children. The language in examiner questions on some items may need to be simplified to ensure understanding.

Group	Level	Publisher
Teacher-made criterion referenced tests for sight vocabulary and reading comprehension	All ages	

Evaluation: These are tests that individual teachers make up for their own classes. There is no way to identify or evaluate them all.

diagnostic instruments for the detection of brain damage. They are but one of the many kinds of data, including neurological examinations, electroencephalograms, CAT scans, and medical histories, that are necessary for conclusive findings. Exceptions, of course, are cases in which the damage is gross, such as hemiplegias, cerebral palsies, and pronounced chronic brain syndromes.

Relationships between a behavioral deficit and the brain area(s) that give rise to

TABLE 10.6. Psychoneurological Tests

Tests	Age	Publisher
Bender-Gestalt Test (Bender 1938)	Childhood through adulthood	New York: Psychological Corporation

Evaluation: Primarily a screening device for visual-motor perceptual problems related to brain damage. It is useful for this purpose. It can be scored quantatively and has been used in research with deaf subjects (Keough, Vernon, & Smith, 1970; Vernon, 1969). With young deaf children or with retarded persons it is difficult to distinguish developmental and intellectual deficits from visual motor pathology of other etiology. For these reasons, it's easiest to use with those 9 years or older and of IQ above 80. The Bender-Gestalt also can be used to get a rough measure of IQ.

Benton Visual Retention Test (Benton, 1974)	8 years to adult	New York: Psychological Corporation

Evaluation: A useful test of visual motor coordination and visual memory across direct copying and immediate and delayed memory administrations.

Developmental Test of Visual Motor Integration (Berry & Buktenica, 1967)	2–15 years	Chicago: Follett

Evaluation: A good test of visual motor coordination and copying skills that require a graphomotor response.

Color Span Test (Richman & Lindgren, 1978)	5–16 years	Available from authors

Evaluation: A measure of visual sequential memory and verbal mediation skills involving different administration and response modes. This test is presently being normed on a hearing-impaired sample.

Digit Span (WISC-R) (Wechsler, 1974) and (WAIS) (Wechsler, 1955).	6 years to adulthood	New York: Psychological Corporation

Evaluation: These subtests may be used with some hearing-impaired persons to assess short-term memory for digits. Digit strings should be presented in total communication. Because Digits Forward and Backward assess verbal and visual-spatial memory, separate norms should be used. The Gaddes and Crockett (1975) norms are recommended for severely and profoundly hearing-impaired children. These subtests are not recommended for deaf people who cannot use sign language.

Auditory Verbal Learning Test (Rey, 1964) Visual-Verbal Learning Test (Taylor, 1959)	5–15 years	None: Easily constructed from details presented in Lezak (1976) or Taylor (1959)

Evaluation: These tests measure immediate memory span for words or pictures, provide a learning curve, and elicit proactive and retroactive interference tendencies. They can be easily adapted for use with children from oral and total communication instructional methodologies.

Three-Dimensional Test of Constructional Praxis (Benton, 1974)	7 and older (adult level of performance is reached at about 9 years)	Iowa City, IA: Department of Neurology, University of Iowa Hospitals

Evaluation: A measure of visuopractic constructional abilities that may be used with all hearing-impaired children.

TABLE 10.6. (continued)

Tests	Age	Publisher
Visual Retention Test: Multiple Choice Form I (Benton, Hamsher, & Stone, 1977)	5 years to adult	Iowa City, IA: Department of Neurology, University of Iowa Hospitals

Evaluation: This is a good measure of visual memory for forms that does not require a graphomotor response. It may also be employed as a measure of visual discrimination.

| Reitan-Indiana Neuropsychological Test Battery for Children (Reitan, 1969) | 5–8 years | Neuropsychology Laboratory, 1925 38th Ave. East, Seattle, WA 98112 |

Evaluation: This battery contains tests that may be adapted for use with the hearing impaired. The Category and Aphasia Screening Test are not recommended because of their emphasis on verbal/language skills.

the deficit are often not direct. Ideally, the aim of a neuropsychological analysis is to identify the component parts of a behavior to assist in locating the cerebral locus uniquely responsible for it (Kinsbourne, 1976).

The relatively high prevalence of brain damage or dysfunction in the hearing-impaired population is a fact (Vernon, 1969, 1976). The development of effective educational programs for these youngsters is contingent upon the identification and delineation of specific areas of deficit. Table 10.6 lists some tests relevant to this purpose. Unfortunately, none of the recommended tests has been normed on hearing-impaired samples. Therefore results are dependent on face validity and extrapolation.

COMMUNICATION/LANGUAGE ASSESSMENT

Because hearing impairment presents its major handicap in the realm of communication, a comprehensive psychological evaluation should include an assessment of communication skills, including speech, speechreading, English language skills (receptive and expressive), and sign language competence. Formal speech and language assessment should be undertaken by a speech/language pathologist with specialized training in deafness, but some basic information in these areas should be provided by the psychologist. For example, can the individual's speech be understood, is the writing comprehensible, and so on.

For a deaf person, the first and most important form of communication is the ability to read and write. It has been found in research (Schein & Delk, 1974) that this is the modality most widely used by them in both school and job settings. Thus it is obviously important to determine how effective the client is in exchanging ideas in written language. His degree of skill will go a long way toward determining the type and level of occupational and educational opportunities open to him. (see chapters 5 and 11).

Speech and speechreading are other key aspects of communication to be evaluated. These skills have considerable potential value to a deaf person in the world of work. To be able to speak intelligibly is especially important and helpful. Speechreading ability is an asset, but even the most skilled lipreader generally finds this an inadequate way to obtain important information. When one remembers that 40 to 60 percent of the sounds of English look just like some other sound on the lips, it is understandable that a deaf person will usually prefer writing. (see Chapter 5).

It is important for psychologists who can to assess the deaf person's sign language competence. Such assessment is highly indicative of factors such as basic linguistic competence, affectivity, acceptance of deafness, and basic capacities to interact with others.

One final point must be made regarding evaluating of communication skills. Many extremely bright and capable deaf individuals lack the ability to speak and lipread. It is of critical importance that the psychologist not confuse difficulty in reading, writing, speaking, or lipreading with lack of intelligence. It is possible that a congenitally deaf person may have a very high IQ yet have written language that is grammatically unsophisticated. The psychologist must be keenly aware of these factors if he is to be fair and helpful to deaf people.

LANGUAGE TESTS

It is important that the psychologist critically review the existing language tests before using them with hearing-impaired children.

For example, the Illinois Test of Psycholinguistic Abilities (ITPA) is not recommended. Serious questions have been raised about the validity of the ITPA as a measure of psycholinguistic functions, the trainability of psycholinguistic dimensions, the adequacy of intervention techniques, and methodological inadequacies in efficacy studies which support its use (Newcomer & Hammill, 1976). Newcomer and Hammill (1976) have described it as being useful with blind and deaf children for nothing more than demonstrating what the examiner already knew: that blind children have visual deficits while deaf children have auditory ones.

The Peabody Picture Vocabulary Test (Dunn, 1965), although commonly used, is only a fair estimate of receptive vocabulary in the hearing impaired. The hearing norms are of limited generalizability (Salvia & Ysseldyke, 1978). More important, the signs for fail items are not similar visually or cheremically (units of gesture that convey meaning). Therefore, the PPVT may tap visual associative rather than receptive vocabulary skills.

Two written syntax tests have been developed and standardized on a hearing-impaired population: The Test of Syntactic Abilities (Quigley, Steinkamp, Power, & Jones, 1978) and The Written Language Syntax Test (Berry, 1981). The Test of Syntactic Abilities (TSA) consists of 20 individual diagnostic tests containing 70 multiple choice items. It was constructed for use with profoundly, prelingually deaf students between the ages of 10 and 19. The TSA measures comprehension and use of nine major syntactic structures of English; negation, conjunction, determiners, question formation, verb processes, pronominalization, relativization, complementation, and nominalization. It has a screening test containing 120 items from the diagnostic battery. The TSA is somewhat impractical to administer because of the amount of time it takes to complete even parts of it. Also, with the multiple choice format, deaf students tend to rush through and guess rather than respond thoughtfully.

The other test that measures syntax, The Written Language Syntax Test (Berry,

1981), is for students with basic language skills from preschool to the secondary levels. The Berry Test has a screening test with three levels of test difficulty, each of which takes about 20 minutes. The total test battery has 69 instructional objectives which allow the tester to measure current levels of written language performance. The student looks at a picture, then sequences a random list of words into an English sentence. The Berry Test is easy to administer, less cumbersome to grade than the TSA, and eliminates guessing of answers.

Another method of language assessment is to take a language sample (Luetke-Stahlman, 1987; Lund & Duchan, 1983). Either oral/sign expression or written expression may be used. In the oral/sign expression, the students are videotaped as they interact with a peer or discusses some picture, movie, filmstrip, experience, or object. The videotape is then transcribed into written form and then analyzed for semantic, syntactic, and pragmatic content. If the students write about a topic, then the written language sample can be similarly analyzed. This type of sampling is very time consuming but provides much information to the examiner.

READING TESTS

The two most commonly used tests to measure reading achievement with deaf students are the Stanford Achievement Test (SAT-HI) and the Metropolitan Achievement Test (MAT) (Brill, 1974, cited in Ewoldt, 1987). The validity of standardized reading achievement tests for deaf children has been seriously questioned (Ewoldt, 1982, 1987). It is argued that deaf children do not do well on these tests because of their lack of experience with the topics and their lack of understanding of the test-taking situation (Ewoldt, 1987). Instead of administering standardized tests, descriptive evaluative techniques have been recommended. One is simply to observe the child reading different kinds of materials (environmental print, recipes, road signs, magazines, books). Other informal techniques include the cloze procedure, in which the child fills in deleted words; a miscue analysis, in which the child's reading errors are described; and the retelling procedure, in which the child retells a story or a passage that has been read (Ewoldt, 1987). These qualitative techniques are believed to be a truer indication of what the child is actually doing during the reading process.

VOCATIONAL, INTEREST, AND APTITUDE TESTING

COMPONENTS

A basic part of a complete psychological evaluation is aptitude testing, that is finding out the particular abilities that a client may have. Because there are hundreds of such tests on the market, it is not feasible to list or discuss them individually. However, certain information about the following general areas is often of value because these aptitudes are directly related to the types of work most deaf people do (Schein & Delk, 1974).

Manual dexterity
Mechanical aptitudes
Spatial relations

It is important, in selecting from the many measures of aptitude available, to choose tests that are not primarily dependent on language for either their directions or administration.

Interest tests are, almost without exception, highly verbal and therefore they can generally not be used effectively with a deaf person. There are pictorial tests designed for clients who are deaf, but these are narrow in scope and offer limited data to a psychological evaluation. Among these are the Geist Picture Interest Inventory and the Wide Range Interest Opinion Test (WRIOT). The letter is preferable, but basically suitable only for those of average or better IQ who are 16 older. The Geist is not recommended.

CASE HISTORY DATA

The past is still the one best predictor of the future. For this reason, complete background information on individuals is of extreme importance, especially if they are deaf and may not have been accurately evaluated with regular psychological procedures. Illustrative of just how essential case history data are is the fact that the best psychiatric and psychological evaluations are often based 75 percent upon background information.

Some factors to consider are the individual's past performance, whether or not he has habitually demonstrated any particular problems or assets, what kinds of circumstances have led to his success or failure, and what specific educational or vocational skills he has mastered.

In the case of young deaf persons from residential or large day schools, it is often possible to obtain complete and insightful information from their school. Integrated or mainstreamed educational programs, that is, facilities where the deaf and hearing attend together, may also offer valuable data if they have teachers or consultants who are qualified to work with deaf youth.

COMPONENTS OF A COMPLETE EVALUATION

The following is the information that should be collected or procedures that should be followed in a comprehensive assessment of hearing-impaired persons.

1. Case history data including type of loss, age of onset, and etiological components (if available).
2. Report of a current medical examination and audiological evaluation.
3. A measure of intelligence.
4. An evaluation of personality structure and/or behavior status.
5. A measure of educational achievement.
6. An appraisal of communication/language skills.
7. A neuropsychological assessment to identify cognitive styles, learning strengths and weaknesses, memory, and processing skills.
8. Aptitude and interest testing.
9. The identification of additional handicapping conditions (if any).
10. Multidisciplinary team staffing and parent-teacher conference.

In many cases all of these data may not be needed or, if needed, they can be obtained in part from school records or sources other than the psychological examination.

REFERENCES

Achenbach, T. M. (1978). *Child behavior profile.* New York: Laboratory of Developmental Psychology, National Institute of Mental Health.

Alpern, G. D., & Boll, T. J. (1972). *Developmental profile.* Indianapolis: Psychological Development Publications.

Anderson, R. J., & Sisco, F. H. (1977). *Standardization of the WISC-R performance scale for deaf children* (Series T, Number 1). Washington, DC: Gallaudet College Office of Demographic Studies.

Arthur, G. (1952). *The Arthur Adaptation of the Leiter International Scale.* Chicago: Stoelting.

Balthazar, E. E. (1971). *Balthazar Scales of Adaptive Behavior.* Champaign, IL: Research Press.

Bayley, N. (1969). *Bayley Scales of Infant Development.* New York: Psychological Corporation.

Bellak, L., & Bellak, S. (1974). *Children Apperception Test.* Larchmont, NY: C.P.S., Inc.

Bellak, L., & Bellak, S. (1975). *Children Apperception Test (Human Figures).* Larchmont, NY: C.P.S., Inc.

Bender, L. (1938). *A visual motor Gestalt test and its clinical use.* New York: The American Orthopsychiatric Association.

Benton, A. (1974). *Benton visual retention test manual.* New York: Psychological Corporation.

Benton, A., Hamsher, K., & Stone, F. B. (1977). *Visual Retention Test: Multiple Choice Form I.* Iowa City, IA: Division of Behavioral Neurology.

Berry, S. R. (1981). *Written Language Syntax Test.* Washington, DC: Gallaudet College Press.

Berry, T. M., & Buktenica, C. L. (1967). *Developmental Test of Visual Motor Integration.* Chicago: Follett.

Brill, R. G. (1977). *Brill Educational Achievement Test for Secondary Aged Deaf Students.* Northridge, CA: Joyce Media.

Brunschwig, L. (1936). A study of personality aspects of deaf children. *Teachers College Contributions to Education,* No. 687.

Buck, J., (1948, 1949). The H.T.P. technique, a qualitative and quantitative scoring manual. *Journal of Clinical Psychology 4, 5.*

Cain, L. F., Levine, S., & Elzey, F. F. (1963). *Cain-Levine Social Competency Scale.* Palo Alto, CA: Consulting Psychologist Press.

Conley, J. (1976). Role of idiomatic expressions in the reading of deaf children. *American Annals of the Deaf, 121,* 381–385.

Connolly, A., Nachtman, W., & Pritchett, E. (1971). *Key Math Diagnostic Arithmetic Test.* Circle Pines, MN: American Guidance Service.

Cox, B. P., & Lloyd, L. (1976). Audiologic considerations. In L. Lloyd (Ed.), *Communication, assessment and intervention strategies* (pp. 123–193). Baltimore: University Park Press.

Doll, E. (1953). *The measurement of social competence.* Minneapolis: Educational Testing Bureau.

Du Bose, R., & Langley, D. B. (1977). *Developmental Activities Screening Inventory.* New York: New York Times Teaching Resources Company.

Dunn, L. M. (1965). *Peabody Picture Vocabulary Test.* Circle Pines, MN: American Guidance Service.

Dunn, L. M., & Markwardt, F. C. (1970). *Peabody Individual Achievement Test.* Circle Pines, MN: American Guidance Service.

Durost, W. N., Bixler, H. H., Wrightstone, J. W., Prescott, G. A., & Belaw, I. H. (1971). *Metropolitan Achievement Test.* New York: Harcourt Brace Javanovich.

Ewoldt, C. (1982). Diagnostic approaches and procedures and the reading process. *Volta Review, 84,* 83–94.

Ewoldt, C. (1987). Reading tests and the deaf reader. *Perspectives for Teachers of the Hearing Impaired, 5*(4), 21–24.

Federal Register. (1977). 42 (163).

Gaddes, W. H., & Crockett, D. J. (1975). The Speen-Benton Aphasia Tests: Normative data as a measure of normal language development, *Brain and Language, 2,* 257–280.

Gates, A. I., & MacGinitie, M. L. (1972). *Gates-MacGinitie Reading Tests.* New York: Teachers College Press.

Giorcelli, L. (1982). The comprehension of some aspects of figurative language by deaf and hearing subjects. Unpublished doctoral dissertation. University of Illinois, Urbana.

Goulder, T. J. (1976). The effects of the presence or absence of being labeled emotionally/behaviorally disturbed on classroom behaviors of hearing-impaired children ages 7–13. Unpublished doctoral dissertation. American University.

Goulder, T. J., & Trybus, R. J. (1977). *The classroom behavior of emotionally disturbed hearing-impaired children.* Washington, DC: Office of Demographic Studies, Gallaudet College.

Graham, E. E., & Shapiro, E. (1963). Use of the Performance Scale of the WISC with the deaf child. *Journal of Consulting Psychology, 17,* 396–398.

Grant, W. D. (1978), The Brill Educational Achievement Test: A review. *American Annals of the Deaf, 123,* 522–523.

Hardy, M. (1970). Speechreading. In H. Davis & S. R. Silverman, (Ed.), *Hearing and Deafness* (pp. 335–345). New York: Holt Rinehart & Winston.

Harris, D. (1963). *Children's drawings as measures of intellectual maturity.* New York: Harcourt Brace Jovanovich.

Hess, D. W. (1960). *The evaluation of personality and adjustment in deaf and hearing children using a non-verbal modification of the Make-A-Picture Story (MAPS) Test.* Unpublished Doctorial Dissertation, University of Rochester, Rochester, NY.

Hiskey, M. S. (1966). *Hiskey-Nebraska Test of Learning Aptitude.* Lincoln, NE: Union College Press.

Jastak, J. F., & Jastak, S. R. (1978). *The Wide Range Achievement Test* (rev. ed.). Wilmington, DE: Jastak Associates.

Karchmer, M. A. (1985). A demographic perspective. In E. Cherow, N. Matkin, & R. Trybus (Eds.), *Hearing-impaired children and youth with developmental disabilities: An interdisciplinary foundation for service.* Washington, DC: Gallaudet College Press.

Keogh, B. K., Vernon, M., & Smith, C. E. (1970). Deafness and visual-motor function. *Journal of Special Education, 4,* 41–47.

Kinsbourne, M. (1976). The neuropsychological analysis of cognitive deficit. In R. G. Granell & S. Gabay (Eds.), *Biological foundations of psychiatry* (pp. 527–589). New York: Raven Press.

Kirk, S. A. (1938). Behavior problem tendencies in deaf and hard-of hearing children. *American Annals of the Deaf, 83,* 131–137.

Levine, E. S. (1960). *Psychology of deafness.* New York: Columbia University Press.

Levine, E. S. (1974). Psychological tests and practices with the deaf: A survey of the state of the art. *The Volta Review, 76,* 298–319.

Levine, E. S. (1981). The ecology of early deafness: In *Guides to fashioning environments and psychological assessments.* New York: Columbia University Press.

Levine, E. S., & Wagner, E. E. (1974). Personality patterns of deaf persons: An interpretation based on research with the Hand Test. *Perceptual and Motor Skills Monograph, 39* (Suppl. 4).

Lezak, M. D. (1976). *Neuropsychological assessment.* New York: Oxford University Press.

Luetke-Stahlman, B. (1987). A method for assessing the language development of students who use signed-and-spoken English. *Perspectives for Teachers of the Hearing Impaired,* 6(1), 11–14.

Lund, N. J., & Duchan, J. F. (1983). *Assessing children's language in naturalistic contexts.* Englewood Cliffs, NJ: Prentice-Hall.

Machover, K. (1949). *Personality projection in the drawing of the human figure.* Springfield, OH: Charles C Thomas.

Madden, R., Gardner, E. F., Rudman, H. L., Karlsen, B., & Merwin, J. C. (1972). *Stanford Achievement Tests special edition for hearing-impaired students.* Washington, DC: Gallaudet College, Office of Demographic Studies.

Matkin, N. D., Hook, P. E. & Hixson, P. K. (1979). A multi-disciplinary approach to the evaluation of hearing-impaired children. In *Audiology: An audio journal of continuing education.* New York: Grune & Stratton.

McCraken, R. A. (1966). *The Standard Reading Inventory.* Klamath Falls, OR: Klemath Printing Co.

Miller, L. C. (1974). *School Behavior Checklist Manual.* Louisville, KY: University of Louisville Press.

Moores, D. F. (1987). *Educating the deaf: Psychology, principles and practices* (3rd ed.). Boston: Houghton Mifflin.

Myklebust, H. (1962). Guidance and counseling for the deaf. *American Annals of the Deaf,* 107, 370–415.

Newcomer, P. L., & Hammill, D. D. (1976). *Psycholinguistics in schools.* Columbus, OH: Charles E. Merrill.

Nihira, K., Foster, R., Shellhaas, M., & Leland, H. (1974). *Adaptive behavior scales: Manual.* Washington, DC: American Association of Mental Deficiency.

Payne, J. (1982). A study of the comprehension of verb-particle combinations among deaf and hearing subjects. Unpublished doctoral dissertation. University of Illinois, Urbana.

Quay, H. C., & Peterson, D. R. (1967). *Behavior problem checklist.* Champaign, IL: University of Illinois Press.

Quay, H. C. & Peterson, D. R. (1983). *Revised Behavior Problems Checklist.* Coral Gables, FL: University of Miami.

Quigley, S., Steinkamp, M., Power, D., & Jones B. (1978). *Test of Syntactic Abilities.* Beaverton, OR: Dormac, Inc.

Rainer, J. D., Altshuler, K. Z., Kallmann, F. J., & Deming, W. E. (Eds.). (1963). *Family and mental health problems in a deaf population.* New York: New York State Psychiatric Institute.

Raven, J. (1948). *Progressive matrices.* New York: Psychological Corporation.

Reed, M. (1970). Deaf and partially hearing children. In P. Mittler (Ed.), *The psychological assessment of mental and physical handicap.* London: Menthen.

Reitan, R. M. (1969). *Manual for administration of neuropsychological test batteries for adults and children.* Indianapolis: Indiana University Medical Center, Neuropsychology Laboratory.

Rey, A. (1964). *L'examen clinique en psychologie.* Paris: Presses Universitaires de France.

Richman, L., & Lindgren, S. (1978). *The Color Span Test.* Iowa City, IA: University of Iowa Hospitals, Pediatric Psychology.

Rorschach, H. (1942). *Psychodiagnostics.* Berne, Switzerland: Hans Huber.

Rosen, A. (1967). Limitations of personality inventories for assessment of deaf children and adults as illustrated by research with the MMPI. *Journal of Rehabilitation of the Deaf, 1,* 47–52.

Ross, M. (1976). Amplification systems. In L. Lloyd (Ed.), *Communication, assessment, and intervention strategies,* (pp. 295–324). Baltimore: University Park Press.

Salvia, J., & Ysseldyke, J. E. (1978). *Assessment in special and remedial education.* Boston: Houghton Mifflin.

Schein, J. D., & Delk, M. T., Jr. (1974). *The deaf population of the United States.* Silver Spring, MD: National Association of the Deaf.

Schneidman, E. (1951). A manual for the MAPS Test. *Projective Techniques Monograph 1,* 2.

Smith, A. J., & Johnson, R. E. (1977). *Smith-Johnson Noverbal Performance Scale.* Los Angeles: Western Psychological Corp.

Spivak, G., & Spotts, J. (1966). *Devereux Child Behavior Rating Scale.* Devon, PA: Devereux Foundation Press.

Spivak, G., Spotts, J., & Haines, P. (1967). *Devereux Adolescent Behavior Rating Scale.* Devon, PA: Devereux Foundation Press.

Spivak, G., & Swift, M. (1966). *Devereux Elementary School Behavior Rating Scale.* Devon, PA: Devereux Foundation Press.

Sullivan, P. M., & Vernon, M. (1979). Psychological assessment of hearing-impaired children. *School Psychology Digest, 8,* 271–290.

Stutsman, R. (1931). *Mental measurement of pre-school children.* Yonkers-on-Hudson, NY: World Book Co.

Taylor, E. M. (1959). *Psychological appraisal of children with cerebral defects.* Cambridge, MA: Harvard University Press.

Terman, L., & Merrill, M. (1973). *Stanford-Binet Intelligence Scale* (1972 Norms Ed.). Boston: Houghton Mifflin.

Thompson, J. M., & Jones, R. A. (1973). *Education Apperception Test.* Los Angeles: Western Psychological Services.

Vernon, M. (1969). *Multiply handicapped deaf children: Medical educational and psychological considerations* (p. 124). Reston, VA: Council of Exceptional Children.

Vernon, M. (1972). Mind over mouth: A rationale for total communication. *Volta Review, 74,* 529–540.

Vernon, M. (1976). Psychologic evaluation of hearing-impaired children. In L. Lloyd (Ed.), *Communication, assessment, and intervention strategies* (pp. 195–223). Baltimore: University Park Press.

Vernon, M., Blair, R., & Lutz, S. (1979). Psychological evaluation and testing of children who are deaf-blind. *School Psychology Digest, 8,* 291–295.

Vernon, M., & Brown, D. W. (1964). A guide to psychological tests and testing procedures in the evaluation of deaf and hard-of-hearing children. *Journal of Speech and Hearing Disorders, 29,* 414–423.

Vernon, M., & Coley, J. (1978). Violation of constitutional rights: The language-impaired person and the Miranda warnings. *Journal of Rehabilitation of the Deaf, 11,* 1–8.

Vernon, M., & Green, D. (1980). A guide to the psychological assessment of deaf-blind adults. *Visual Impairment and Blindness, 6,* 229–230.

Wachs, O. D., & Vaughn, M. A. (1976). *Wachs Analysis of Cognitive Structures.* Los Angeles: Western Psychological Services.

Walker, H. M. (1976). *Walker Problem Behavior Identification Checklist.* Los Angeles: Western Psychological Services.

Wechsler, D. (1955). *Wechsler Adult Intelligence Scale.* New York: Psychological Corporation.

Wechsler, D. (1967). *Wechsler Preschool and Primary Scale of Intelligence.* New York: Psychological Corporation.

Wechsler, D. (1974). *Wechsler Intelligence Scale for Children—Revised.* New York: Psychological Corporation.

Zieziula, F. R. (1982). *Assessment of hearing-impaired people: A guide for selecting psychological, educational, and vocational tests.* Washington, DC: Gallaudet University Press.

CHAPTER 11
Helping Deaf Children Learn: A Bilingual/Bicultural Approach

The school is a creche of living where people can still be changed and where creative activities are agents of this change.
Sylvia Ashton-Warner, Teacher, 1963

Helping children to learn in order to live in two cultures is a common educational enterprise. One example is in New Zealand. Sylvia Ashton-Warner rejected the unsuccessful European methods used in the Maori schools. Instead, she employed an approach that used the Maori culture while incorporating English language skills.

Such a bilingual/bicultural educational approach may be useful to American deaf children who will live in two societies—deaf and hearing. This approach was proposed as early as 1968 in a case study by Judith Williams (Stokoe, 1980) and more recently recommended in the United States (Kannapell 1974, 1985; Luetke-Stahlman 1986; Quigley & Paul, 1984; Reagan 1985; Vernon 1985; Woodward, 1982), in France (Bouvet, 1983), and in England (Kyle, 1986.) Experimental programs with deaf children have been set up with bilingual/bicultural components (Bernstein & Goodhart, 1985; Bouvet, 1983).

Can deaf children be considered bilingual, with two languages? In fact, 90 percent of the deaf school-age population have hearing and speaking parents who know little sign language. Thus they come to school with neither ASL competencies, nor experience with a deaf culture, nor English skills.

According to Grosjean (1982), deaf children can be considered to be bilingual. He writes:

> Contrary to general belief, bilinguals are rarely equally fluent in their languages: some speak one language better than another, others use one of their languages in specific situations, and others still can read or write one of the languages they speak. And yet, what characterizes all of them is that they interact with the world around them in two or more languages.

According to this definition one needn't be proficient in both languages but simply be functioning (however competently) in two cultures (Grosjean, 1982). Thus deaf people can be considered functioning as bilinguals in ASL and English even though their levels of competence in one or both may be underdeveloped. For example, we can easily agree that the deaf children of deaf parents are bilingual because they have competencies in both ASL and English. It is more difficult to view the deaf children of hearing parents as bilingual, because they may have only a small sign vocabulary and may be able to read and write only few words. Yet both are functioning in the two systems, with different degrees of competence. According to Grosjean, most deaf children (with the exception of those who are exclusively orally trained) are bilingual.

This chapter focuses on a bilingual/bicultural perspective in helping deaf children to learn within a deaf and hearing society. It incorporates knowledge of the deaf community—its values and language—into a curriculum that enables deaf children to learn to read and write English. Before outlining the goals of this curriculum, we will consider how hearing loss affects communication competence and learning as these variables critically affect academic achievement.

HOW HEARING LOSS AFFECTS COMMUNICATION COMPETENCE

As we mentioned in chapter 5, deafness has its most devastating effects on the development of communication skills. Hearing loss alters the mode, decreases the amount, and drastically changes the quality of input. An understanding of how language is normally acquired is necessary in order for one to understand the effects of hearing loss on language acquisition.

FIRST-LANGUAGE ACQUISITION

To learn language, children must actively interact with conversational partners in highly affective and social contexts. Language learning is a creative and rule-governed process and unfolds in predictable stages (Gleitmen & Wanner, 1986). These stages are not always dependent on hearing, as in the case of deaf children of deaf parents.

Hearing Children

With all babies, cries are first reflexes which take on communicative intent at about the second or third month. Vocalizations of hearing babies will increase as people respond to them. Infant studies of conversations show that mother–infant exchanges occur as early as 4 months, with mothers responding to burps, smiles, yawns, gestures, and gazes as part of conversations. At this time, turn-taking skills emerge. Mothers will orient their speech to the baby's verbal and nonverbal behavior using a simplified speech register called "motherese" during daily routines such as eating, dressing, and washing (Snow, 1972).

Cooing sounds or vowel repetitions come at about 5 months and the babbling of consonants at 6 months. Before 6 months, babbling is primarily a motor reflex. At 8 or 9 months, babbling decreases when babies become more attentive to what other people say. Vocalizations then increase again toward the end of the first year as babies begin to babble in conversation. While this "gibberish" may sound like sentences, it is not until the end of the second or third year that the baby will map these intentions onto the corresponding English form. Nonetheless, infants are capable of using intonations in their babblings to convey feelings, commands, or questions. This is a precursor of later syntax development. Besides vocalizations, hearing infants use gestures such as waving, pointing, and nodding to communicate.

They point to objects and events, and interact by giving and taking objects. This communicative gesturing precedes speech and provides the framework for the development of language. The acquisition of speech, then, is a gradual transfer from a visual-gestural mode of communication into the auditory-spoken mode.

At about 12 months, babies begin to symbolize and attach their speech sounds to single words, typically in the context of some activity. Single words take on more meanings as they are used in the holophrastic sense. Lexical development is slow initially until about 50 words are acquired. A spurt in vocabulary development occurs when babies start combining words into two-word utterances to express a variety of semantic-syntactic relations. This telegraphic speech later is filled in with grammatical morphemes (Brown, 1973). Typically, by age 4 most of children's utterances are adultlike (Menyuk, 1977) with expanded noun and verb phrases. By the age of 8, children's receptive vocabulary is said to be between 6,000 to 8,000 words while their expressive vocabulary ranges between 2,500 and 2,800 words (Berry, 1969, cited in Bernstein & Tiegerman, 1985).

Deaf Children of Deaf Parents

Deaf children of deaf parents show these same developmental stages but with American Sign Language (Newport & Meier, 1985). Deaf infants are able to share in communication by participating in "gaze" and body movement proto-conversations with mother. Deaf babies will vocalize up to 6 months as a motor reflex but will cease babbling at the stage when auditory feedback would become important for babbling development. Whereas the hearing children's vocalizations, gazes, and gestures develop into spoken language, deaf infants will develop language out of their gestural system.

Deaf mothers have been observed using "motherese" with their deaf babies by simplifying signs and using repetition (Erting & Marlborough, 1986). They often will mold their baby's hands to make a sign and then guide the movement patterns to make signs on the parent's or baby's bodies (Maestas y Moores, 1980). Deaf mothers will read semantic intentions into their baby's hand configurations just as hearing mothers do with their hearing baby's babbling. Deaf babies acquire hand shapes in an orderly fashion much as hearing infants learn the speech sounds of words (McIntyre, 1977). Deaf babies will often "finger babble" before acquiring complex hand shapes (McIntyre, 1977; Maestas y Moores, 1980), much in the same way that hearing babies will babble sounds before pronouncing words.

Parents who use ASL with their deaf or hearing infants will use signs earlier than the age at which children learn to speak their first words (Bonvillian, Charrow, & Nelson, 1973). For example, hearing children learn their first words at about one year whereas deaf babies use their first signs at about 9 months. Furthermore, a sign vocabulary is acquired at a faster rate than a spoken vocabulary. Also deaf children are reported to acquire the same range of semantic relations as that acquired in spoken language, and they acquire ASL syntax (Newport & Meier, 1985).

Studies of interactions of deaf mothers with deaf preschoolers compared with hearing mothers of hearing preschoolers show similar richness of communicative content, long periods of sustained interaction, focus on symbolic referents rather than present objects, and the ability to carry on conversations about themselves (Meadow, Greenberg, Erting, & Carmichael, 1981). Thus ASL, like voice input, promotes prelinguistic, linguistic, and social development.

Deaf Children of Hearing Parents

Formal longitudinal studies are not available of the stages deaf children of hearing parents go through in acquiring language with only oral input. Neither are longitudinal studies available of younger deaf children of hearing parents acquiring sign language, because identification does not occur until age 2 or 3 and also hearing parents do not have knowledge of sign language at that time. However, information is available from case studies, early mother–child interaction studies, and early intervention studies. Overall, this research suggests that while language can be acquired through bimodal input (sign and speech), the development is slower and the rate more delayed than with language development of deaf children with deaf parents (see chapter 5 for discussion of bimodel communication). While bimodal communication cannot replicate the exact natural processing of either total oral or total signing, described above, it is nonetheless much more effective than only the oral input because of the ambiguity of speechreading.

Conditions for Bimodal Input

Providing a bimodal system must begin early and be consistent for the full development of prelinguistic and linguistic behaviors to unfold. While a common language of eye contacts, smiles, and frowns will be established early, a common symbolic language typically will not develop at about age 2 (Wedell-Monnig & Lumley, 1980) unless language intervention takes place. If it does not develop, a breakdown in the mother–child interaction pattern will occur with detrimental and negative effects on the child's psychological, social, and linguistic development. Mothers typically respond to this situation by becoming more controlling and intrusive of the child's behavior (Greenberg, 1983). As the child grows older, the parents become more frustrated with the minimal involvement of their children in the interaction and begin to communicate with them less.

Studies show that an early bimodal system of communication can lead to more positive parent–child interactions (Greenberg, 1983). Early intervention programs which include the teaching of sign language, counseling for parents, and home visits can promote satisfying mother–child interactions that more closely approximate the experiences of deaf mothers of deaf children and hearing mothers of hearing children (Greenberg, Calderon, & Kusché, 1984). Families who participated in such interventions communicated more with their children. Additionally, mothers were less didactic and less controlling, asked more questions, and had longer conversations with their children. The deaf children in response used more linguistically mature utterances than children who had not participated in such intervention (Greenberg, 1983).

However, it must be realized even with bimodal intervention, deaf children of hearing parents show delays in vocabulary development (Howell, 1984) and in the syntactic development of English (Moog, Geers, & Schick, 1984). These studies reiterate the fact that hearing loss has a devastating effect on language development.

OTHER CHARACTERISTICS THAT AFFECT LEARNING

Besides the delayed language development, there are other characteristics that affect learning and achievement for the deaf child.

Learner Characteristics

Learner variables include extent of hearing loss, age of onset, etiology, cultural background of the parents, and hearing status of parents.

The 70,000 school-age deaf children enrolled in special programs in the United States (Ries, 1986) do not make up a homogeneous group but are widely diverse in characteristics, many of which dramatically affect academic achievement. Deaf children, for example, will vary on how much usable (residual) hearing they have to use for communication and language development. Hearing loss is typically expressed as a range across decibel losses, but these ranges do not always indicate how much hearing the child is able to use to hear speech sounds (see chapter 12 for a discussion of audiological considerations). Teachers need to know how much residual or usable hearing a child has within the speech range for classroom instruction. Table 11.1 shows ranges of decibel losses with the child's speech understanding capabilities along with educational recommendations.

TABLE 11.1. Hearing Loss with Educational Recommendations

Average Hearing Level (ANSI, 1969) for 500, 1000, and 2000 Hz in the Better Ear	Category Description	Ability to Understand Speech	Educational Recommendations
0–15 dB	Normal range	No difficulty understanding speech	Regular education
16–25 dB	Slight	Difficulty in perceiving some speech sounds	May need hearing aid, lipreading instruction, auditory training, speech therapy, and front seat in regular classroom
26–40dB	Mild	Hears only some of speech sounds	All of the above
41–65 dB	Moderate	Does not hear most speech sounds at normal conversational level	All of the above. Special education placement
66–90 dB	Severe	Hears no speech sound at normal conversational level	Severe speech problems, language delays. Special educational placement, probably at a self-contained class for the hearing impaired or a state residential school
90 dB and above	Profound	Hears only environmental sounds	Placement in state residential school

Another variable that affects learning is when the hearing loss occurred. If it occurred at birth (congenital) or prior to age 2 and before language was acquired, it is a prelingual loss. If it occurred after language was acquired, it is postlingual loss. The two groups present different kinds of teaching situations. For example, children who are born deaf need intensive instruction in concept, speech, and language development whereas children who lose their hearing at age 7 may need only lipreading instruction and auditory training to regain what language was lost.

The type of hearing loss has educational implications too. Hearing loss can be permanent, temporary and correctable by surgery, fluctuating, or progressive—all of which affect educational programming.

Hearing loss can be classified as sensorineural, conductive, or mixed or can be a central hearing loss. *Sensorineural losses* are permanent and are caused by damage to the cochlea or inner ear section. A *conductive loss* is remedied by surgery and is usually caused by an infection in the outer or middle ear. Many children will get fluid in the middle ear and experience fluctuating hearing losses during allergy season or the winter months. This temporary hearing loss can be especially problematic during the time young children are developing language. It is treatable with medicine or surgery but the child may also require speech and language therapy. Children can have both a sensorineural and a conductive loss; this condition is called a *mixed loss.*

Another type of loss is a *central hearing* impairment, caused by injury to the eighth auditory nerve up to the cortex. Permanent hearing loss can be progressive, the child gradually losing hearing over time. This condition is particularly traumatic for children and families who may have difficulty getting a reliable diagnosis, going through the grief process, and obtaining realistic information for planning the child's future (see chapter 6).

Etiology or cause of deafness also influences the teaching situation because many of the causes of deafness also cause brain damage, learning disabilities, and other handicaps. We discussed the educational effects of various etiologies in chapters 2 and 3.

Deaf children from non-English speaking homes have the double handicap of minority group discrimination and deafness. Minority deaf children—those from Hispanic, black, Native American, Oriental, and other minority populations—make up about 7 percent of the total deaf school-age population. Furthermore, about 51 percent of minority deaf children have handicaps in addition to deafness (Delgado, 1984). Such high prevalence figures have been attributed to lack of valid and reliable assessment, late intervention because parents were not aware of services, teachers' prejudices, the dearth of minority teachers who could function as role models, and lack of understanding of cultural values from the home (Maestas y Moores & Moores, 1984). As the numbers of these hearing-impaired children from nonnative language speaking homes are increasing, specialized programming needs to be expanded to meet their needs.

Hearing status of the parents is important from an educational viewpoint, because it influences what type or types of language input the child receives from infancy and parental attitudes toward deafness. About 10 percent of deaf children have deaf parents who, for the most part, provide them with a complete language system in American Sign Language from infancy. These children have an advantage and generally do better academically and are better adjusted psychologically and socially than deaf children with hearing parents (see chapter 4).

Setting Characteristics

Parents may choose a state residential school or an integrated program in a public school for their deaf child. Because deafness is a low-incidence handicap, occurring in only about 1 per 1,000 children, large numbers of deaf children traditionally have been educated at state residential schools in order to centralize their special needs in education. (There are a few private residential schools which use the oral method only.) These institutions provide comprehensive services generally from preschool to high school at no cost to the parents. Many of these programs also have outreach programs whereby teachers go into the homes to teach communication and social skills to parents and their babies from point of diagnosis, which could be at birth or soon afterwards. However, typically, most students transfer from other programs as teenagers or before.

The disadvantage of this placement is that the child is away from the home environment. However, since many parents cannot communicate with their deaf child, this disadvantage is usually offset by the numerous advantages. These include full academic, vocational, and pre-occupational programming; the services of a psychologist, social worker, trained teachers, audiologists, and speech therapists; and athletic and social programs. Perhaps the best advantage—in terms of long-term effects on the child's psychosocial, emotional, and linguistic development—is having a community of deaf adults and peers with whom the deaf child can identify, establish meaningful relationships (Furth, 1973), and learn American Sign Language. This interaction helps deaf persons to accept and understand their deafness as well as to learn lifelong coping skills in the hearing world (Vernon & Ottinger, 1980).

In integrated programs, the child can be placed in classes with normal hearing children and given hearing aids and front seats with a resource teacher available. Or a child can be placed in a self-contained classroom for deaf children in a public school and mainstreamed for some periods such as lunch, physical education, and art. Still another variation is for the child to be placed in a day-school program in a self-contained classroom for the elementary years but mainstreamed into regular classrooms in junior and senior high school (Vernon & Prickett, 1976).

Children are typically selected for integration programs on the basis of their academic achievement, their communication ability, and their social adjustment (Kindred, 1980). The advantages of the integrated programs is that children can stay home with their parents. A disadvantage is that children are not homogeneously placed with their age group. Often too they must spend most of the day with children who are learning disabled or mentally retarded. Furthermore, children in the mainstream are often isolated from other deaf peers and adults; they are unable to participate fully in social and athletic events because of the communication handicap.

In the past, children in the profound and severe-to-profound ranges typically went to a residential school for the deaf while the children with lesser hearing losses were educated in public schools. However, with the enactment of P.L. 94–142, more children across all ranges of hearing loss are being mainstreamed into the public schools.

The National Association of the Deaf (NAD) believes that not all public schools have the resources to meet the deaf child's needs and that the better educational placement may be day and residential schools for deaf children (NAD Executive Board, 1986). They hold that while integration places deaf children with hearing children in the same geographic location, token services such as occasional help from a speech therapist or resource teacher fail to provide services the children really need, such as interpreters, tutors, curriculum modifications, and counseling (Vernon & Ottinger, 1980).

BILINGUAL/BICULTURAL APPROACH

To address the educational needs of deaf children, we recommend a bilingual/bicultural approach. This approach uses the natural language of the deaf as the base upon which English skills are superimposed. A linguistic environment is set up at home and at school where the child at an early age learns to communicate with deaf as well as hearing persons. The deaf child's language is allowed to evolve and develop naturally as he or she interacts with peers, hearing adults, and deaf adults in meaningful conversational contexts and learns from a curriculum which stresses a cognitive, linguistic, and experiential base (Bernstein & Goodhart, 1985; Bouvet, 1983; Livingston, 1986). Six goals are stressed.

GOAL 1: CONSIDER ASL/PIDGIN AS A FIRST LANGUAGE

A major task of childhood for deaf children is to acquire a language system for receiving and expressing thoughts, feelings, and experiences. In other words, the child needs to develop a receptive and expressive communication system.

What form of inner language do deaf children acquire? Is it oral English, ASL, some manual code of English, or a combination? The answer to this question has yet to be determined by research. Clearly, for the 10 percent who have deaf parents who used ASL with them since birth, the first language is ASL. But for the majority of deaf children, the remaining 90 percent who have hearing parents, some of whom used oral English or manual coded English or "home signs," the question is less clear. The question is further clouded by the fact that we don't know precisely how much English language is actually internalized at home in either oral or manual codes of English. The low success rate of oral students (Quigley & Paul, 1984) and the limited competence achieved by those exposed to four years of Signed English (Bornstein, Saulnier, & Hamilton, 1980, Bornstein & Saulnier, 1981) raise questions about these approaches as primary linguistic systems for most deaf children.

What is clear is that many deaf children do learn sign language when they establish contact with other deaf children, even in the absence of deaf adult linguistic models (Livingston, 1986). Further, this rich language competence carries them into adulthood, where they hold jobs, marry, raise families, and pay taxes even with minimal English skills. Thus it can be assumed that visual rather than auditory languages are the natural communicative modes for a majority of deaf children. Further, it is reasonable to assume that ASL or an English-based sign system like Pidgin sign language could very well be the first complete language system that many deaf children are able to internalize, and it is thus their first language.

In this approach, the child is introduced to and engages in conversations with deaf adults, other deaf children, and signing hearing people at an early age (Bouvet, 1983; Bernstein & Goodhart, 1985). Since parents and teachers have difficulty learning ASL, they can use a Pidgin sign language which uses ASL expression but in English word order. This is a more natural form of language than the artificial manual codes of English and will permit the language acquisition process to occur.

Opportunities should arise for many conversations with real-world use of language rather than stereotypic responses which have traditionally been drilled in many classrooms for deaf children. The teacher and parent need to focus on the meaning of the utterances rather than the correct grammatical form.

GOAL 2: CONSIDER ENGLISH AS A SECOND LANGUAGE

Another major goal of the bilingual/bicultural approach is for deaf children to learn how to use English—spoken, signed, reading a text, and writing a message. The difficulties deaf children have in acquiring literacy skills are well documented. In chapters 3, 5, and 10 we described the low achievement scores of deaf children on standardized tests in communication, reading, and writing.

How can English skills be taught? The literature on research with various theoretical frameworks for the past 100 years has repeatedly documented that a hearing loss causes delays and deficits in language development across all components—phonological, semantic, syntactic, and pragmatic in spoken, reading texts, and written forms (see reviews by Kretchmer & Kretchmer, 1986). These studies report low academic achievement scores, indicating that classroom and clinical intervention procedures have produced meager results in view of deaf children's intellectual potential (Vernon, 1967).

The goal of deaf students' acquisition of English must be grounded in realistic terms. For deaf children who have significant mental handicaps such as brain damage, the learning of English will be minimal. Even for the average deaf child, achievement levels in language and reading after 11 or more years of formal schooling often plateau at about the third- or fourth-grade level.

Bilingual and English as a second language (ESL) methods used with minority children in the United States have been proposed for deaf children (Bernstein & Goodhart, 1985; Bouvet, 1983; Reagan, 1985). Some types of these model bilingual programs are outlined by Fillmore & Valadez (1986). While there is controversy in the field of bilingualism as to which approach is better, it is generally agreed that school programs that recognize, accept, and use the minority children's language and culture in the school do facilitate their acquisition of English as a second language (Fillmore & Valadez, 1986). These techniques need to be utilized in programs for deaf children.

GOAL 3: GIVE DEAF TEACHERS AN IMPORTANT ROLE

This goal considers deaf adults as co-equal partners in educational decision making (Reagan, 1985; Vernon, 1970). Deaf adults function as role models from which deaf children can form their identity. Additionally, they serve as linguistic models who provide mature American Sign Language input to all deaf children, especially those with minimal signing skills. Additionally, deaf adults provide knowledge to hearing educators about how deafness affects day-to-day living and working as well as the learning of English.

Unfortunately, discriminatory practices in schools and universities impede the participation of capable deaf adults in educational programs. Only about 12 percent of teachers in programs in the United States who responded to a 1985 survey were deaf (Craig & Craig, 1986). Those who do make it into programs are seldom promoted to administrative positions (Vernon, 1970). These discriminatory practices may result from authoritarian personalities in hiring positions who have negative attitudes toward minority populations such as the deaf community (see chapter 9).

At the university level, deaf persons face obstacles in earning a teaching certificate because of negative attitudes from professors and lack of support services such as notetaking and interpreting. Deaf adults are typically penalized because of poor speech and hearing skills—areas where their capabilities are limited. Instead, teacher-training programs need to focus on areas where they can contribute, such as in communication, psychosocial development, language, reading, and other academic areas.

For the small minority of capable hearing-impaired and deaf adults who persist and receive their teacher certification, employment is difficult to obtain. Even after being hired, deaf teachers experience great frustration in public schools because of the lack of awareness about deafness. One deaf teacher's frustrations in a self-contained classroom in a public school are expressed as follows:

> I have one awful time understanding him [her hearing principal]. He doesn't move his upper lip. He is very patient with me and scribbles notes when he is utterly incomprehensible. He does not have a PA system and sends a written announcement sheet around every morning. Dandy! But I must get a light installed in our room for the emergency bell. We have been left behind a few times.

The concessions a school system may make to accommodate deaf teachers for hearing-impaired and deaf children are amply repaid in the services these adults provide. A mixture of hearing and deaf teachers in a school can provide a rich cognitive and linguistic environment where deaf children are exposed to mature language models—ASL and English—from which they can extract rules and generate their own language. Over time, with repeated use in interactions with communicating adults and peers, the child's language will naturally evolve into adult forms. Hearing adults help the deaf child learn the conversational function of speech that, when supported by sign, will help them communicate more effectively with their hearing parents.

GOAL 4: INCLUDE THE HISTORY, CULTURE, AND LITERATURE OF DEAFNESS IN THE SCHOOL CURRICULUM

In order for deaf children to form a positive self-concept, it is important to bring into the classroom information about the history, culture, and literature about deafness. Chapters 1 and 4 cover some of this information. Publishing companies such as Gallaudet University Press, the NAD, and T. J. Publishers provide numerous books, periodicals, and curriculum materials. Deaf children of all ages need to be exposed to the experiences of deaf adults who have made valuable contributions to society and have coped with their hearing loss. Biographies of deaf leaders, authors, inventors, scientists, and artists, for example, could be covered. The student protest in support of a deaf president for Gallaudet University would make an excellent reading and history lesson for a classroom of deaf students.

GOAL 5: GROUND CLASSROOM PRACTICE IN LEARNING THEORY

Cognitive psychology offers insights on how students learn. One current theory—the cognitive information processing view—states that learning and behavior emerge from an interaction of the environment and the learner's previous experiences and knowledge. Rather than just looking at the learner's behavior, this theory examines the learner's mental processes (Phye & Andre, 1986). Cognitive processes for learning that have been identified include attention, short-term memory, long-term memory, and metacognitive skills.

Attentional processes involve how the student is attending to the teacher's presentation. Teachers with deaf students need to make decisions on how to maintain and focus their attention. Techniques that focus on visual displays of information via signs, pictures, films, videotapes, or acting out of ideas could be used in such a classroom.

Two other cognitive processes involve short-term and long-term memory. Helping deaf children with rehearsal techniques after studying math facts is an example of the short-term process. Making sure the lesson in appropriately paced so as not to overload the student with information is another. Long-term memory processes include helping the student build "schemes, scripts or frames" about concepts and principles. Teachers can build up the students' background knowledge to expand their conceptual knowledge.

Another cognitive process relates to metacognition. Metacognitive skills refers to how students know what they have to learn and how they go about learning this information. For example, what strategies would they use to read a passage for pleasure as opposed to reading a passage to pass an exam. Another example is how they are monitoring their reading comprehension.

Knowledge of these cognitive processes enables teachers to make changes in students' mental processes as they go about carrying out instructional tasks in the classroom, rather than just altering the environment (Phye & Andre, 1986).

GOAL 6: PROMOTE INTERACTIVE LEARNING STRATEGIES

Teachers need to have the communication skills to interact manually and orally with deaf children. As was mentioned before, we recommend a combination of ASL, Pidgin Sign English, and the addition of the 14 Signed English markers.

With these communication skills, teachers can set up an environment that emphasizes interaction between the teacher and student. Just as children naturally learn language through conversations with mother in a highly affective and social context, teachers need to set up classroom situations that replicate this process.

Traditionally, language instruction in many programs for deaf children has been limited to written language. One reason is that many teachers do not have the communication skills to converse manually with deaf children (Maxwell, 1984). Classroom methods have been didactic, relying on drill, the Fitzgerald key, other procedures using symbols for grammatical categories, a slot grammer approach, programmed instruction, transformational grammar, or behavior modification (Clarke & Stewart, 1986). These approaches generally start with an adult model of language competency and do not take into account child developmental levels. Another problem is that these methods emphasize the role of correcting "bad

English" despite the fact that child language research reveals that correction plays a limited role in language learning.

A DEVELOPMENTAL PERSPECTIVE

Reading and writing instruction, like natural language development, is best viewed as a process (Hartse, Woodward, & Burke, 1984). Rather than focusing on the weaknesses and deficiencies of deaf children using the adult model, recent attempts have been made to document what strengths deaf children do have that lead to conventional knowledge and performance of reading and writing. Research methodology has increasingly shifted from tasks such as answering comprehension questions or making a grammatical judgment about a sentence, to simply performing whole reading and writing tasks in the best way they can (Hartse, Woodward, & Burke, 1984).

There is an emergent data base which examines deaf childrens' strengths in reading and writing abilities. Many relevant studies show how deaf children build literacy skills upon their already existing sign language. Some of these studies will be reviewed here.

HOME LITERACY

In a longitudinal reading acquisition study hearing parents were interviewed as to what their kindergarten or first-grade children knew about environmental print (words on labels, street signs, etc.), printed letters, words, and stories and how parents supported reading activities at home (Andrews & Mason, 1986a, 1986b). Parents reported that their kindergarten children often pointed out letters on environmental signs using fingerspelling. With other labels, they showed a progression from first focusing on a picture or a logo on a label to focusing on the actual print. For example, Trix breakfast food was identified with the signs RABBIT CEREAL. Other children incorporated fingerspelling and numerals into their reading of labels. For instance, McDonald's was frequently signed "M" with the arch sign, and alphabet soup was A-B-C-1-2-3. Other children were reading addresses on family mail, other food and clothing labels, and road signs but were pairing print with their knowledge of sign language.

In this same study parents reported a variety of book-sharing behaviors they used with their children. Some parents would just sign pictures in storybooks. Others would condense the story plots, using what signs they knew. One exceptional mother, a former teacher of French and skilled user of ASL, reported she approached reading to her deaf son as if she were reading in a second language. She translated English words, idioms, and sentences into Pidgin Sign English, making sure he understood the meanings of the English structures. She often would bracket groups of words in pencil, then explain the meaning in context and conceptually in signs.

Other case studies describe young deaf children beginning to read when their parents tie sign language communication to print. For example, Marie began to read books at age 4 years, 5 months when she transferred her fingerspelling games used with her mother to reading material (Schlesinger & Meadow, 1972). Another deaf child, Mark, began to read at age 5 years, 6 months when his parents pointed out that printed words can have corresponding manual signs (Henderson, 1976). Maxwell (1984) reports on Alice, a deaf girl with deaf parents, who was videotaped from age 2 years, 3 months to 6 years, 3 months as she was read storybooks by her parents. Alice began attending to her father's sign movements as he read her books. From age 21 months on, Maxwell reports, books were the source of stimulating social interaction between Alice and her parents. She learned about the conventions of front and back, directionality, and page turning. She learned how meaning could be referenced to signs made by her parents, to sign illustrations in books, and to printed words.

Teachers can encourage parents to foster literacy in the homes by pointing out and discussing environmental print, helping children print their names, label drawings with letters, and reading storybooks to their deaf children. These informal home intervention procedures can lead the child into literacy acquisition based on their knowledge of fingerspelling and signs.

EARLY LITERACY

Several studies have examined deaf children's literacy knowledge in kindergarten and the first grade (Andrews & Mason, 1986; Booth & Hall, 1985; Conway, 1985; Ewoldt, 1985).

Booth and Hall (1985) designed a six-week classroom intervention program in which deaf children were introduced to print that had a communicative purpose. Classroom activities included increased awareness of environmental print and awareness that print conveys a message, that it is useful, and that it can be interesting. Teacher strategies included walking around the neighborhood to read environmental print, taking photographs of street and store signs, going to the public library, reading magazines and newspapers, setting up a cafe in the classroom, writing letters to friends, having the teacher demonstrate administrative paper work, and increasing the amount of storytelling. The children responded with increased interest in literacy activities during and after the intervention.

Another classroom intervention focused on storybook reading in kindergarten and the first grade (Andrews, 1988; Andrews & Mason, 1986a). Twenty-three deaf children in groups of five to six participated in a weekly story-reading session over a nine-month period. The teacher used a technique called *reciprocal teaching*, which is an interactive dialogue between students and teacher. The teacher models reading a story, (i.e., pointing to the title, page turning, reading from left to right), discusses the story content, guides the children as they read, and supervises them as they hold and read books, play act, and recite the stories. The students then take turns being the teacher. After a full year of participation in this routine, the deaf children made gains in storybook reading, fingerspelling, word recognition, and story reciting. Additionally, they showed self-monitoring behaviors such as predicting story outcomes for familiar stories and initiating asking questions about story titles.

Ewoldt (1985) examined literacy development over a three-year time frame of 10 preschool deaf children of deaf parents. She studied the children's school writing, reading, art, and sign production as related to the *language experience* approach to writing, a strategy in which the teacher writes a child's story as the child signs it. Also the children were provided with library books and daily experiences for reading of writing. Ewoldt reported that the children's free writing typically had a message behind it, demonstrating that they knew that writing was a communicative act. The children's writing developed from scribbling as a motor activity to unanalyzed wholes to analysis of salient features. Deaf children showed evidence of invented spellings. Teachers gave them extensive input on how printed language works through reading to them and taking their sign dictation.

Conway (1985) described the purposes of free-choice (in contrast to teacher-directed) writing in a class of hearing-impaired kindergarteners. In his 23 classroom visits, he used a naturalistic approach, incorporating observing classrooms, compiling field notes, videotaping the children while they wrote, collecting their written products, and interviewing the children and teachers. A table was set up in the classroom with writing materials, and Conway observed the children in their free-choice writing activities. He identified seven purposes in the children's writing: to preserve or recall experiences, to convey personal information, to organize general information, to interact with a specific audience, and to entertain, plus nonmessage-related purposes of practicing skills and exploring the mechanics of creating writing. For the children in his study, writing emerged early and was evolving as a purposeful activity that could be used to fulfill personal and cultural needs.

Deaf children need to be introduced to the purpose or communicative function of print during the early school years or before. Storybook reading should be a daily activity in the classroom, with the children encouraged to retell and play act the plots. Teachers need to make explicit the connection between the manual sign and printed forms through classroom activities. The above studies give suggestions on how the teacher can accomplish these goals.

School Literacy

Other studies have focused on elementary and high school deaf youth's attempts to read and write.

Ewoldt (1985) videotaped four deaf children to determine how they were reading whole stories or passages using sign language. She identified several strategies they were using to get meaning from print: fingerspelling strategies, context clues, and rereading strategies. All four students were able to retell stories using sign language; Ewoldt believed this to be a good measure of their comprehension.

Yurkowski & Ewoldt (1986) suggest other instructional activities based on their work with deaf readers: matching story characters with their characteristics, finding similarities among stories, using the DRTA—Directed Reading-Thinking Activity (predicting the next event) (Stauffer, 1970) combined with retelling of the story and discussion. Ewoldt stresses preparing the deaf child for the text rather than preparing the text (by rewriting) for the deaf child. She encourages teachers to use simpler texts as a way to build background knowledge in deaf readers before exposing them to more difficult texts.

Ewoldt (1977) and Gormely and Franzen (1978) have suggested the use of whole stories on topics familiar to the readers, enabling them to bypass more difficult syntax. Ewoldt cautions teachers that rewriting materials or avoiding difficult syntactic passages may inhibit rather than promote reading growth, because deaf children need the exposure to difficult structures to use strategies.

Another area of reading development for elementary and secondary students is training in metacognitive strategies, those strategies used by skilled readers to help themselves over difficult spots (Baker & Brown, 1984). In reading cloze passages from expository text, five deaf high school readers across various reading levels from a residential school were found to use such strategies as background knowledge, context clues, looking ahead in the passage, looking back at previous sentences, and rereading difficult words, phrases, or sentences in the passage (Andrews & Mason, 1986b). These findings suggest that deaf students may profit from direct instruction of what to do when they encounter difficult print. Using the strategies used by skilled deaf readers teaching them to unskilled deaf readers is a promising area of research. Recent self-monitoring training studies have shown that direct instruction of these cognitive skills does increase reading comprehension of underachieving readers (Palinscar, 1984).

Educators who hold a developmental view in the teaching of literacy suggest several ideas for teachers. Staton (1984) described the Gallaudet College Research Institute's Dialogue Journal Projects, developed for elementary and secondary hearing-impaired students. A student notebook or journal was used to generate interactive dialogue, which consisted of frequent and continuous written conversations carried on by students and teachers over an extended period. Each student wrote an entry each day and gave it to the teacher for a response. These encounters resembled face-to-face conversation rather than the formal writing assignments given in school. Writing lessons became reading lessons too, as the student had to read the teacher's response. Although language input was not grammatically sequenced in advance, grammatical structures emerged and were used naturally by teachers in response to the students' written language competence, thus giving them the input in a conversational way from which to extract the rules of English.

Another writing study involved the effects of complementary training in sign language and simultaneous communication on the literacy skills. In complementary instruction, a student receive instruction consisting of linguistic analysis of sign language or sign systems and practice translation from the student's preferred sign language/system into written English (Akamatsu, 1986). Deaf high school students received instruction during the two 10-week intervention periods. The experimental group achieved higher scores than the control groups on guided writing and sign comprehension. No difference was found in spontaneous writing. The author attributed this to insufficient time and input for internalizing the rules. The lack of effect of grammatical instruction on grammaticality in spontaneous writing was also noted.

TECHNOLOGY

Technology over the last decade has impacted classroom teaching. TDD and TV captions have made telephones and television accessible to deaf persons. TV captioned programs have been used successfully to improve interest, vocabulary, and comprehension in young deaf readers (Koskinen, Wilson, & Jensema, 1986).

Computer technology holds promise especially for deaf children with additional disabilities (Andrews, Haas, Weller, 1987; Andrews & Sinclair, 1989). Children with motor difficulties, short attention spans, and learning disabilities can benefit from peripheral devices such as enlarged keyboards or joysticks. Students whose handwriting is illegible because of a motor handicap feel pride when they can print their work on a word processor. Many computer games have speed controls to slow down the rate of programming. The microcomputer is a promising tool, not to replace but to assist the teacher.

These studies only review a segment of the emerging data base on how to teach reading and writing by using the strengths of the deaf child. Literacy is believed to take place within dialogue or communication between teacher and student. Like hearing children, deaf children learn language best through conversational exchanges, interactive storytelling, interactive writing, and genuine dialogue in educational contexts.

Deaf children and youth can learn to read and write if they are given ample opportunity in the classroom to explore the processes of reading and writing. Many may never achieve the levels of proficiency of their hearing counterparts because of multiple handicaps. Nevertheless, they need to be exposed to literacy activities from an early age. A bilingual approach to literacy instruction allows the teacher to use what sign language skills the child has on which to build English skills.

FUTURE RESEARCH

Educational ethnography holds valuable tools and techniques to direct and evaluate learning outcomes in classrooms for deaf children. Educational ethnography analyzes and describes what goes on in the classroom, taking into account the cultural background of the teachers and students, their values and beliefs, the communities they come from, their ways of interacting, and their use of language and communication (Goetz & LeCompte, 1984; Heath, 1983). By taking into account the social and cultural contexts of learning, educators and researchers can determine more fully what are the language and learning habits of deaf children (Maxwell, 1985).

REFERENCES

Akamatsu, C. T. (1986, April). The effects of instruction in sign language on writing and sign comprehension in deaf students. Paper presented at the American Educational Research Association, San Francisco.

Andrews, J. F. (1988). Deaf children's acquisition of prereading skills using the reciprocal teaching procedure. *Exceptional Children, 54*(4), 349–355.

Andrews, J. F., Haas, D., & Waller, J. (1987). How to use the microcomputer with multihandicapped hearing impaired students. *Perspectives for Teachers of the Hearing Impaired, 5*(3), 15–19.

Andrews, J. F., & Mason, J. M. (1986a). How do deaf children learn about prereading? *American Annals of the Deaf, 131*(3), 210–217.

Andrews, J. J., & Mason, J. M. (1986b, April). How do deaf, hearing and reading disabled youths comprehend expository texts? Paper presented at the American Educational Research Association, San Francisco.

Andrews, J. F., & Sinclair, J. (1989). Software with graphics: A language motivator for high school students who are deaf. *Teaching Exceptional Children 21,* (3), 16–18.

Ashton-Warner, S. (1963). *Teacher.* New York: Simon & Schuster.

Baker, L., & Brown, A. (1984). Metacognitive skills and reading. In D. Pearson (Ed.), *Handbook of reading research.* New York: Longman.

Bernstein, D., & Tiegerman, E. (1985). *Language and communication disorders in children.* Columbus, OH: Charles Merrill Publishing.

Bernstein, M., & Goodhart, W. (1985). *Demonstration project evaluation report.* Philadelphia: The Pennsylvania School for the Deaf.

Bonvillian, J. D., Charrow, V. R., & Nelson, K. E. (1973). Psycholinguistic and educational implications of deafness. *Human Development, 16,* 321–345.

Booth, E., & Hall, N. (1985). Making sense of literacy. In D. Hustler (Ed.), *Action-research in classrooms and schools.* London: Allen and Unwin.

Bornstein, H., & Saulnier, K. (1981). Signed English: A brief follow-up to the first evaluation. *American Annals of the Deaf, 126,* 69–72.

Bornstein, H., Saulnier, K., & Hamilton, L. (1980). Signed English: A first evaluation. *American Annals of the Deaf, 125,* 467–481.

Bouvet, D. (1983, July). Bilingual education for deaf children. In W. Stockoe & V. Volterra (Eds.), *Proceedings of the III. International Symposium on Sign Language Research,* Rome.

Brown, R. (1973). *A first language: The early stages.* Cambridge, MA: Harvard University Press.

Clarke, B. R., & Stewart, D. A. (1986). Reflections on language programs for the hearing impaired. *Journal of Special Education, 20*(2), 153–165.

Conway, D. (1985). Children (re)creating writing: A preliminary look at the purposes of free-choice writing of hearing-impaired kindergarteners. In R. Kretchmer (Ed.), Learning to write and writing to learn. *The Volta Review, 87*(5), 91–107.

Craig, W. N., & Craig, H. B. (1986). Programs and services for the deaf in the United States. *American Annals of the Deaf, 131*(2), 134–135.

Delgado, G. L. (1984). Hearing-impaired children from non-native language homes. In G. Delgado (Ed.), *The Hispanic deaf: Issues and challenges for bilingual education.* Washington, DC: Gallaudet College Press.

Erting, C., & Marlborough, C. (1986). Deaf mothers' communication with deaf infants. *Research at Gallaudet,* Fall, p. 11.

Ewoldt, C. (1977). A psycholinguistic description of selected deaf children reading in sign language. Unpublished Doctoral Dissertation, Wayne State University, Detroit.

Ewoldt, C. (1985). A descriptive study of the developing literacy of young hearing-impaired children. In R. Kretchmer (Ed.), Learning to write and writing to learn. *The Volta Review, 87*(5), 109–126.

Furth, H. (1973). *Deafness and learning: A psychological approach.* Belmont, Calif.: Wadsworth Publishers.

Fillmore, L. W., & Valadez, C. (1986). Teaching bilingual learners. In M. Wittrock (Ed.), *Handbook of research on teaching.* (pp. 648–685). New York: Macmillan.

Gleitman, L. R., & Wanner, E. (1986). Language acquisition: The state of the art. In E. Wanner & L. Gleitman (Eds.), *Language acquisition: The state of the art.* London: Cambridge University Press.

Goetz, J. P. & LeCompte, M. D. (1984). *Ethnography and qualitative design in educational research.* New York: Academic Press.

Gormely, K., & Franzen, A. (1978). Why can't the deaf read? *American Annals of the Deaf, 123,* 542–547.

Greenberg, M. T. (1983). Family stress and child competence: The effects of early intervention for families with deaf infants. *American Annals of the Deaf, 125*(9), 407–417.

Greenberg, M. T., Calderon, R., & Kusche, C. (1984). Early intervention using simultaneous communication with deaf infants: The effect on communication development. *Child Development, 55,* 607–616.

Grosjean, F. (1982). *Life with two languages: An introduction to bilingualism.* Cambridge, MA: Harvard University Press.

Hartse, J. C., Woodward, V. A., & Burke, C. L. (1984). *Language stories and literacy lessons.* Portsmouth, NH: Heinemann Educational Books.

Heath, S. B. *Ways with words.* (1983). London: Cambridge University Press.

Henderson, J. M. (1976). Learning to read: A case study of a deaf child. *American Annals of the Deaf, 121,* 502–506.

Howell, R. F. (1984). Maternal reports of vocabulary development in four-year-old deaf children. *American Annals of the Deaf, 129*(6), 459–465.

Kannapell, B. (1974). Bilingual education: A new direction in the education of the deaf. *The Deaf American, 26*(10), 9–15.

Kannapell, B. (1985). Language choice reflects identity choice: A sociolinguistic study of deaf college students. Unpublished doctoral dissertation, Georgetown University, Washington, DC.

Kindred, E. (1980). Mainstream teenagers with care. *American Annals of the Deaf, 125,* 1053–1056.

Koskinen, P. S., Wilson, R. M., & Jensema, C. J. (1986). Using close-captioned television in the teaching of reading to deaf students. *American Annals of the Deaf, 131*(1), 43–46.

Kretchmer, R., & Kretchmer, L. (1986). Language in perspective. In D. Lutterman (ed.) *Deafness in perspective.* San Diego; College-Hill Press.

Kyle, J. G. (1986). Deaf people and minority groups in the U.K. In B. Trevort (Ed.), *Signs in life.* Amsterdam: Dutch Foundation for the Deaf.

Livingston, S. (1986). An alternative view of education for deaf children: Part 1. *American Annals of the Deaf, 131*(1), 21–25.

Luetke-Stahlman, B. (1986). Building a language base in hearing-impaired students. *American Annals of the Deaf, 131*(3), 220–228.

Maestas y Moores, J. (1980). Early linguistic environment: Interaction of deaf parents with their infants. *Sign Language Studies, 26,* 1–30.

Maestas y Moores, J., & Moores, D. (1984). The status of Hispanics in special education. In G. Delgado (Ed.), *The Hispanic deaf: Issues and challenges for bilingual education.* Washington, DC: Gallaudet College Press.

Maxwell, M. (1984). A deaf child's natural development of literacy. *Sign Language Studies, 44,* 191–224.

Maxwell, M. (1985). Introduction: Ethnography & education of deaf children. *Sign Language Studies, 47,* 97–108.

McIntyre, M. L. (1977). The acquisition of American sign language hand configurations. *Sign Language Studies, 16,* 247–266.

Meadow, K. P., Greenberg, M. T., Erting, C., & Carmichael, H. (1981). Interactions of deaf mothers and deaf preschool children: Comparisons with three other groups of deaf and hearing dyads. *American Annals of the Deaf, 126,* 454–468.

Menyuk, P. (1917). *Language and maturation.* Cambridge, MA: MIT Press.

Moog, J., Geers, A., & Schick, B. (1984). Acquisition of spoken and sign of English by profoundly deaf children. *Journal of Speech and Hearing Disorders, 49*(4), 378–388.

National Association of the Deaf Executive Board. (1986, April). Public Law 94-142 and the least restrictive environment: A position paper of the National Association of the Deaf. *The Broadcaster.*

Newport, E., & Meier, R. (1985). The acquisition of American Sign Language. In D. Slobin. *The crosslinguistic study of language acquisition. Volume 1: The Data.* Hillsdale, N.J.: Lawrence Erlbaum.

Palinscar, A. (1984). The quest for meaning from expository texts: A teacher guided journey. In G. Duffy, L. Roehler & J. Mason (Eds.), *Comprehension instruction: Perspectives and suggestions.* New York: Longman.

Phye, G., & Andre, T. (Eds.). (1986). *Cognitive classroom learning: Understand, thinking, and problem solving.* New York: Academic Press.

Quigley, S. P., & Paul, P. P. (1984). *Language and deafness.* San Diego: College Hill Press.

Reagan, T. (1985). The deaf as a linguistic minority: Educational considerations. *Harvard Educational Review, 55*(3), 265–277.

Reich, P., & Bick, M. (1977). How visible is visible English? *Sign Language Studies, 14,* 59–72.

Ries, P. (1986). Characteristics of hearing impaired youth in the general population and of students in special education programs for the hearing impaired. In A. Schildroth & M. Karchmer (Eds.), *Deaf children in America.* San Diego: College Hill Press.

Schlesinger, H. S., & Meadow, K. P. (1972). *Sound and sign: Childhood deafness and mental health.* Berkeley: University of California Press.

Snow, C. (1972). Mothers' speech to children learning language. *Child Development, 43,* 549–565.

Staton, J. (1984). Using dialogue journals for developing thinking, reading, and writing with hearing-impaired students. In R. R. Kretchmer (Ed.), Learning to write and writing to learn. *The Volta Review, 87*(5), 127–154.

Stauffer, R. (1970). *The language experience approach to the teaching of reading.* New York: Harper and Row.

Stokoe, W. C. (Ed.). (1980). *Sign and culture: A reader for students of American Sign Language.* Silver Spring, MD: Linstok Press.

Vernon, M. (1967). Relationship of language to the thinking process. *Archives of General Psychiatry, 16,* 325–333.

Vernon, M. (1970). The role of the deaf teachers in the education of deaf children. *Deaf American, 22,* 17–20.

Vernon, M. (1985, August). Controversy within sign language. Paper presented at the Learning Vacation Camp of Deaf Children's Society, British Columbia.

Vernon, M., & Ottinger, P. (1980). Counseling the hearing impaired child in a mainstreamed setting. In L. Benjamin and G. Walz (Eds.), *Counseling exceptional people.* Ann Arbor, MI: ERIC Counseling and Personnel Services Clearinghouse.

Vernon, M., & Prickett, H. (1976, February–March). Mainstreaming: Issues and a model plan. *Audiology and Hearing Education, 2,* 5–10.

Wedell-Monnig, J., & Lumley, J. (1980). Child deafness and mother–child interaction. *Child Development, 51,* 766–774.

Woodward, J. (1982). Some sociolinguistic problems in the implementation of bilingual education for deaf students. In J. Woodward (Ed.), *How you gonna get to heaven if you can't speak with Jesus.* Silver Spring, MD: T. J. Publishers.

Yurkowski, P., & Ewoldt, C. (1986). A case for the semantic processing of the deaf reader. *American Annals of the Deaf, 131*(3), 243–247.

CHAPTER 12
Partial Hearing

They have ears but they hear not.   Psalm 115:5–6

The hard-of-hearing person is probably the least understood and most neglected of all handicapped individuals. This is especially true for those with early onset (from birth to age 3). The public's lack of understanding is somewhat ironic considering the size of the hard-of-hearing population. For example, 7 out of 1,000 schoolchildren have a bilateral hearing loss (500–20000Hz) of 26 dB or more (Berg, 1971). This means there are about four times more people who are hard-of-hearing than who are deaf (Schein & Delk, 1974, p. 19; Ross 1976). As we mentioned in the introduction, on a national level, hearing loss is the most prevalent of all chronic diseases.

AUDIOLOGICAL CONSIDERATIONS

DEFINITION OF HARD-OF-HEARING

The definition of hard-of-hearing that has the greatest significance for psychological purposes is, "an auditory loss in which the individual can hear sufficiently (with or without amplification) to understand most, but not all, conversation in a quiet one-to-one situation in which he is looking at the speaker. In group situations or where there are background noises, the hard-of-hearing person understands some to none of what is said." Those with only unilateral losses would not be considered hard-of-hearing because one good ear is adequate in most normal communication situations.

Most other definitions of hard-of-hearing are expressed in decibel ranges. While these have value audiologically, they generally fail to indicate in clear operational terms the functional hearing a person has for speech sounds. Part of the problem of a definition in terms of decibels is the poor correlation between pure tone audiograms and the ability to hear and understand speech. However, in every definition of hard-of-hearing there remains a gray area between being deaf or hard-of-hearing and between being hard-of-hearing or having enough hearing to communicate essentially as a normally hearing person.

PSYCHOLOGICAL IMPLICATIONS OF AUDIOLOGICAL PRACTICES

One problem that has contributed tremendously to the failure to understand the hard-of-hearing person's psychological and educational problems is the manner in which hearing is frequently measured and reported. Often testing is done in elaborately sound-treated rooms which eliminate all ordinary environmental noises. The only sounds present are the beeps of the audiometer or the words spoken for the comprehension tests. Obviously the results of such testing would generalize primarily to other sound-treated audiological suites, not to the real world. The hard-of-hearing person's actual environment is the noisy nursery, the acoustically reverberating classroom, the clangs and bangs of a factory, buzzing offices, a family room dominated by the blare of television, or a restaurant with 85 dB level of background conversation and clattering utensils.

Predicting the functional hearing that a person has for everyday life from a test of performance in a sound-treated audiometric chamber can be almost as inaccurate as forecasting weather from whether or not the groundhog sees his shadow (Yanick, 1976). For example, the individual who understands 80 percent of the words on a speech comprehension test taken in a sound-treated booth may not be able to understand *a single word* the teacher says in an average classroom. The teacher who has been told by the audiological report that the child has a speech discrimination score of 80 percent will expect the child to hear almost everything said in the classroom, but the child actually may be hearing little or nothing. Tremendous problems can develop as a result of differences between expectation and level of performance. Frequently the teacher concludes that the child is stupid, a view then shared by other students and, subsequently, by the child himself. The child may even be transferred to a class for slow learners. This kind of tragic error is perpetrated yearly upon thousands of hearing-impaired schoolchildren in the United States. The effects on the children are devastating.

Good audiological clinics avoid many of the above problems by using tapes of environmental sounds as background noises during testing. Use of this more realistic environment permits the hard-of-hearing person's functional hearing for speech sounds to be assessed under conditions similar to what he will face in the real world and greatly improve the understanding and prediction of actual auditory potential for aural communication. However, just as the best IQ testing has limitations for predicting school schievement, audiometric findings are still far from perfect as predictors of the degree of speech comprehension in everyday life.

Apart from the technicalities of audiologic assessment, the crucial fact is that many hard-of-hearing people are unable to understand what is being said in the classroom, nursery, home, office, theater, and other settings where communication occurs (Bradley & Bryant, 1978; Conrad, 1979). This obvious but frequently ignored fact has tremendous significance for the hard-of-hearing person and those with whom they come in contact. Their perception of, and therefore their exposure to, oral language is in many cases minimal and inconsistent (Conrad, 1979). Instead of hearing complete sentences and words, they get a fragmented input which is syntactically and phonetically incorrect (Conrad, 1979; Vernon & Billingslea, 1973). They are inevitably far more linguistically deprived than would be expected from superficial interaction with them, especially in a quiet one-to-one setting (Graham, 1975). A general assumption that these people understand far more than they actually do leads to grossly unrealistic expectations for linguistic development, educational achievement, and socialization (Hine, 1970a,b, & c). In fact, many prelingually hard-of-hearing persons often have a linguistic development character-istic of congenitally deaf individuals (Conrad, 1979). This surprising fact is of absolutely premium importance for an understanding of psychological function-ing.

Special Problems of the Hard-of-Hearing Person

The reasons underlying the differences between audiometric test results and functional hearing outside the audiometric room are of such crucial psychological significance that they need even further elaboration. First, hearing aids distort sound. For example, they tend to amplify background noises disproportionately. These background sounds are frequently low pitched and intense, masking or blocking out the acoustic parameters that make speech understandable. As a result, the hearing aid does not facilitate speech comprehension in normal environments as effectively as it does in the sound-treated room when hearing is being tested.

Second, for the normally hearing individual, as background noises increase, the ability to comprehend speech declines gradually. For the hard-of-hearing person, the decline tends to be precipitous (Yanick, 1976). Hence, in schoolrooms, with their normal high levels of noise, the hard-of-hearing student may understand little or nothing of what teacher or classmates say.

Third, those with hearing losses have a particularly difficult time understanding speech if the background sounds are also speech (Carhart & Tillman, 1970). For example, group discussion, classroom discourses, cocktail party conversation, church sermons, or conversation with television or radio in the background would be disproportionately difficult for the hard-of-hearing person to understand (Carhart & Tillman, 1970). In fact, most hard-of-hearing persons are "communicatively lost" in these settings.

A fourth consideration is that a hard-of-hearing person's ability to hear in natural situations relates to whether or not the loss is sensorineural. Generally, amplification distorts sound far less for those whose loss is conductive in nature rather than sensorineural (Graham, 1975). They also have less of a problem distinguishing speech sounds from background noises (Carhart & Tillman, 1970). In the case of otitis media and allergic reactions, individuals' hearing levels often vary tremendously according to the state of their nasal aural congestion. This variation creates still another problem, and resulting language retardation is common (Holm & Kunze, 1969).

Two basic auditory problems of the hard-of-hearing, then, are discrimination and consistency of input. While most people understand that the hard-of-hearing person's ability to make distinctions between speech and background sounds is inferior to that of the normally hearing person, even under ideal conditions (Wilcox & Tobin, 1974), few realize how precipitously discrimination falls as the signal-to-noise ratio drops (Yanick, 1976). For those whose hearing loss varies because of changing middle ear conditions, the basic problem is further compounded.

A final point needs to be made. Many sensorineural hearing losses that in the past were assumed to be stable are now regarded as progressive and irreversible. Also chronic conductive losses can cause permanent damage to audition. Long-range planning for patients must take these facts into consideration. Ironically, parents are often told by physicians and other professionals that their child "will grow out of it" (Graham, 1975). The rehabilitation and educational planning required in the case of progressive hearing loss is drastically different from that required for a static or correctable loss. Thus, whenever possible, the prognosis must be established and fully communicated to the patient and family.

Amplification and auditory training can help many hard-of-hearing people. Tremendous advances have been made enabling many who once would have functioned as deaf to now communicate aurally with adequacy. Unfortunately, the enthusiasm of some proponents of these approaches has led to unrealistic, unproven claims for their value (Grammatico, 1975; Griffiths, 1975; Pollack, 1974, 1975). Testimonials or case histories are often presented which suggest that "hearing is restored by amplification." Sometimes highly unreliable hearing tests on extremely young infants are compared with later tests and the differences are used to support claims of improved hearing through amplification. The alleged improvement is often no more than an indication of invalid infant test scores (Griffiths, 1975). Actually there is considerable evidence that high levels of amplification, especially if used early, can impair hearing and that auditory training does not improve speech (Conrad, 1979).

The false promises of "professionals" concerning the value of amplification are destructive. They feed the parent's, the public's, and the professional's needs to deny the unpleasant realities of the hard-of-hearing individual's life situation. As a result of such denial, the misguided will set unrealistic goals instead of facing and coping constructively with the problem. Psychological, social, and educational damage (often irreversible) is the consequence. However, false claims such as these should not deter us from expecting reasonable results from amplification nor should they blind us to the progress that audiology, medicine, and technology have made in the improvement of hearing aids and surgical procedures. It should also be recognized that technology has its limitations and that such limits may have been reached relative to hearing aid development (Conrad, 1979).

PROBLEMS IN SCHOOL AUDIOLOGICAL SERVICES

Frequently hearing screening programs and support services for hard-of-hearing children that look good on paper may be failures in practice. The following example from a fairly typical Eastern school system illustrates the problem (Vernon & Billingslea, 1973). According to school policy:

> Audiometric screening by state trained technicians was done on all children in the second, fourth, and sixth grades. Results were entered on the child's folder. If hearing losses were identified, parents were notified. Follow-up was the parents' responsibility.

These kinds of programs, which abound in the United States, may sound adequate, but when they are examined closely, several facts become clear. One is that many parents take no action, even after receiving two or three notifications (Vernon & Billingslea, 1973). In cases where the classroom teacher aggressively pursues the matter with the school nurse, further diagnosis and therapy may result, but these instances are the exception.

Second, regardless of whether or not there is parental follow-up, the educational program provided to the child is often the same as it would otherwise have been. Either the regular classroom teacher is left to cope with the student on her own, or, more commonly, the child is forced to contend with the identical situations he would have had were he not identified as hard-of-hearing. The only exception may be that he now has a hearing aid, *if* his parents provided it. In rare cases a speech therapist may see a hard-of-hearing child for 30 minutes every two or three weeks. With each speech therapist serving an average of 5,000 children, this is the extent of therapy possible.

Third, although many school programs do audiometric screening, school officials are frequently unable to provide a list of the names of their hard-of-hearing children. Often schools will refer inquiries about such names to the Health Department, which, just as often, will not have the data either. Persistent investigators are likely to be sent to the school principals, whose only way of finding the information is to go through each child's records, a tedious task they invariably delegate to the inquiring person, if this person can get clearance to read confidential files.

The point to be made is that even though a school system does audiometric screening, it often has no accessible records of the results and thus no way of identifying the scope or nature of the hearing loss problem among pupils (Davis, Shepard, Stelmachowicz, & Gorga, 1981; Shepard, Davis, Gorga, & Stelmachowicz, 1981). This is a common problem nationally.

"Variety" best describes the systems used to record the audiometric data in the different schools. Some have hearing and vision cards on all children in a single file. Others have the information recorded in such files for certain grades and in the child's individual folder for other grades. A few list hard-of-hearing children on their rosters of the handicapped, others do not. Some school nurses neglect to send their lists of the hearing impaired to the principals, so there are no records available to the teachers. In some schools the principal's list includes only the hard-of-hearing students identified in that particular year. For example, in four schools in a Maryland County where there were over 1,200 students, the principals naively stated that they had no hard-of-hearing children, a statement that defies probability, considering the prevalence of hearing impairment among children (Berg & Fletcher, 1970). Usually if asked about hard-of-hearing children in a school, the administrators are polite and cooperative, but incredulous that anyone should want information about these children.

SUMMARY

The problems encountered in audiological assessment, amplification, different types of hearing losses, and school programs form the basis for many psychological difficulties faced by hard-of-hearing people. They are practical issues which need to be grapsed as a base for understanding how the hard-of-hearing person copes in life. In some communities and schools the pitfalls described here are avoided and the services delivered are excellent. Unfortunately, such settings tend to be the exception. The fault is not necessarily with the audiologist or speech pathologist, because inordinate demands for service frequently preclude the full diagnostic procedures and follow-ups needed to serve hard-of-hearing students appropriately.

PSYCHO-SOCIAL FACTORS

INTELLIGENCE

Intelligence is essentially normally distributed in the hard-of-hearing population (Mindel & Vernon, 1971). This point must be emphasized, because the linguistic, speech, and educational problems of hard-of-hearing children frequently cause them to be misdiagnosed as mentally retarded or slow in comparison with normally hearing children (Sullivan & Vernon, 1979). However, hearing impairment has a retarding effect on language development. Thus, the results of verbal IQ scales to measure intelligence are more of an indication of the hard-of-hearing person's linguistic limitations than of his actual intelligence (see chapter 10). The situation is somewhat analogous to giving a Spanish-speaking Puerto Rican child, who has heard little English, an English form of the Standford-Binet. It is not uncommon for a congenitally hard-of-hearing child to score in the 70's on the verbal scale of an IQ test and 110 on the performance scale. Hence, for the hearing-impaired child, verbal tests are often invalid (Ross, 1982). (See Chapter 10).

The tragic result of this testing procedure is that hard-of-hearing students are frequently labeled dull and grouped in classes for slow learners or mentally retarded children. This treatment can have a destructive effect on the child's total future (Vernon & Billingslea, 1973). In other instances the hearing problem is simply ignored by the schools. The result, either way, is an educational approach totally inappropriate to the child's needs.

LANGUAGE DEVELOPMENT

From what has been said about the effects of hearing loss in the hard-of-hearing, it is obvious that they are markedly deprived in their perception of oral language (Conrad, 1979). Thus they frequently have severely limited vocabularies (Davis, 1974) and a deficient knowledge of syntax (Davis & Blasdell, 1975). This problem is usually profound when the onset of hearing loss is prelingual. These difficulties manifest themselves with special severity in reading, writing, spelling, and academic courses that depend on language arts. Most of the public and many professionals are blind to these basic linguistic problems in the prelingually hard-of-hearing because their oral language seems essentially normal (Ross, 1976). The characteristic yes's, hmm's and short answers these persons learn to give to cover up the fact that they do not understand most of what is said conceal their language problem. Hence the difference between their perceived linguistic skill and their actual lack of basic English competence goes undetected.

It is essential to understand the language problem of prelingually hard-of-hearing people because it tends to create major educational, interpersonal, and vocational difficulties of great psychological significance. The failure to recognize this language problem is one of the primary reasons other educational, psychological, and social difficulties of hard-of-hearing children are largely ignored. Linguistically, hard-of-hearing persons are often more similar to deaf people than to the normally hearing.

SPEECH

Hard-of-hearing persons, especially those in whom the hearing loss is severe and prelingual, will usually speak differently than normally hearing people. For example, if they have a high-frequency deficit, they will not hear or pronounce sounds such as *sh, r,* or *s.* In fact, speech production is a good guide to speech comprehension (Montgomery, 1966).

Unfortunately, the lay public associates certain speech defects with mental retardation, atypical sexual orientation, cleft lip and palate, and other conditions which are the butt of crude humor and deprecatory attitudes. For example, comedians will often mimic retarded or homosexual people by using certain speech patterns. This type of humor is especially common among children, adolescents, and insecure adults looking for somebody upon whom to project their anxieties and hostilities.

Thus, psychologically, hard-of-hearing people are frequently perceived as being mentally retarded or effeminate because of their speech problems. The effects of this attitude can be devastating. They may include rejection, scapegoating, and other negative behaviors destructive to the self-image of hard-of-hearing persons and to the social-vocational roles and opportunities open to them.

EDUCATION

On the average, hard-of-hearing children are one year or more behind in academic achievement (Trybus & Karchmer, 1977). Over one-third of hard-of-hearing children fail one or more grades (Berg, 1971). This educational retardation *increases* as they get older, resulting in many academic dropouts and serious behavioral problems (Hine, 1970b; Payne & Payne, 1970), representing an unnecessary waste of human potential.

The more sensitive teachers realize the hard-of-hearing child's frustration. They know that in classes of 30 or 40 there is no real way they can properly serve the child. Standard procedures, such as moving them to the front, tutoring, and writing, are attempted but frequently prove insufficient (Wilcox & Tobin, 1974). The youngsters who do succeed usually do so despite school, not because of it (Vernon & Billingslea, 1973).

Some hard-of-hearing children wind up in classes or schools for deaf youngsters. While such an arrangement may not be ideal, it is far better for many of these youths than the educational failure they face in regular public schools, a fact not realized by most professionals. They decry the placement of a hard-of-hearing child with deaf children, claiming the youngsters will grow up in "a deaf world," that speech will not develop, and that other dire consequences will result. These concerns are, for the most part, unwarranted. There is clear evidence that, given specialized instruction in classes with deaf children, the hard-of-hearing individual can successfully complete school and often attend college (Conrad, 1979).

It is also important to realize that exposure to both the deaf and hearing communities provides the hard-of-hearing person with a choice of social environments and friends to which he is entitled. Too often professionals arbitrarily decide hard-of-hearing people belong with the normally hearing, socially and educationally, despite the fact that they are often cruelly rejected and that they fail academically. The whole problem of educational placement has been compounded by P.L. 94–142, The Education for All Handicapped Children Act of 1975. Essentially, this Federal law mandates a free and appropriate education for handicapped children in the least restrictive environment. The law has been interpreted to mean hard-of-hearing children should be taught in regular classes; however, it has frequently failed to provide the support services needed for such placement.

Obviously, the ideal arrangement for most hard-of-hearing students is a specialized academic program or adequate supplementary services in regular schools. Britain has progressed in this area and has numerous special facilities for those they term partially hearing (Hine, 1971). Results have been favorable (Hine,

1971). A key consideration is the degree of functional hearing. Obviously a child with a 30 dB loss correctable with amplification is wrongly placed in a program for the deaf. When the loss is 60 dB and no adequate special program in the public school exists, a special class or school for the deaf is far better than placement in a class with 40 hearing children and insufficient support services.

One final point must be made with regard to education and the hard-of-hearing child. Programs that on paper seem adequate or even excellent can in practice be horribly deficient.

VOCATIONAL EFFECTS

There are no data on the vocational adjustment of the hard-of-hearing, except where they have been a subgroup in studies of the deaf (Schein & Delk, 1974). However, it is obvious from their educational retardation, communication problems, and employer attitudes that the occupational level of the hard-of-hearing is significantly lower than that of the general population. The level of unemployment is also higher among the hard of hearing than among the normally hearing.

The first author's clinical judgment, based on some 30 years of experience with hard-of-hearing persons in educational, vocational, and hospital settings, is that as a group they are grossly underemployed relative to their intellectual potential. Like deaf workers, they are disproportionately represented in unskilled and semiskilled manual work. Personality problems are often a major impediment in peer and supervisor relationships. In fact, some employers prefer deaf workers because with them the expectations for communication are usually less ambiguous and attitudes less troublesome.

PERSONAL ADJUSTMENT IN SCHOOL AND IN SOCIETY

The educational retardation of hard-of-hearing persons is usually severe, especially if the onset of auditory loss is early. Even more disturbing are the behavior problems. Many of these individuals are withdrawn. Often they are reported as isolates and thought by others to be stupid. Their speech is frequently mimicked in a deprecating way. In fact, teachers themselves are sometimes guilty of this attitude (Vernon & Billingslea, 1973). The following case study illustrates how serious the problem can become.

> John, a hard-of-hearing junior high school student, age 16, slashed his wrists and threatened to try to kill himself again if forced to return to school. When interviewed, he reported his teachers often became angry when he did not understand. They blamed him for not wanting to learn. At recess he was teased mercilessly. Classmates mimicked his speech and called him stupid. The bus ride to and from school was of such trauma that he sat directly behind the bus driver for protection. Even then, spitballs and verbal abuse made the ride miserable. At home John played with much younger children. His favorite game was "school," in which he was always the teacher.
>
> Despite a performance IQ of 115, John's hearing loss (corrected to an average of 60 dB in his better ear) had resulted in a 2.5 grade academic retardation, the repeating of two grades, and more important, terrible unhappiness. Subsequently John was hospitalized as a mental patient. (Vernon & Billingslea, 1973)

Many hard-of-hearing children cope by being overly aggressive instead of withdrawn. Frequently they bully younger children and are disruptive in class. The "acting out" tends to increase in adolescence and contributes to a high dropout rate in high school. Poor study habits and negative attitudes are common and understandable. Most hard-of-hearing children in regular public school have significant adjustment problems (Berg & Fletcher, 1970).

The first author has observed in his clinical work that a healthy adjustment by the hard-of-hearing child who has been placed in a program for deaf children is usually contingent upon two factors—his acceptance of his hearing loss and his avoidance of exploiting deaf children. The hard-of-hearing youngster who psychologically denies his hearing impairment or uses it for unfair advantage faces severe rejection and abuse from deaf children. Deaf youngsters are deeply hurt by the air of superiority hard-of-hearing children tend to assume, and they extract a price for this hurt.

Often the hard-of-hearing child comes to a program for the deaf with a history of having been teased and abused by hearing children. Perceiving that deaf children are even lower on the totem pole than he, he vents his frustrations, anger, and inadequacy on them. At an even deeper psychological level, the hard-of-hearing child often finds deafness psychologically threatening, an extension of his own area of weakness, and his response is to treat deaf children in a hostile and authoritarian manner.

The problem is further compounded because teachers of deaf children often favor the hard of hearing. Somewhat analogous to "the one-eyed man in the kingdom of the blind," the hard-of-hearing child is usually easier to teach and to communicate with than his deaf classmates. Not infrequently teachers will use hard-of-hearing children to interpret in sign language to their deaf classmates. This deprecates the deaf child and tends to magnify his envy and dislike of the hard-of-hearing youngster.

Relevant to this basic problem is the fact that the hard-of-hearing child of average ability or below will often excel in a program for deaf children because of his communication advantage and the individual attention he receives in a class of six to ten students. Consequently, hard-of-hearing youths with IQs of 90 to 100 may pass entrance examinations to postsecondary programs for the hearing impaired, while deaf applicants with IQs of 120 or 130 fail. Whereas the hard-of-hearing child's intelligence and overall ability tend to be underestimated in a setting with normally hearing youngsters, the reverse occurs when placement is with deaf youths.

In both educational programs and social organizations, hard-of-hearing children or adults who accept their hearing loss and without feeling the need to flaunt their residual hearing before their deaf counterparts generally find an acceptance among deaf people they do not get from the hearing. For the severely hard-of-hearing, in particular, a close contact with the deaf community offers many social and psychological advantages.

A significant percentage of hard-of-hearing people, especially those in whom onset of hearing loss was early, have their closest identification with others who are hearing impaired. They use sign language as well as speech. They are involved in the deaf community, go to clubs for the deaf, and may have a deaf or hard-of-hearing spouse. At the same time they also have normally hearing friends (often neighbors, co-workers, or long-time family friends).

This form of adjustment is generally the most satisfying and psychologically healthy for hard-of-hearing people. It gives them the largest possible range of social contacts while meeting their communication needs in the most effective way. The person who makes this type of adjustment has usually come to accept the implications of his hearing loss. This acceptance makes possible an open, constructive interaction with both deaf and hearing people.

ADJUSTMENT TO LATE ONSET HEARING LOSS

For the individual whose onset of hearing loss is in adulthood, the problem of psychological adjustment is often traumatic. Several major factors are relevant. First, one's career is often jeopardized. For the salesman, the attorney, the secretary, the teacher, the nurse, the clerk, the physician, and most job holders, hearing loss threatens financial survival. Often it strikes during the peak years of earning power. Compounding the problem is the fact that many of these hearing losses are progressive, but rarely can an accurate prognosis be given. Thus the individual who may have just enough hearing to get by professionally has no idea how long he will be able to continue to communicate adequately for the demands of the job.

A second traumatic dimension to late onset hearing loss is its effect on marriage and social life. For the couple whose lifestyle is primarily dependent on extensive social interaction, the effect of hearing loss can be shattering. To illustrate:

> Mr Gold, a successful attorney, married shortly after college. He taught school for several years to save money to enter law school. Throughout his legal education Mrs. Gold worked to support them. After years of financial sacrifice, Mr. Gold started a practice in the town where he and his wife had been teaching. His genuine interest in people, his competence, and his social and civic commitment brought Mr. Gold immediate professional success and a social calendar full of parties and meetings. The Golds also started a family.
>
> By this time Mr. Gold's initially mild hearing loss had begun to progress. Clients started to complain that he was not responsive, that he did not listen to them, and that he would sometimes walk out of the room when they were still talking. Socially, people began avoiding him. Although invited out frequently because of his still high social status in town, once at the party no one wanted to be "stuck" with Mr. Gold because it meant shouting, repeating, and misunderstanding. Sensing the social stress, Mr. Gold started having an extra cocktail or two and eating too much food as ways of coping with his anxiety. While he was being avoided, people paid attention to his wife, thereby arousing feelings of envy and suspicion.
>
> Eventually the problem became worse. His practice and income dropped dramatically and invitations for social events were rare.
>
> Mr. Gold could get no prognosis for his hearing. He does not know if he will become deaf or whether, and when, his loss will stabilize. Should he change careers or specialize in some form of legal research? The latter option would require moving out of town. Both alternatives would demand more education. Financial stresses combined with the loss of social life around which their marriage had revolved leave them considering divorce.

The Gold case illustrates some of the stresses found by persons with late onset hearing losses. Psychologically these problems are more difficult in many ways than the adjustments that must be made by those whose hearing impairment began in childhood. The latter have an early opportunity for career selection, marriage, and lifestyle that can accommodate a hearing loss.

The kind of problems characterized by Mr. Gold are not easily resolved. Rarely are there any services for the psychosocial dimensions of his problem. Because his loss is sensorineural, there is no effective medical treatment. A hearing aid may help some. If Mr. Gold lives in a large city, there is probably a hearing and speech clinic that has some kind of program for the hard-of-hearing. Most of its members are probably senior citizens, and Mr. Gold may not find it interesting. Since he does not know sign language, deaf people do not want to bother with him.

If Mr. Gold seeks psychological or psychiatric help, he faces two basic problems. One is communication: in addition to undergoing the stresses inherent in psychotherapy, the hard-of-hearing person may have trouble understanding the therapist's speech. However, more important is the second problem. Only a minutia of psychologists, psychiatrists, and social workers have any concept of how an individual can effectively cope with hearing loss. Hence Mr. Gold may get sophistocated diagnostic labels for his problems and some extremely helpful insights into his psychodynamics, but he will get little practical help in how to cope careerwise and socially.

Similarly, he can get medical, auditory, and communication information from physicians, audiologists, and speech pathologists, but these specialists almost never know much about the deaf community. Generally they see deaf people as inappropriate companions, socially and linguistically, for the hard-of-hearing person whose loss was of late onset. Ironically, research data indicate that most of the friendships of hard-of-hearing people are with others who have a hearing loss (Myklebust, 1954).

Hence, if we regard as representational the sort of professional counsel that a person with Mr. Gold's type of hearing loss would receive, we can understand why about 99 percent of such persons would not identify with deaf people. They may identify to some extent with other hard-of-hearing people, if they live in a large city where such groups exist. In the United States there are few such groups and very limited programs; professionals have essentially ignored these people. Great Britain, by contrast, has an extensive social and service network to serve its partially hearing adults.

MARRIAGE

There is a high rate of unmarried persons among the hard of hearing (Schein & Delk, 1974). This fact is very revealing of the public's rejection. It is when the issue of marriage and physical intimacy arises that attitudes become most transparent. For these reasons, and because they share a problem in communication, hard-of-hearing people marry each other far more often than would be expected by chance (Schein & Delk, 1974).

MARGINALITY

Hard-of-hearing persons are marginal in the sense that they rest somewhere between being deaf and having normal hearing. Inherent in this marginality is often a confusion about self-identity relative to hearing.

As was indicated above, some adapt by identifying primarily as a deaf person. They may have a deaf spouse, participate in clubs for the deaf, and use sign language. Others handle marginality differently. They want an identity as a hearing person, and they want hearing friends. Some, mostly those with mild hearing losses and good social skills, can function effectively this way. Usually such persons are flexible and easygoing. They communicate their fondness for people.

Others have a tolerance or preference for more than average isolation. They choose careers and hobbies requiring little social interaction. Most have not attended special schools or programs for the deaf, and they are acquainted with few others who have hearing problems. In general they cope with their auditory deficit by satisfactory social contacts with a few close friends and family, by other minimal but adequate forms of interaction, and by much inner-directed nonpeople-oriented activity.

Many hard-of-hearing individuals who seek to identify with hearing people face rejection. Nobody wants to bother with them. Their odd speech, the hearing aid, and the endless need to repeat stigmatize them. This difficult situation engenders a hurt, defensive person who may try to cope in ways that frequently intensify the rejection. If such people had contact with deaf people during the school years, they often turn to deaf people in desperation. However, as a result of their rejection by hearing people (and sometimes by parents), their self-image often is related to "hearing loss as bad, as terribly negative." Even though they have turned to hearing-impaired people out of desperation, their attitude toward them tends to be deprecatory. The negative feelings they have about themselves and their hearing problem are projected onto the others, whom they desperately need for companionship. The result is a hostile dependency. Once these dynamics become apparent, the individuals will be rejected not only by other hearing-impaired people but also by the normally hearing.

COPING MECHANISMS

Denial

In chapter 6 the mechanism of denial was discussed at length. It is seen frequently among the hard-of-hearing. It is not a denial of the fact of auditory deficit but of the implications of the deficit. It is, at the deepest level, rejection of an integral aspect of self. To deny and reject an important integral part of oneself is to be seriously maladjusted. The following case illustrates the problem:

> Mrs. Apple has always been hard of hearing. Her brother is deaf and attended a school for deaf children. Because his more severe problem symbolized her own hearing loss, the implications of which she rejected, Mrs. Apple has always been ashamed of her brother. When hearing friends visited, she tried to make sure that they did not meet him or know that she had a deaf brother.
>
> As a child she started in regular public school but had problems because of her hearing loss. Finally, in middle school, she transferred to the State School for the Deaf. Immediately she impressed on all her classmates that she was not deaf. She refused to use sign language even though it was the only way the other students could understand. Needless to say, they responded to this behavior

with anger (and envy). She never missed an opportunity to vaunt her speech and hearing in front of deaf people and never signed for them when hearing people were present.

Whenever she referred to deaf and hard-of-hearing people, it was always "they," never "us." When with deaf people, she always spoke of her "hearing friends" and the "hearing world" in which she claimed to live. However, she was rejected by the hearing community and really had no close hearing friends. Thus she was driven, in desperation for social life, to deaf and hard-of-hearing people. The more this happened, the more psychologically threatened and defensive she became. Soon she was offensively paternalistic to hearing-impaired people, referring to them in terms of their deficits and their need for "hearing" people such as herself.

Because no hearing man would marry her, she found a deaf husband for whom she symbolized the hearing he lacked. However, she was ashamed of his deafness. She forced him to wear conspicuous bilateral hearing aids, despite their uselessness to a person with his profound hearing loss. She would take him with her only when they were to socialize with deaf people. Even then she referred to the deaf man as her "hearing-impaired" husband, a denial in which he feebly participated. When dining out with him, she refused to use sign language, despite this being the only way they could communicate.

The pattern represented by Mrs. Apple is present primarily among hard-of-hearing people whose onset was before or during school years and who at one time were in an educational program for the hearing impaired or who have deaf family members.

In those whose onset of hearing loss is in adulthood, denial will often appear first in reaction to the hearing loss itself. For example, on the average it is five years after first experiencing a hearing loss that he seeks professional help. Frequently he will blame others for mumbling or otherwise speaking indistinctly, for turning the TV too low, and so on *ad infinitum,* rather than acknowledge that he no longer hears well.

This delay in dealing with the problem is terribly destructive. (It results in people's being unnecessarily alienated for five years.) It deprives the individual of the opportunity to learn to use amplification during the desirable people when he has maximum residual hearing. In some cases it causes loss of job and family discord, even divorce.

DOMINATING CONVERSATION

Hard-of-hearing people generally have understandable speech, but they often have difficulty comprehending what is said to them. One way to cope with such a situation is to dominate the conversation, that is, to do all the talking. This common coping mechanism saves the hard-of-hearing person from the embarrassment and struggle of trying to grasp what is being said from the incompletely perceived sounds and lip movements of the speaker. He is saved from the humiliation of not understanding, of replying irrelevantly, and of asking the person to repeat.

Unfortunately, nobody enjoys the company of someone who does all the talking. Therefore, this way of coping is highly counterproductive. Yet it is a common ploy, and the hard-of-hearing person frequently adopts it without being consciously aware of doing so.

NEUTRAL RESPONSES

Almost every hard-of-hearing person becomes the master of the "smile and nod," the neutral response, and the affirmative statement. In a sense they use the techniques of the nondirective counselor, responding with a variety of "Hmm's," "Yes's," smiles, and nods which are sufficiently neutral so that the speaker feels he has been understood and accepted. This technique can be extremely effective because it encourages the speaker to talk on and on. The redundance in most conversations of this sort enables the hard-of-hearing person to eventually get the idea of what is being said. However, it is extremely stressful to the hard-of-hearing listener. Of equal importance, when the topic of conversation is complex or significant, the speaker eventually realizes that he has been deceived—that the listener, by neutral responses, has only feigned understanding. Once this discovery is made, the hard-of-hearing person may face anger and rejection.

INVOLVEMENT IN ACTIVITIES OF COMMON INTEREST

The hard-of-hearing person who has a hobby or professional interest in which the communication required is minimal will often find social satisfaction through friends who share the hobby or interest. For example, if two people share an intense interest in stamps, tennis, real estate, or other activity, they are often willing to tolerate a communication problem they would avoid at a more general gathering such as a party or Rotary Club meeting. Thus the hard-of-hearing person can often maximize chances for positive social contacts by emphasizing activities of strong mutual interests with the hearing person and by avoiding the more generalized social settings.

SUSPICIOUSNESS AND PARANOID RESPONSES

A person who cannot hear all that is being said is at a tremendous disadvantage. Defective hearing sometimes results in misunderstandings. Others, realizing that they can say things without the hard-of-hearing person understanding them, may talk about this person in a negative way. If an unpleasant job assignment is given a group orally, those with normal hearing may discuss it and delegate it to the hard-of-hearing person who never heard the assignment to start with.

These types of experience, and the feelings of isolation, rejection, and vulnerability, all combine to make some hard-of-hearing people overly suspicious, and in some cases paranoid. It is not the modal pattern, the pattern that appears most often, for persons who are hard-of-hearing. Furthermore, hearing people do take advantage of the hard-of-hearing sufficiently often to justify a certain amount of reality-based suspiciousness on the part of the latter.

For those whose onset of hearing loss was early in life, there are undoubtedly many memories of other children making fun or taking advantage of them. The feelings that develop from such cruelties persist and intensify as the individual grows older and experiences similar incidents. The result is a reality-based hostility and suspicion which, regardless of its foundation in fact, can impair human relationships.

President Carter's observation that "Life is full of injustice" has special relevance for hard-of-hearing people.

CONCLUSION

There are approximately one million hard-of-hearing school-age children and approximately 5 million adults, most of whom have special psychological and educational needs which are rarely met. Consequently the majority are significantly retarded educationally and are beset by psychological problems which are compounded by their speech and communication impairments. As these youngsters grow into adulthood, their school problems often become chronic, leading to employment, family, and social failure and frustration. Part of the tragedy is that these problems are largely preventable at costs that are within reason. The key is early identification and therapy followed by adequate support services in the educational system.

REFERENCES

Berg, F. S. (1971). The school years. *Hearing and Speech News, 39,* 14–20.

Berg, F. S., & Fletcher, S. G. (Eds.). (1970). *The hard of hearing child.* New York: Grune & Stratton.

Bradley, L., & Bryant, P. E. (1978). Difficulties in auditory organization as a possible cause of reading backwardness. *Nature, 271,* 746–747.

Carhart, R., & Tillman, T. W. (1970). Interaction of competing speech signals with hearing loss. *Archives of Otolarngology, 91,* 273–279.

Conrad, R. (1979). *The deaf school child.* (pp. 287, 299, 300, 311). London: Harper & Row.

Davis, J. (1974). Performance of young hearing-impaired children on a test of basic concepts. *Journal of Speech and Hearing Research, 17,* 342–351.

Davis, J., & Blasdell, R. (1975). Perceptual strategies employed by normal-hearing and hearing impaired children in the comprehension of sentences containing relative clauses. *Journal of Speech and Hearing Research, 18,* 281–295.

Davis, J., Shepard, N., Stelmachowicz, P., & Gorga, M. (1981). Characteristics of hearing-impaired children in the public schools. Part II: Psycho-educational data. *Journal of Speech and Hearing Disorders, 46,* 130–137.

Goetzinger, D. P. (1962). Effects of small perceptive losses on language and speech discrimination. *Volta Review, 64,* 408–414.

Graham, A. B. (1975). Counseling parent and teacher regarding the effects of mild hearing loss. *Transactions of the American Academy of Ophthalmology and Otology, 80,* 73–78.

Grammatico, L. F. (1975). The development of listening skills. *Volta Review, 77*(5), 303–308.

Griffiths, C. (1975). The auditory approach: Its rationale, techniques and results. *Audiol. Hear. Educ., 1*(1), 35–39.

Hefferman, A. (1955). A psychiatric study of fifty children referred to a hospital for suspected deafness. In B. Caplan (Ed.), *Emotional problems of childhood* (pp. 98–120). Basic Books.

Hine, W. D. (1970a). The ability of partially hearing children. *British Journal of Educational Psychology, 40,* 171–178.

Hine, W. D. (1970b). The attainments of children with partial hearing loss. *Teacher of the Deaf, 68,* 129–135.

Hine, W. D. (1970c). Verbal ability and partial hearing loss. *Teacher of the Deaf, 68,* 450–459.

Hine, W. D. (1971). The social adjustment of partially hearing children. *Teacher Deaf, 69*(405), 5–13.

Holm, V. A., & Kunze, L. H. (1969). Effect of chronic otitis media on language and speech development. *Pediatrics, 43,* 833–839.

Kodman, F. (1963). Educational status of hard of hearing children in the classroom. *Journal of Speech and Hearing Disorders, 28,* 297–299.

Ling, D. (1959). *The education and general background of children with defective hearing in reading.* Cambridge, England: Institute of Education Library.

Macrae, J. H. (1968). Deterioration of the residual hearing of children with sensorineural deafness. *Acta Oto-Laryngologica, 66,* 33–39.

Markides, A. (1971). Do hearing aids damage the user's residual hearing? *Sound, 5,* 99–105.

Mindel, E. D., & Vernon, M. (1971). *They grow in silence.* Silver Spring, MD: National Association for the Deaf Press.

Montgomery, G. W. (1966). Relationship of oral skills to manual communication in profoundly deaf students. *American Annals of the Deaf, 111,* 557–567.

Myklebust, H. R. (1954). *Auditory disorders in children, a manual for differential diagnosis.* New York: Grune and Stratton.

Oller, D. K., & Kelly, C. A. (1974). Phonological substitution processes of a hard of hearing child. *Journal of Speech and Hearing Disorders, 39,* 64–74.

Payne, P. D., & Payne, R. L. (1970). Behavior manifestations of children with hearing loss. *American Journal of Nursing, 70,* 1718–1719.

Pollack, D. M. (1974). Denver's acoupedic program. *Peabody Journal of Education, 51*(3), 180–185.

Pollack, D. M. (1975). The development of an auditory function. *Hearing Aid Journal, 28*(7), 6, 40.

Quigley, S. P., & Thomure, R. E. (1968). *Some effects of a hearing-impairment on school performance.* Urbana: University of Illinois, Institute of Research on Exceptional Children.

Ross, M. Amplification systems. (1976). In L. Lloyd (Ed.), *Communication, assessment and intervention strategies* (pp. 295–324). Baltimore: University Park Press.

Ross, M. (1982). *Hard of hearing children in regular schools.* Englewood Cliffs, NJ: Prentice-Hall.

Schein, J. D., & Delk, M. T., Jr. (1974). *The deaf population* (pp. 1–30). Silver Spring, MD: National Association of the Deaf.

Shepard, N., Davis, J., Gorga, M., & Stelmachowicz, P. (1981). Characteristics of hearing-impaired children in the public schools. Part 1: Demographic data. *Journal of Speech and Hearing Disorders, 46,* 123–129.

Sullivan, P. M., & Vernon, M. (1979). Psychological assessment of hearing-impaired children. *School Psychology Digest, 8,* 271–290.

Trybus, R. J., & Karchmer, M. A. (1977). School achievement status of hearing-impaired children: National data on achievement status and growth patterns. *American Annals of the Deaf, 122,* 62–29.

Vernon, M., & Billingslea, H. (1973). Hard-of-hearing children in a public school setting. *Maryland Teacher, 30,* 16–17, 27–28.

Wilcox, J., & Tobin, H. (1974). Linguistic performance of hard of hearing and normal hearing children. *Journal of Speech and Hearing Research, 17,* 286–292.

Yanick, P. (1976). Effects of signal processing on intelligibility of speech in noise for persons with sensorineural hearing loss. *Journal of the American Audiological Society, 1,* 229–238.

SECTION IV SUMMARY

Chapter 10 began with a discussion of how deaf children and adults are frequently misdiagnosed as mentally retarded or psychotic, a misdiagnosis often caused by language-communication difficulties. To prevent misdiagnosis, general principles were given on psychological evaluation and administration of tests. A chart was presented outlining form names and descriptions of specific tests.

Chapter 11 began with a discussion of how student characteristics and educational placements affect deaf children's learning. Since deafness is primarily a communication disability, it discussed how hearing and deaf children acquire communication competence. A bilingual/bicultural approach was recommended for the classroom, with information about deaf culture being infused into the curriculum along with strategies on how to cope in a hearing society. It was emphasized that deaf children need adult deaf role models. Teachers were encouraged to use interactive teaching strategies in the classroom. Finally there was a discussion of educational ethnography as a research tool to guide and evaluate classroom activities.

Chapter 12 covered the psychological and education needs of the hard-of-hearing population. It was pointed out that most hard-of-hearing students are significantly retarded educationally and are beset by psychological problems which are compounded by their speech and communication impairments. As these youths grow into adulthood, their school problems often become chronic and lead to employment, family, and social failure and frustration. This chapter emphasized that the key is early identification and therapy followed by adequate support services in the educational system.

REVIEW QUESTIONS

1. Why are deaf individuals frequently misdiagnosed as mentally retarded or psychotic?
2. What communication model(s) should the psychologist use in administering an intelligence test to a deaf client?
3. What is the rationale behind a bilingual/bicultural approach to educating deaf children?
4. The difficulties of learning language have been cited as the reason deaf children's academic achievement is rarely commensurate with their intellectual potential. Using the information on normal language acquisition, explain *why* and *how* insufficient and inconsistent linguistic input contributes to this problem.
5. Why are the psychological and educational needs of hard-of-hearing individuals frequently misunderstood and neglected?
6. What are some of the predominant coping mechanisms hard-of-hearing persons use?

SECTION V

Deafness: An Experiment in Nature

OVERVIEW

This section introduces the perspective that deafness can be viewed as "an experiment in nature." By providing a control over various major psychological variables that determine the human condition, deafness may contribute to our knowledge of psychology. Some of the profound questions are discussed which deafness can answer. Examples are given from theoretical and applied research which examines deafness from a scientific point of view.

CHAPTER 13

An Experiment of Nature: Research and Theory

The history of science is rich in the example of the fruitfulness of bringing two sets of techniques, two sets of ideas, developed in separate contexts for the pursuit of truth, into touch with each other.   *Oppenheimer*

The study of deaf people, especially those who were born deaf, offers the scientist a tremendous research and theoretical opportunity. Deafness is actually "an experiment of nature" which provides control over a number of major psychological variables that determine the human condition. This scientific perspective, in the final analysis, may yield the most significant dividend to psychological knowledge and humankind.

The potential that is inherent from the study of deafness generalizes far beyond deaf persons themselves. If we understood the role that was played by deafness in the development of deaf people, that is, if we understood the psychology of deafness, we would immediately know the role of hearing in the development of all people. Such knowledge could be the most significant advance in psychology of this century.

This premise can be elaborated with an analogy. Once medicine knew the effects of phenylketonuria (PKU) on victims of this disease, it then knew the role played by the biochemical process using PKU in the development of normal intellectual growth. Similarly, in agriculture, once farmers understood the effects of the absence of potassium on pathological plant development, they then knew the role played by potassium in normal plant growth. Thus, if psychology could understand the variable of hearing in psychological development, this knowledge would be a milestone in the history of science. This is the potential of deafness as an "experiment of nature."

Some of the profound questions that deafness can answer are fairly obvious, yet science has never asked them. This is typical of science, which so often dissipates its energies in the compulsive analysis of minutia while studiously avoiding that which has greater generality and is, in some cases, more apparent. The major reason scientists make this error is that often the ability to ask the profound question intelligently presupposes a rare human trait: the capacity to look at the world from an unconventional frame of reference. Deafness is such an unconventional frame of reference.

Consider Darwin's theory of evolution. Once Darwin rejected the book of Genesis as a frame of reference for creation, his theory of evolution was almost self-evident for a person with a biological background. Similarly, most of Einstein's theoretical contributions in physics did not require that he do extensive experiments. He did not have to undertake the massive data collection that goes into the average doctoral dissertation. What he did have to do was to consider motion from a different perspective than was customary. Once this different perspective was assumed, his theories followed logically and directly because they were the only explanation possible to account for what was observed. Galileo's momentus theories about the solar system were similar in that the basic requirement was that Galileo disregard the geocentric frame of reference which said that the earth was the center of the universe, and look at the solar system from a different frame of reference.

By the same token, if we can reject the egocentric frame of reference that we as hearing people have, and assume the frame of reference of the person born deaf, then some fascinating theory results. What are some of the psychological questions that can be answered or have been answered by our taking the frame of reference of congenital deafness?

Autism: Functional or Organic?

The first is the question of whether or not autism is functional or organic etiology. Is autism due to brain damage or to poor parenting? Chess, Fernandez, and Corn (1972) studied deafness and rubella, and their work answered this fundamental question. When Kanner first described autism back in 1942, learned psychiatrists and psychologists immediately began to expound at length about how this tragic childhood psychosis was due to poor parenting procedures. Descriptions such as "refrigerator parents" were used to describe mothers and fathers of autistic children. These parents were told that their poor parenting had created these frustrating psychotic children. The parents were put into prolonged psychotherapy to cure their pathology. A book dealing primarily with the pathology of these parents and their autistic children was written by Bettelheim (1967).

Chess et al., in their study of rubella deaf children, found that a highly disproportionate percentage of these youngsters were autistic, yet there was no more autism among deaf children in general than there was among the general population of hearing children. Rubella children who were not deaf also had greater probability of being autistic. These studies on deafness demonstrated that a very serious childhood psychosis long thought to be a functional disease resulting from poor parenting was actually an organic psychosis that can occur totally independent of parenting practices.

Thought and Language

Another issue that can be looked at from the perspective of deafness as an experiment of nature regards the relationship between the thinking process and language. The issue of the role played by language in thought processes dates back almost as far as recorded history. It has challenged great minds in almost every generation, as is evidenced by several fascinating quotations.

Samuel Taylor Coleridge said: "I believe that the process of thought might be carried on independent and apart from spoken language. I do not in the least doubt that if language had been denied or withheld from man, thought would have been a process more simple, more easy, and more perfect than at present." He is clearly saying that language interferes with thought.

Thesoledia, a teacher in about the 15th or 16th century, said, "Conceptual thinking is built on visual understanding—visual understanding is the basis of all knowledge." He meant visual understanding independent of language.

Einstein, in describing his own accomplishments, stated: "I very rarely think in words at all. A thought comes and I may try to express it in words afterwards. Words or language as they are written or spoken do not seem to play any role in my mechanism of thought. For me it is not dubious that our thinking goes on for the most part without use of words." A psychiatrist who studied Einstein has concluded: "The lessons from Einstein's story are clear. Our present verbally oriented educational system should include lessons in visual thinking" (Rosen, 1964).

Congenital deafness precludes language development unless language is formally taught (except when parents are deaf and know sign language). Thus, those persons who are born deaf are in essence an "experiment of nature" in which there is a total absence of language—a total control of the variable of language. They therefore provide the opportunity to compare the thought process in human beings having no verbal symbol system (the uneducated deaf) with the thought process in (hearing) people who have sophisticated language development. For example, if we give both of these groups problems to solve, one group has to solve the problem but has no language with which to do so, while the other group (the hearing) will have language to use in solving the problem. We can give the same problems to each group to determine whether both groups solve them with the same degree of efficiency, that is, whether both groups get the same number right in the same amount of time. Furthermore, we can examine the steps by which they solve the problems to determine whether these steps are comparable for both groups. If we discover that this process actually is comparable for a group that has no verbal symbol system at all and one that has a very sophisticated symbol system, then the only conclusion that is possible is that the thought process occurs independent of a verbal symbol system. In other words, we would conclude that the mediating process of thought is not language.

Such experiments have been done by Furth (1966, 1973), Vernon (1967), and Vander Woude (1970). Their findings demonstrate that verbal symbols are not the mediating process of thought. Those subjects with a verbal symbol system (language) and those without language solve the problems with equal effectiveness and they use identical strategies in the problem solving (see Figure 13.1).

This concept of thought without language is difficult to accept. We naturally assume that we think in words. The question to be asked is this: What theoretical model of thought processing can accommodate the information that thought occurs independent of language, that is, what is the nature of the thought process?

First consider a theoretical model of how we might have viewed the thought processes of hearing people. The hearing person first sees the problem, that is, the stimulus. Perhaps it is an algebraic equation or a nonverbal analogy. The nervous system then processes this stimulus to the brain, where the problem is solved. The analysis is made at the highest level: in the brain power. It is at this level of thought that we assume that we use language. After the problem is solved, the solution to the problem is stated or verbalized, as Einstein has indicated. This is the classical model of how psychology used to view the thought process.

Let us turn now to deafness. With deaf children who have no verbal language, we have the stimulus or the problem, that is, the equation or nonverbal analogy. This problem is then transmitted by the nervous system to the brain, where the problem is solved and the solution is demonstrated by the deaf child. The question really being raised is, what happens in the analysis? What happens in the brain where the actual thought process occurs? Unfortunately, nobody knows. However, a study of

FIGURE 13.1.   Mediating process of thought

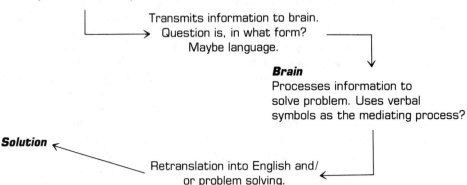

Sensory Nervous System in Hearing People

Stimuli
Problems of various types often
"conceptualized" verbally.

Transmits information to brain.
Question is, in what form?
Maybe language.

Brain
Processes information to
solve problem. Uses verbal
symbols as the mediating process?

Solution

Retranslation into English and/
or problem solving.

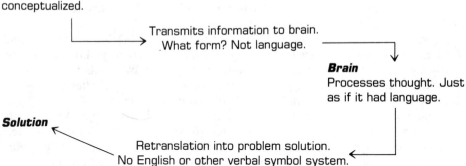

Sensory Nervous System in Prelingually Deaf People

Stimuli
Problems of various types.
(Same as above). Not
conceptualized.

Transmits information to brain.
What form? Not language.

Brain
Processes thought. Just
as if it had language.

Solution

Retranslation into problem solution.
No English or other verbal symbol system.

thought process in deaf people with no language (including no sign language) provides the best theory for the nature of this thought process.

The theory is most clearly explained through an analogy to a computer. In order for a problem to be presented to a computer, some sort of program is needed, perhaps FORTRAN or COBAL or something else. It is the program that transmits the problem to the computer. Regardless of the form, or the program, in which the problem is presented to the computer, the mathematical process that occurs in a computer is always a binary mathematical process. Following the solution of the problem, a program of some type transmits the answer, and the solution to the problem is presented in a printout.

If we look at thought processing in nonverbal deaf children and in hearing children, according to the evidence previously presented (Furth, 1973; Vander

Woude, 1970; Vernon, 1967) we have to conclude that the thought process itself is not mediated by a verbal symbol system. It does not occur in language. Language may or may not be the "program" that transmits the problem to the brain and transmits the answer back to the sheet of paper. However, the thought process itself is independent of the mode in which the problem is transmitted to the brain. It may be presented linguistically, pictorially, or in some other mode or "program." To state this again in terms of congenitally deaf children, even in those children having no verbal symbol system at all, thought goes on in exactly the same way that it does in a person with a full command of the English language (Furth, 1973; Vander Woude, 1970; Vernon, 1967). In other words, language is not the mediating process of thought. Thus this "experiment of nature" presented by congenitally deaf nonverbal children not only tells us a great deal about the nature of the thought process, it also provides data of great value, on encoding, on human learning, and on memory coding.

ATROPHY OF BRAIN TISSUE DUE TO AUDITORY DEPRIVATION

Consider another scientific discovery revealed by deafness as an experiment of nature. Common sense tells us that most of our sensory input (that is, with hearing people) is auditory. If this is true, then huge areas of the cerebral cortex must be devoted to processing this auditory input. If this is accepted as being true, a congenital auditory deprivation—in other words, deafness—could have only one of two possible consequences. First, the cerebral cortex tissue normally devoted to processing auditory input might atrophy. This would mean that in a deaf person there would be large areas of "dead" tissue in the cerebral cortex. The assumed alternative consequence would be that brain tissue normally devoted to processing auditory input would, in the absence of auditory input, be used to process some other form of sensory input. For example, the deaf person would have unusually good vision or a superior tactile sense because cortex normally devoted to processing auditory input would be available for processing visual input.

What research clearly indicates is that neither of the assumed consequences actually occurs. Deaf people's brains do not atrophy, nor do deaf people develop compensatory sensory capability. This finding gives further support to the model described in the previous section and illustrated in Figure 13.1. The only logical explanation to account for the effects of congenital auditory deprivation on brain tissue is that when sensory input reaches the brain, it is processed the same way, regardless of whether it comes in auditorially, visually, tactilely, or through any other modality. In other words, regardless of whether you see it, hear it, or feel it, when the impulse is processed in the cortex it is processed independent of mode of input.

ROLE OF ENVIRONMENT AND GENETICS ON IQ

One of the hottest theoretical issues in psychology today is the role of genetics on intelligence. This is a theoretical issue which can be examined through the study of deafness as an experiment of nature.

Congenital deafness is the single most severe form of cultural deprivation possible. Typically, many young preschool deaf children get no linguistic input at all. Explanations of cause and effect are never given because no one is able to communicate them to the deaf child. In general, congenitally deaf children are denied massive amounts of information about their culture and about the world in which they live, information that is readily available to all who can hear.

If environment plays a significant role in developing IQ, it would be logical to assume that the IQ of deaf children, as a rule, would be grossly deficient. Their scores would be significantly below those of whites, blacks, American Indians, Mexican Americans, and culturally deprived groups.

Surprisingly, this is not the case (Vernon, 1968). The IQ distribution of the congenitally deaf is essentially identical to that of the general population (see chapter 11). In addition, there are the same relationships between IQ and ethnicity among the deaf that exist among the hearing. Furthermore, there is no relationship between the age of onset of deafness (which would be directly related to degree of cultural deprivation) and IQ. In other words, the data from deafness strongly support the idea of genetics as the dominant factor in the determination of intelligence.

LEARNING AND SENSORY MODALITY

Congenitally deaf people, as a group, have great difficulty mastering English. However, they learn sign language rapidly and easily. Part of the difficulty congenitally deaf children have with the English language can be accounted for by their limited exposure to it. However, the problem goes much deeper than this. Stated in experimental terms, lack of exposure to English can account for only a part of the variance that is involved in the deaf person's difficulty in learning English. It is possible that much of their difficulty in learning English is due to the sensory modality involved. Hearing people learn English through audition. Deaf people learn English through vision. English is a sequential, phonetic language, just as are French, German, and most other spoken languages. By contrast, sign language is not phonetic or fully sequential. It is interesting to note that deaf persons who grow up in France, Germany, Israel, and other nations universally have difficulty with the spoken language of their homelands but they universally have no trouble with the sign language of their country.

The theoretical issue raised here relates to how human beings learn. What are the components of spoken language, that is, languages that have developed orally, that make them difficult to learn visually? Is it the lack of iconicity? Is it their sequential nature? What exactly is it? By the same token, what is different about sign language that makes it so easy for deaf people to learn? Why is it possible for a private or a nonverbal trainable mentally retarded person to learn sign language and not a spoken language? If we knew the variables accounting for this difference, the psychology of human learning would be significantly advanced.

OPTIMAL AND CRITICAL STAGE THEORIES

Another issue that can be examined by using deafness as an experiment of nature is one that has been accepted as "fact" for several decades. This is the existence of an optimal or critical period for language development (Greenberg, Vernon, Dubois, & McKnight, 1982). It is stated as being between the ages of 2 and 4. Deaf people are a perfect experiment of nature by which to test this theory, because many of them have little or no exposure to language before 5 or 6. In addition, in our culture and even more so in other cultures, there are some deaf people who reach their teens or even adulthood with no exposure to language, including sign language. When exposed to sign language as adults, these individuals learn to sign so fluently that within two years they cannot be identified as different in skill from deaf people who have been signing since infancy. There is also limited evidence suggesting that those who have no exposure to language until adulthood learn English as well as those exposed to it much earlier.

These data cast a dubious light on critical stage or optimal stage theories of language development. They suggest that one reason 2- to 4-year-olds learn language so well is not simply because they are 2 to 4 years of age, but because they have no existing language to interfere with the learning of a new one. In other words, they do not face the problem of retroactive inhibition. The absence of this problem can account for the fact that deaf people exposed for the first time to language at age 18, 20, or 25 learn sign language so quickly and effectively. They have no other language already established to interfere with their learning of signs.

LATERALITY AND LANGUAGE

Another area in which deafness as an experiment of nature can help us learn is the area of laterality and language, that is, the respective roles of the left and right hemispheres of the brain. The generally accepted theory is that almost all right-handed people have their language function in the left hemisphere. Evidence from stroke victims and people with other brain injuries shows that when the left hemisphere is damaged, speech usually becomes defective or is lost altogether. These same people who have lost the capacity for oral language can often learn sign language with relatively little difficulty (Greenberg et al., 1982), despite their left hemisphere damage, and despite the fact that the left hemisphere is thought to be the hemisphere where language functioning occurs. This phenomenon raises some basic questions about the role of sensory modality in laterality and language function.

MEMORY FUNCTION

Another process to be examined by deafness as an experiment of nature is the function of memory and the very complex issue of how the human brain stores information. Some information theorists who study memory theorize that the way we store information is in terms of the auditory qualities of the data (Greenburg et al., 1982). Obviously, the deaf person has no "auditory quality" to the data he or she remembers. Thus the study of deafness raises questions about current theories of memory.

The examples we have covered only touch the surface of what could be learned if more persons became genuinely interested in deafness from a purely scientific point of view, that is, if they viewed deafness from the perspective of an experiment in nature.

REFERENCES

Bettelheim, B. (1967). *The empty fortress: Infantile autism and the birth of self.* New York: Free Press.

Chess, S., Fernandez, P., & Corn, S. J. (1972). *Psychiatric disorders in children with congenital rubella.* New York: Brunner-Morel.

Furth, H. G. (1966). *Thinking without language: Psychological implications of deafness.* New York: Free Press.

Furth, H. G. (1973). Further thoughts on thinking and language. *Psychological Bulletin,* 79(3), 215–216.

Greenberg, J. C., Vernon, M., Dubois, J. H., & McKnight, J. C. (1982). *The language arts handbook: A total communication approach.* Baltimore: University Park Press.

Rosen, V. H. (1964). Some effects of artistic talent on character styles. *The Psychoanalytic Quarterly, 33,* 1–24.

Vander Woude, K. W. (1970). Problem solving and language. *Archives of General Psychiatry, 23,* 337–342.

Vernon, M. (1967). The relationship of language to the thinking process. *Archives of General Psychiatry, 16,* 325–333.

Vernon, M. (1968). Fifty years of research on the intelligence of deaf and hard of hearing children: A review of literature and discussion of implications. *Journal of Rehabilitation of the Deaf, 1.*

SECTION V SUMMARY

Chapter 13 departed from the previous 12 chapters of book on service issues and instead focused exclusively on a scientific view. It considered deafness as "an experiment in nature" which allows us to examine many psychological questions by using congenital deafness as a point of reference. These questions included: Is autism functional or organic? What is the relationship between thought and language? Is atrophy of brain tissue due to auditory deprivation? What are the roles of environment and genetics in IQ? How do humans learn? Is there an optimal time for language acquisition? What are the roles of the left and right hemispheres of the brain? How does the human brain store information? After each question was posed, its implications for further scientific research were discussed.

REVIEW QUESTIONS

1. What benefits for the scientific community can be gained from taking the view of deafness as "an experiment in nature"?
2. What do the data on congenitally deaf noverbal children tell us about the nature of the thought process?

ORGANIZATIONS, PUBLISHING COMPANIES, PUBLICATIONS, AND INSTITUTIONS SERVING DEAF PEOPLE

Organizations

Alexander Graham Bell Association for the Deaf
3417 Volta Place, N.W.
Washington, DC 20007
Voice/TDD: (202) 337-5220

American Academy of Otolaryngology
—Head and Neck Surgery
1101 Vermont Ave., N.W., Suite 302
Washington, DC 20005
Voice: (202) 289-4607

American Athletic Association of the Deaf
10604 E. 95th St. Terrace
Kansas City, MO 64134

American Deafness and Rehabilitation Association
P.O. Box 55369
Little Rock, AR 77225
Voice/TDD: (501) 375-6643

American Hearing Research Foundation
55 E. Washington St.
Suite 2022
Chicago, IL 60602
Voice: (312) 726-9670

American Society for Deaf Children
814 Thayer Ave.
Silver Spring, MD 20910
Voice/TDD: (301) 585-5400

American Society of Deaf Social Workers
2700 Martin Luther King, Jr. Ave., S.E.
St. Elizabeth's Hospital
Washington, DC 20032
Voice/TDD: (201) 373-7469

American Speech-Language-Hearing Association
10801 Rockville Pike
Rockville, MD 20852
Voice/TDD: (301) 897-5700
 (301) 897-8682
 (800) 638-8255

American Tinnitus Association
P.O. Box 5
Portland, OR 97207
Voice: (503) 248-9985

Better Hearing Institute
P.O. Box 1840
Washington, DC 20013
Voice: (703) 642-0580
Voice: (800) EAR-WELL

Captioned Films for the Deaf
Modern Talking Pictures Service, Inc.
5000 Park St. N.
St. Petersburg, FL 33709
Voice/TDD: (800) 237-6213

Conference of Educational Administrators Serving the Deaf
Gallaudet University
800 Florida Ave., N.E.
Washington, DC 20002
Voice/TDD: (202) 651-5015

Convention of American Instructors of the Deaf
P.O. Box 2163
Columbia, MD 21045
Voice/TDD: (301) 461-9988

Deafness and Communicative Disorders Branch
Office of Special Education and Rehabilitative Services
Department of Education
330 C St., S. W., Room 3316
Washington, DC 20201
Voice: (202) 732-1401, 1398
TDD: (202) 732-1298, 2848

Deafness Research Foundation
9 East 38th St.
New York, NY 10016
Voice: (212) 684-6556
TDD: (212) 684-6559

Deafpride, Inc.
1350 Potomac Ave., S.E.
Washington, DC 20003
Voice/TDD: (202) 675-6700

Episcopal Conference of the Deaf
51 Woodale Rd.
Philadelphia, PA 19118
Voice/TDD: (215) 247-2245, 6454

Gallaudet University Alumni Association
Alumni House, Gallaudet University
Washington, DC 20002
Voice/TDD: (202) 651-5030

Helen Keller National Center for Deaf-Blind
   Youths and Adults
111 Middle Neck Rd.
Sands Point, NY 11050
Voice/TDD: (516) 944-8900

House Ear Institute
256 South Lake
Los Angeles, CA 90057
Voice: (213) 483-4431
TDD: (213) 484-2642

International Catholic Deaf Association
814 Thayer Ave.
Silver Spring, MD 20910
TDD: (301) 588-4009

International Lutheran Deaf Association
1333 S. Kirkwood Rd.
St. Louis, MO 63122
Voice/TDD: (314) 965-9917, ext. 684

Junior National Association of the Deaf
NAD Branch Office
445 N. Pennsylvania St., Suite 804
Indianapoilis, IN 46204
Voice/TDD: (317) 638-1715

National Association of Speech and Hearing
   Action (NASHA)
10801 Rockville Pike
Rockville, MD 20852
Voice: (301) 897-8682

National Association of the Deaf
814 Thayer Ave.
Silver Spring, MD 20910
Voice/TDD: (301) 587-1788

National Black Deaf Advocates, Inc.
175 Remsen St.
Brooklyn, NY 11201
Voice/TDD: (718) 855-1004

National Captioning Institute, Inc.
5203 Leesburg Pike
Falls Church, VA 22041
Voice/TDD: (703) 998-2400

National Catholic Office of the Deaf
814 Thayer Ave.
Silver Spring, MD 20910
Voice/TDD: (301) 587-7992

National Center for Law and the Deaf
Gallaudet University
800 Florida Ave., N.E.
Washington, DC 20002
Voice/TDD: (202) 651-5373

National Congress of Jewish Deaf
4960 Sabal Palm Blvd.
Building 7, Apartment 207
Tamarac, FL 33319
Voice: (305) 763-8177

National Cued Speech Association
P.O. Box 31345
Raleigh, NC 27622
Voice/TDD: (919) 828-1218

National Fraternal Society of the Deaf
1300 W. Northwest Highway
Mt. Prospect, IL 60056
Voice: (312) 392-9282
TDD: (312) 392-1409

National Hearing Aid Society
20361 Middlebelt Rd.
Livonia, MI 48152
Voice: (313) 478-2610
         (800) 521-5247 Hearing Aid
            Helpline

National Information Center on Deafness
Gallaudet University
800 Florida Ave., N.E.
Washington, DC 20002
Voice/TDD: (800) 672-6720
ext. 5051 Voice ext. 5052 TDD

The National Rehabilitation Information
  Center
8455 Colesville Rd.
Suite 935
Silver Spring, MD 20910
Voice/TDD: (301) 588-9284
                (800) 34-NARIC

National Technical Institute for the Deaf
P.O. Box 9887
Rochester, NY 14623
Voice: (716) 475-6400
TDD: (716) 475-2181

The National Theatre of the Deaf
The Hazel E. Stark Center
Chester, CT 06412
Voice: (203) 526-4971
TDD: (203) 526-4974

Oral Deaf Adults Section
Alexander Graham Bell Association of the
  Deaf
3417 Volta Place, N.W.
Washington, DC 20007
Voice/TDD: (202) 337-5220

Professional Rehabilitation Workers with
  the Adult Deaf
814 Thayer Ave.
Silver Spring, MD 20910
(301) no number (but see National
  Association of the Deaf)

Quota International, Inc.
1420 21st St., N.W.
Washington, DC 20036
Voice/TDD: (202) 331-9694

Registry of Interpreters for the Deaf, Inc.
1 Metro Square
51 Monroe St., Suite 1107
Rockville, MD 20850
Voice/TDD: (301)   279-0555, 6
                279-6773

Self Help for Hard of Hearing People
  (SHHH)
7800 Wisconsin Ave.
Bethesda, MD 20814
Voice: (301) 657-2248
TDD: (301) 657-2249

Telecommunications for the Deaf, Inc.
814 Thayer Ave.
Silver Spring, MD 20910
Voice: (301) 589-3786
TDD: (301) 589-3006

Tripod
955 North Alfred St.
Los Angeles, CA 90069
Voice/TDD: (213) 656-4904
                (800) 362-8888
                (800) 346-8888
                (CA only)

U.S. Deaf Skiers Assoc., Inc.
Box USA
Gallaudet University
800 Florida Ave., N.E.
Washington, DC 20002
TDD: (202) 651-5255

World Recreation Association of the Deaf
P.O. Box 7814
Van Nuys, CA 91409
(818) no number

Publishing Companies

Gallaudet University Press
Kendall Green
800 Florida Ave., N.E.
Washington, DC 20002
Voice: (202) 651-5488

National Association of the Deaf
814 Thayer Ave.
Silver Spring, MD 20910
Voice: (301) 587-1788

T. J. Publishers, Inc.
817 Silver Spring Ave.
Suite 206
Silver Spring, MD 20910
Voice: (301) 585-4440

Publications

American Annals of the Deaf
Gallaudet University
KDES, PAS 6
800 Florida Ave.
Washington, DC 20002
Voice: (202) 651-5488

American Athletic Association of the Deaf
  Bulletin
1313 Tanforan Dr.
Lexington, KY 40502
Voice/TDD: (816) 765-5520

Clarke Today
Clarke School for the Deaf
Center for Oral Education
Northampton, MA 01060-2199
Voice: (413) 584-3450

The Deaf American
National Association of the Deaf
814 Thayer Ave.
Silver Spring, MD 20910
Voice/TDD: (301) 587-1788

The Deaf-Blind American
American Association of the Deaf-Blind
814 Thayer Ave.
Silver Spring, MD 20910
Voice: (301) 459-2121

Deaf Counseling, Advocacy, and Referral
  Agency (DCARA)
125 Parrott St.
San Leandro, CA 94577
Voice: (415) 351-3937

Deaf Spotlight
American Atheletic Association of the Deaf
125 Parrott St.
San Leandro, CA 94577

The Endeavor
American Society for Deaf Children
814 Thayer Ave.
Silver Spring, MD 29910
Voice/TDD: (301) 585-5400

The Frat
National Fraternal Society of the Deaf
1300 W. Northwest Highway
Mt. Prospect, IL 60056
Voice/TDD: (312) 392-9282

Gallaudet Alumni Newsletter
Gallaudet University
800 Florida Ave., N.E.
Washington, DC 20002
Voice/TDD: (202) 651-5030

Gallaudet Today
Gallaudet University
800 Florida Ave., N.E.
Washington, DC 20002
Voice/TDD: (202) 651-5671

GA-SK
Telecommunications for the Deaf, Inc.
814 Thayer Ave.
Silver Spring, MD 20910
Voice: (301) 589-3786
TDD: (301) 389-3006

Hispanic-Deaf Newsletter
Department of Learning, Development and
  Special Education
Northern Illinois University
DeKalb, IL 60115
Voice: (815) 753-1000

Interpreter Views
RID, Inc.
51 Monroe St.
Suite 1107
Rockville, MD 20850
Voice: (301) 279-0555

Journal of Rehabilitation of the Deaf
American Deafness and Rehabilitation
  Association
P.O. Box 55369
Little Rock, AR 72226
Voice/TDD: (501) 663-4617

NAD Broadcaster
National Association of the Deaf
814 Thayer Ave.
Silver Spring, MD 20910
Voice/TDD: (301) 587-1788

NAD Youth Program
Junior National Association of the Deaf
814 Thayer Ave.
Silver Spring, MD 20910
Voice/TDD: (301) 587-1788

Newsounds
Alexander Graham Bell Association for the
   Deaf, Inc.
3417 Volta Place, N.W.
Washington, DC 20007-2778
Voice/TDD: (202) 337-5520

NTID Focus
National Technical Institute for the Deaf
1 Lomb Memorial Dr.
P.O. Box 9887
Rochester, NY 14623
Voice/TDD: (716) 475-6753

Perspectives for Teachers of the Hearing
   Impaired
Pre-College Programs
Gallaudet University
800 Florida Ave., N.E.
Washington, DC 20002
Voice: (202) 651-5342

Preview
Pre-College Programs
Gallaudet University
Washington, DC 20002
Voice: (202) 651-5342

The Progress Report
Pre-College Programs
Gallaudet University
Washington, DC 20002
Voice: 651-5342

Research at Gallaudet
Gallaudet Research Institute
800 Florida Ave., N.E.
Washington, DC 20002
Voice: (202) 651-5575

SHHH
Self Help for Hard of Hearing People, Inc.
7800 Wisconsin Ave.
Bethesda, MD 20814
Voice/TDD: (301) 657-2248

Sign Language Studies
Linstok Press, Inc.
9306 Mintwood St.
Silver Spring, MD 20901-3599

Silent News, Inc.
Williamsville Branch
P.O. Box 830
Buffalo, NY 14221
Voice/TDD: (716) 626-0986

Voice
11931 N. Central Expwy., No. 11
Dallas, TX 75243
No number

Volta Review
Alexander Graham Bell Association for the
   Deaf
3417 Volta Place, N.W.
Washington, DC 20007
Voice/TDD: (202) 337-5220

The World Around You
KDES Box 5N
Gallaudet University
800 Florida Ave., N.E.
Washington, DC 20002
Voice/TDD: (202) 651-3361

Institutions:

Gallaudet University
800 Florida Ave.
Washington, DC 20002
Voice: (202) 651-5488

National Technical Institute for the Deaf
Rochester Institute of Technology
1 Lomb Memorial Drive
Rochester, NY 14623
Voice: (716) 475-6400
TDD: (716) 475-2181

Source: National Information Center on Deafness, Gallaudet University

Index

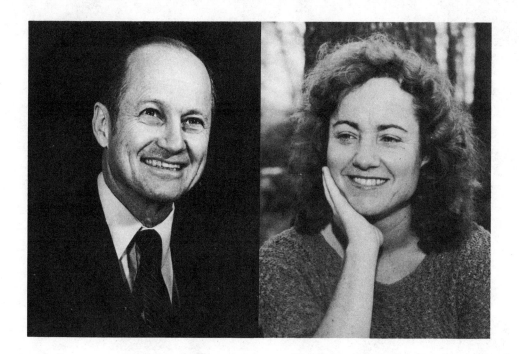

About the Authors

McCay Vernon, PhD, received his doctorate in Psychology from the Claremont Graduate School and University Center in 1966. Currently a Professor of Psychology at Western Maryland College, psychological consultant at Springfield Hospital, and Fellow in the American Psychological Association, Dr. Vernon has authored seven books and over 200 other professional publications on deafness and partial hearing. His writings and speeches have had a profound effect on an entire generation of hearing impaired children and adults. Dr. Vernon's research interests in deafness include mental illness, psychodiagnostics, test development, neuropsychology, deaf-blindness, and forensics. For the last twenty years he has been editor of the *American Annals of the Deaf.* He is the recipient of an honorary doctorate from Gallaudet University, and he has won major awards from the National Association of the Deaf, World Federation of the Deaf, and the British Deaf Association. His marriage of 33 years to a deaf woman (Mrs. Vernon is a published scientist in the field of microbiology) imparts to Dr. Vernon's background an in-depth knowledge not derived from scholarship alone.

Jean F. Andrews, PhD, received her doctorate in Speech and Hearing Science from the University of Illinois, Champaign-Urbana, in 1983. Currently, she is an Associate Professor at Lamar University where she trains teachers of deaf children and youths. Her research interests include: improvement of teacher-training, reading assessment, parent-child bookreading, reading acquisition, reading comprehension and using the microcomputer to improve literacy skills. She is on the editorial board of the *American Annals of the Deaf.* Dr. Andrews has managed federal projects to train teachers and educational interpreters to work with deaf children. Recently, Dr. Andrews has published juvenile fiction in magazines and two novels for the 9- to 12-year age group.

Deafened adults

Paranoid ideation   170

Age – on set   178

Warped personality   189

Continually faces promblem
– must learn to Cope   190

Musical hallucinations   176

Positive self concept –
accept deafness – non   190
authorian